Stroke Revisited

This authoritative book series presents state of the art knowledge on the pathophysiology, prevention, diagnosis, and treatment of stroke, highlighting the many very important advances that have been achieved in recent years. Current issues in management are addressed in detail, equipping readers with an understanding of the rationale for particular approaches in different settings and with a sound knowledge of the role of modern imaging methods, surgical techniques, and medical treatments. The inclusion of numerous high-quality illustrations facilitates understanding of practical aspects and rapid retrieval of fundamental information. The series will be of value for stroke physicians, surgeons, other practitioners who care for patients with stroke, and students.

More information about this series at http://www.springer.com/series/15338

Seung-Hoon Lee
Editor

Dong-Wan Kang
Associate editor

Stroke Revisited: Hemorrhagic Stroke

Sponsored by
Korean Cerebrovascular Research Institute

Springer

Editor
Seung-Hoon Lee
Department of Neurology
Seoul National University Hospital
Seoul
South Korea

Korean Cerebrovascular Research Institute
Seoul
South Korea

ISSN 2522-5588 ISSN 2522-5596 (electronic)
Stroke Revisited
ISBN 978-981-10-1426-0 ISBN 978-981-10-1427-7 (eBook)
https://doi.org/10.1007/978-981-10-1427-7

Library of Congress Control Number: 2018949945

This Springer imprint is published by the registered company Springer Nature Singapore Pte Ltd.
The registered company address is: 152 Beach Road, #21-01/04 Gateway East, Singapore 189721, Singapore

Preface

It has already been a year since the publication of the first volume of the Stroke Revisited series under the title *Volume 1: Diagnosis and Treatment of Ischemic Stroke*. As promised, the second volume has now been published under the title *Volume 2: Hemorrhagic Stroke*. I have tried to publish the second volume as early as possible with the help of the experiences gained from the previous publication. However, since it is an edited book for which manuscripts are gathered from many physicians, professors, and scientists around the world, the publication has been made much later than anticipated. I would like to apologize to readers who have shown great interest in the first volume and have waited for the second one.

As its title suggests, this book is a textbook that summarizes hemorrhagic stroke. Stroke can be largely divided into ischemic and hemorrhagic stroke. Although it is common to find books on ischemic stroke, not many books deal with hemorrhagic stroke. Even experts assume that the topic of stroke concerns ischemic stroke; this shows how the perception of hemorrhagic stroke is low while it is often misunderstood. Ischemic stroke accounts for 85% of all stroke cases, whereas hemorrhagic stroke accounts for 15%. In other words, the incidence rate of hemorrhagic stroke is less than 1/5 of that of ischemic stroke. However, since hemorrhagic stroke has a mortality of 40–50%, it has a much higher severity. Moreover, hemorrhagic stroke shares the same pathophysiology as ischemic stroke, particularly lacunar infarction caused by small vessel occlusion, and numerous patients have both types of stroke. Therefore, it is necessary to understand ischemic and hemorrhagic stroke in a comprehensive manner. Although there is no systematic classification system for hemorrhagic stroke, it is largely classified into intracerebral hemorrhage (ICH) occurring within the brain parenchyma and subarachnoid hemorrhage (SAH) occurring within the subarachnoid space surrounding the brain. In ICH, arteriolosclerosis occurs in penetrating arteries due to risk factors such as long-standing hypertension within the brain parenchyma, and these arteries rupture suddenly. In SAH, aneurysm (frequently caused by congenital defects) in large intracranial arteries bursts. Causes of two types of hemorrhagic strokes, ICH and SAH, are clearly different, and most books have explained the two diseases separately. Moreover, although healthcare systems differ in each country, ICH is often treated by physicians related to neurology while SAH is often treated by neurosurgeons, further adding to the understanding of the two diseases as separate. However, this textbook seeks to explain the following aspects of these two diseases under the classification of hemorrhagic stroke: causes, pathophysiology, clinical manifestations, diagnosis, treatment, and prevention. As the editor of this book, I recommend readers to read this book cover to cover while understanding the overall organization of the book rather than reading certain chapters only. This will enable the readers to comprehensively understand all clinical aspects of hemorrhagic stroke while also learning the newest findings on diagnosis and treatment.

Not many textbooks deal with stroke even until today. I used two or three books during my residency and fellowship although these were not sufficient to deliver the knowledge in stroke care that improved greatly in 1990–2000. Owing to brain MRI and CT imaging, it has become possible to gain an immediate understanding of a patient's pathophysiology changing moment by moment. Nevertheless, most textbooks published previously strived to explain the outdated neurological examinations, being unable to support the advances made in the practice field. Moreover, most textbooks listed minute details about research findings that often conflicted and lacked appropriate diagrams and sufficient explanation of the core concepts. Although it would have also been true for other areas, studying stroke required great perseverance then.

With the developments of smartphones and tablets, all people around the globe are now communicating through social media and are living in a previously inexperienced wealth of information. Along with recent technological advances, textbooks that deliver medical knowledge should change to be able to deliver information in a concise yet precise way. Moreover, it is necessary to minimize the amount of contents in each chapter, use many visual diagrams to deliver concepts, refrain from listing unnecessary research findings, and deliver information while considering practice guidelines serving as standards of clinical practice nowadays. I was determined to write a textbook reflecting such changes and contacted Springer Nature. Springer Nature has been very cooperative with my requests and planned a new textbook series under the title *Stroke Revisited*. In fact, it is not easy to publish a textbook series while communicating from Korea with a publisher based in Europe due to various obstacles, including language. I would like to thank the many staff members of Springer Nature who have nevertheless helped with the publication of this book.

This textbook targets trainees, such as residents and fellows, physicians, and scholars in their early career majoring in stroke, as well as other physicians and researchers in other fields who aim to study stroke. The relatively shorter chapters concern one subject at a time whenever possible; in this regard, I have strived to organize them concisely in order for the readers to be able to read them in one sitting. I have minimized unnecessary descriptions and inserted at least one conceptual figure or diagram per chapter to aid the readers' understanding. The textbook consists of two parts as follows. Part I—General facts on hemorrhagic stroke—explains the epidemiology, classification, risk factors, and pathophysiology of hemorrhagic stroke. Part II—Diagnosis and treatment of hemorrhagic stroke—explains the latest findings in diagnosis and treatment of hemorrhagic stroke. Since most textbooks are organized according to the traditional academic formats, it is difficult to obtain knowledge required in clinical settings. I have put my utmost efforts to deliver clinical knowledge from real clinical settings in a concise manner. Meanwhile, since this is a textbook on hemorrhagic stroke, I have strived to put together the best academic expertise and latest findings. I sincerely hope that such efforts would come across to the readers effectively.

In order to organize the textbook with full details of the newest knowledge, each chapter was written by the best medical scientists from around the world. I wholeheartedly thank all authors from around the globe who have participated in this process. I hope that this textbook will be evaluated highly and act as a good example for future textbooks.

Seoul, South Korea Seung-Hoon Lee
April 2018

Acknowledgement

Although I had an ideal model for a textbook in my brain, I rarely had an active conversation with publishers about my idea. This textbook was conceived in an e-mail proposal of the textbook after an unplanned meeting with Ms. Lauren Kim, the editor of Springer Nature. The editorial team and I have obtained manuscripts from renowned medical experts in the world and have edited the manuscripts according to the principles we have set for this textbook. Therefore, the contents of this book were completed only after tremendous efforts from the editorial team. I would like to especially thank Dr. Dong-Wan Kang as associate editor, Ms. Eun-Sun Park, and other colleagues for their enormous efforts to complete this book. In addition, I would like to thank the executive members of the publisher, Springer Nature Inc., who agreed with the philosophy behind this textbook and provided the title for this textbook series—*Stroke Revisited*. Finally, I greatly appreciate the financial and technical support of the Korean Cerebrovascular Research Institute.

Throughout my research career, I focused on publishing papers as an author and becoming a famous, prosperous scientist. I rarely thought of writing a textbook. I would like to express my love toward my wife and my kids for changing my selfish thoughts and helping me understand my responsibilities, that is, to help others and provide education to future medical doctors.

April 2018

Seung-Hoon Lee
Department of Neurology
Seoul National University Hospital
Seoul, South Korea

Korean Cerebrovascular Research Institute
Seoul, South Korea

Contents

Contributors

Alessandro Biffi Divisions of Stroke, Memory Disorders and Behavioral Neurology, Department of Neurology, Massachusetts General Hospital and Harvard Medical School, Boston, MA, USA

Won-Sang Cho Department of Neurosurgery, Seoul National University Hospital, Seoul, South Korea

Jae H. Choi Center for Unruptured Brain Aneurysms, Neurological Surgery, P.C., Lake Success, NY, USA

Department of Neurology, State University of New York, Downstate Medical Center, Brooklyn, NY, USA

Hybernia Medical, LLC, Uniondale, NY, USA

Brandon R. Christophe Columbia University Medical Center, Columbia University, New York, NY, USA

Edward S. Connolly Jr Department of Neurological Surgery, Columbia University, New York, NY, USA

Wuwei Feng Medical University of South Carolina, Charleston, SC, USA

Duk Ho Gho Department of Neurosurgery, Seodaegu Hospital, Busan, South Korea

Tarun Girotra Medical University of South Carolina, Charleston, SC, USA

Dae Hee Han Department of Neurosurgery, Cerebral and Cardiovascular Disease Center, National Medical Center, Seoul, South Korea

Jeong-Ho Hong Department of Neurology, Keimyung University Dongsan Medical Center, Daegu, South Korea

Chae Wook Huh Department of Neurosurgery, Inje University Haeundae Paik Hospital, Busan, South Korea

Sung-Chul Jin Department of Neurosurgery, Inje University Haeundae Paik Hospital, Busan, South Korea

Dong-Wan Kang Gangjin Public Health Center, Gangjin, South Korea

Department of Neurology, Seoul National University Hospital, Seoul, South Korea

Korean Cerebrovascular Research Institute, Seoul, South Korea

Seung-Ki Kim Department of Neurosurgery, Seoul National University Hospital, Seoul National University College of Medicine, Seoul, South Korea

Yun-Hee Kim Department of Physical and Rehabilitation Medicine, Sungkyunkwan University School of Medicine, Seoul, South Korea

Center for Prevention and Rehabilitation, Heart Vascular Stroke Institute, Samsung Medical Center, Seoul, South Korea

Samsung Advanced Institute for Health Science and Technology, Sungkyunkwan University, Seoul, South Korea

Natalie Kreitzer Department of Emergency Medicine and Division of Neurocritical Care, University of Cincinnati, Cincinnati, OH, USA

Ji Yeoun Lee Department of Anatomy, Seoul National University College of Medicine, Seoul, South Korea

Department of Neurosurgery, Seoul National University Hospital, Seoul, South Korea

Seung-Hoon Lee Department of Neurology, Seoul National University Hospital, Seoul, South Korea

Korean Cerebrovascular Research Institute, Seoul, South Korea

Si-Hyun Lee Korean Cerebrovascular Research Institute, Seoul, South Korea

Shyle H. Mehta Columbia University Medical Center, Columbia University, New York, NY, USA

Bruce Ovbiagele Department of Neurology, Medical University of South Carolina, Charleston, SC, USA

Eun-Sun Park Seoul National University Hospital and Korean Cerebrovascular Research Institute, Seoul, South Korea

Marco Pasi Hemorrhagic Stroke Research Program, Department of Neurology, Massachusetts General Hospital Stroke Research Center, Harvard Medical School, Boston, MA, USA

John Pile-Spellman Center for Unruptured Brain Aneurysms, Neurological Surgery, P.C., Lake Success, NY, USA

Hybernia Medical, LLC, Uniondale, NY, USA

Josephine U. Pucci Columbia University Medical Center, Columbia University, New York, NY, USA

Tanvir Rizvi Neuroradiology Division, Department of Radiology, University of Mississippi Medical Center, Jackson, MS, USA

Yong Sam Shin Department of Neurosurgery, College of Medicine, Seoul St. Mary's Hospital, The Catholic University of Korea, Seoul, South Korea

Sook Young Sim Department of Neurosurgery, College of Medicine, Seoul Paik Hospital, Inje University, Seoul, South Korea

Anand Viswanathan Hemorrhagic Stroke Research Program, Department of Neurology, Massachusetts General Hospital Stroke Research Center, Harvard Medical School, Boston, MA, USA

Kyu-Chang Wang Department of Neurosurgery, Seoul National University Hospital, Seoul National University College of Medicine, Seoul, South Korea

Max Wintermark Neuroradiology Division, Department of Radiology, Stanford University, Stanford, CA, USA

Daniel Woo Department of Neurology and Rehabilitation Medicine, University of Cincinnati, Cincinnati, OH, USA

Part I

General Facts on Hemorrhagic Stroke

1 Introduction on Hemorrhagic Stroke

Seung-Hoon Lee

1.1 Introduction

Stroke is a disorder that represents abrupt focal neurological symptoms resulting from brain tissue damage from the vascular origin. The vascular origin referred to here is divided into occlusion and rupture of the cerebral vessels, which cause ischemic and hemorrhagic strokes, respectively. For ischemic stroke, we have a widely used classification system such as Oxfordshire Community Stroke Project (OCSP) and Trial of ORG 10172 in Acute Stroke Treatment (TOAST), but there has not been such an agreed classification system for hemorrhagic stroke. The reason for classifying stroke subtypes is to distinguish the pathophysiology of strokes and to establish appropriate treatment and prevention methods accordingly. In ischemic stroke, it is not easy to distinguish its pathophysiology of the disease in the early stage, and the classification systems are quite beneficial. In contrast, with brain computed tomography, in hemorrhagic stroke, it is relatively easy to identify its pathophysiology even in the early stage, and the classification system has not generally been needed. However, for a better understanding and treatment of hemorrhagic stroke, it is necessary now to have a proper classification system.

1.2 Definition, Classification, and Epidemiology of Hemorrhagic Stroke

Hemorrhagic stroke refers to a disorder in which hemorrhages occur in the brain parenchymal area, subarachnoid space, or intraventricular space spontaneously due to abrupt rupture of intracranial blood vessels. Hemorrhagic conditions must occur spontaneously or primarily without effects of trauma and include intracerebral hemorrhage (ICH), subarachnoid hemorrhage (SAH), intraventricular hemorrhage (IVH), subdural hemorrhage (SDH), and epidural hemorrhage (EDH). EDH, which is induced by head trauma in most cases, generally does not meet the criteria of hemorrhagic stroke, but spontaneous subacute or chronic cases of SDH can be included. Hemorrhagic stroke predominantly occurs in the form of ICH or SAH. Because IVH usually accompanied ICH or SAH, isolated IVH is quite rare accounting for 3% of the total intracranial hemorrhage [1]. Hemorrhagic stroke can be classified according to the pathophysiology as follows: (1) ICH, (2) SAH, and (3) other intracranial hemorrhages – primary IVH, spontaneous SDH, etc. (Fig. 1.1). Classification of

S.-H. Lee
Department of Neurology, Seoul National University Hospital, Seoul, South Korea

Korean Cerebrovascular Research Institute, Seoul, South Korea
e-mail: sb0516@snu.ac.kr

S.-H. Lee (ed.), *Stroke Revisited: Hemorrhagic Stroke*, Stroke Revisited,
https://doi.org/10.1007/978-981-10-1427-7_1

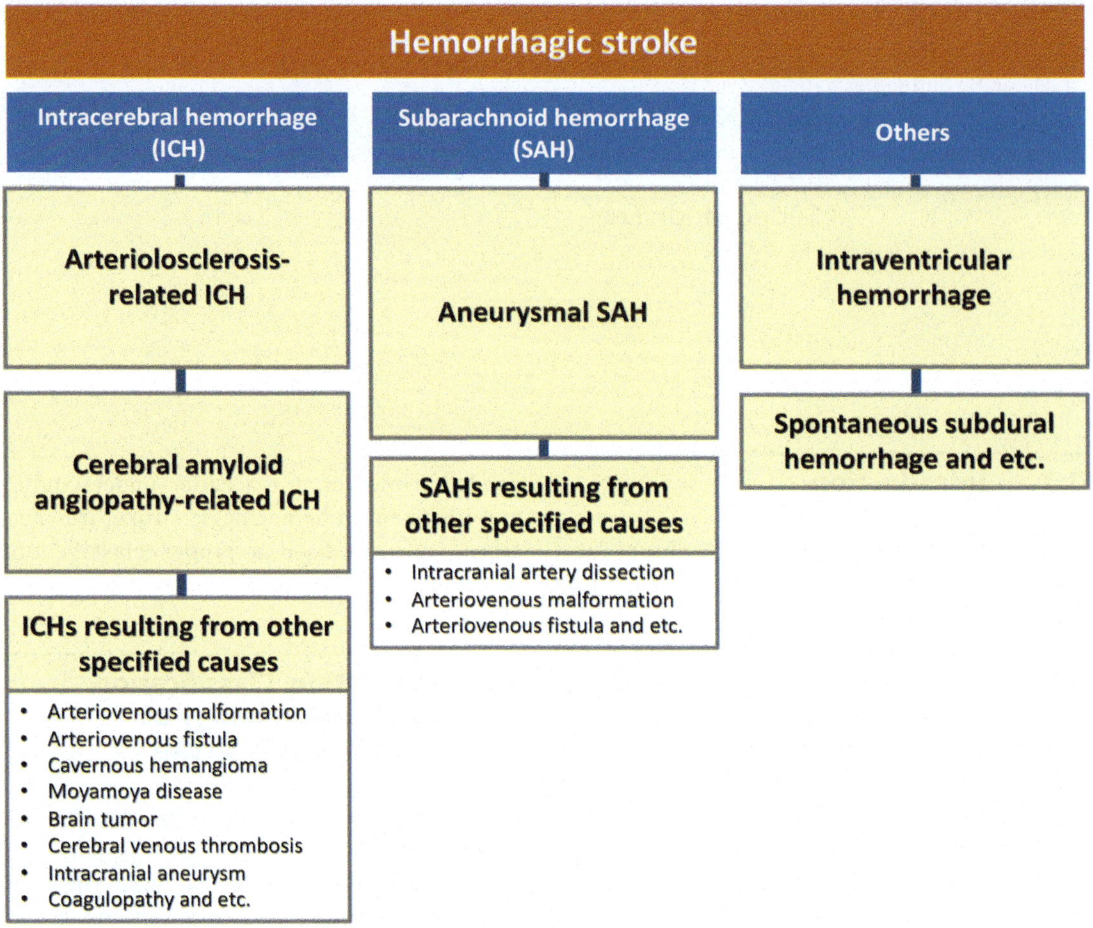

Fig. 1.1 Classification of hemorrhagic stroke

hemorrhagic stroke may be often confused when it occurs as a mixed type (e.g., ICH with SAH). In this case, I determine the classification under the basic rule that it should be based on the primary site of blood vessel rupture.

The overall incidence of hemorrhagic stroke is 15–40 per 100,000 individuals of the population. While ischemic stroke represents approximately 85% of total stroke, hemorrhagic stroke accounts for approximately 15% (ICH, 10–15% vs. SAH, about 5%) [2, 3]. In terms of ICH, the incidence varies widely among ethnic groups with the highest in Asia. According to a meta-analysis of 36 studies from 1983 to 2006, the incidence of ICH in races per 100,000 population was 24.2 for white, 22.9 for black, 19.6 for Hispanic, and 51.8 for Asian [4]. In the Global Burden of Disease 2010 study, which included a variety of studies published from 1990 to 2010, the number of hemorrhagic stroke patients worldwide increased by 47%; compared with an 8% reduction in incidence of hemorrhagic stroke and a 38% reduction in mortality in high-income countries, middle- and low-income countries showed a 22% increase in incidence and a 23% reduction in mortality [5]. With regard to SAH, the incidence is about 9 per 100,000 people, and the prevalence increases with age. Ethnicity is known to be relatively high in Japan [6]. Compared with a lower incidence than ICH's, the prognosis of SAH is much worse. Approximately 15% of SAH patients die before arriving at the hospital, with a case fatality of approximately 50% and a posttreatment failure of 20%. Despite advances in therapy, case fatality was only slightly reduced [7].

1.3 General Facts About ICH

ICH can be defined as a disease representing sudden neurological symptoms caused by a spontaneous bleeding in the brain parenchymal area without trauma and is associated with hypertension, cerebral amyloid angiopathy (CAA), arteriovenous malformation (AVM), cavernous hemangioma, moyamoya disease, brain tumor, cerebral venous thrombosis, intracranial aneurysm, coagulopathy, etc. For convenience of practice, ICHs are often divided as supratentorial (lobar, putaminal or thalamic ICH) and infratentorial ICH (pontine or cerebellar ICH) depending on location, which may be helpful for the patient's treatment. On the other side, as described in other chapters of this book (Chaps. 2 and 3), hypertension- or CAA-related ICH often refers to "primary" ICH, and the other ICHs are regarded as "secondary" ICH, accordingly. However, I do not consider this classification as appropriate because pathophysiologic consideration is limited. What is the reason why hypertensive arteriolosclerosis or amyloid angiopathy are denied as primary lesions? I claim that concepts using primary or secondary ICH are not valid on the basis of pathophysiology. Here, I present a new classification system for ICH as follows: (1) arteriosclerosis-related ICH, (2) CAA-related ICH, and (3) ICHs resulting from other specified causes – AVM, arteriovenous fistula, cavernous hemangioma, moyamoya disease, brain tumor, cerebral venous thrombosis, intracranial aneurysm, coagulopathy, etc. (Fig. 1.1).

Arteriolosclerosis-related ICH, classified here, has been generally referred to as hypertensive ICH. Arteriolosclerosis is a chronic cerebral microangiopathy occurred in penetrating small arteries and leptomeningeal arteries as a direct pathological finding leading to hemorrhage. Although hypertension is the most important risk factor for this type of hemorrhage, arteriosclerosis can be induced by aging, smoking, and other risk factors, in addition to hypertension. Four major types of arteriolosclerosis are (1) lipohyalinosis, (2) microaneurysm, (3) microatheroma, and (4) fibrinoid necrosis. Among them, both lipohyalinosis and microaneurysm are responsible for ICH, but lipohyalinosis is more frequently found as background pathologic findings in patients with ICH. Moreover, lipohyalinosis is the most common underlying pathologic findings of lacunar infarctions, and this lesion should be understood as a main cause of both ischemic and hemorrhagic stroke. All of the arteriolosclerosis findings are also closely related to white matter lesions (also known as leukoaraiosis) and microbleeds [8]. These lesions are predominantly found in the deep brain structure (basal ganglia and thalamus) where blood pressure is the largest in brain. CAA is a disease that causes vessel dilatation and focal wall fragmentation due to accumulation of congophilic amyloid protein in small- and medium-sized arteries and arterioles located in the cortex and its surrounding leptomeningeal space. CAA-related ICH occurs mostly in the cerebral cortex or cerebellum because these CAA findings mainly involve blood vessels around the cortex. In AVM or AVF, bleeding may occur due to high-flow shunt in anomalous connections between arteries and veins. In moyamoya disease, complication of ischemia-induced angiogenesis due to progressive stenosis of distal internal carotid arteries may cause ICH. Here, I do not use the terms primary or secondary in our classification. Because the hemorrhagic stroke including ICH is defined as "spontaneous (or primary)" bleeding, there is a risk of confusion if ICHs are divided into primary and secondary. In addition, since ICH occurs basically in vascular pathology, differentiation of primary or secondary ICH is not scientific. Risk factors for ICH will be covered in more detail in Chap. 2.

1.4 General Facts About SAH

SAH refers to neurologic conditions resulting from a rupture of the cerebral large arteries in the subarachnoid space between the pia mater and the arachnoid mater of three membranes surrounding the brain, leading to blood extravasation to the subarachnoid space. Except for traumatic SAH, 85% of spontaneous SAH is caused by a rupture of intracranial aneurysms, and direct causes are not found in approximately

10% of SAH. In addition, intracranial artery dissection, AVM, and AVF may be rare causes of SAH. The classification of SAH is described in Fig. 1.1.

Most frequently ruptured aneurysms in the intracranial arteries are 2.5–4 mm in size. Rupture of aneurysm causes bleeding in various subarachnoid spaces such as suprasellar cistern, sylvian fissure, ambient cistern, and quadrigeminal cistern depending on the location of the rupture. The bleeding may extend to the ventricular spaces. The shape of the aneurysm is varied, with saccular aneurysm being the most common, with various forms such as fusiform aneurysm, bleb formation in cerebral aneurysm, and blood blister aneurysm. Bleb formation or blood blister aneurysm has a greater risk of rupture. High SAH amount, consciousness impairment, and hydrocephalus due to ventricular obstruction are the poor prognosis factors. In contrast, if the patients have alert consciousness, or mild headache without neurologic symptoms, the prognosis will be better. Thus, a fast and appropriate diagnosis with severity grading is required in practice. For more information, see Chap. 7.

1.5 Other Intracranial Hemorrhage

IVH refers to conditions with acute hemorrhage in the ventricle. Major causes of IVH are as follows: (1) hemorrhage in the ventricle secondary to ICH, (2) a rupture of anterior communicating artery aneurysm, (3) hemorrhage from choroidal plexus around the brain parenchyma (usually caudate nucleus) around the ventricle, and (4) hemorrhage in the ependymal wall, such as AVM. Secondary IVH has a worse prognosis than primary IVH, especially in case of hydrocephalus caused by obstruction of the third ventricle or fourth ventricle.

SDH occurs as a rupture of the bridging veins in the subdural space, and EDH is caused by a rupture of the middle meningeal artery or a branch of the maxillary artery in the epidural space. These diseases are usually caused by trauma and are generally not included in the hemorrhagic stroke category. However, without a history of apparent head trauma, spontaneous SDH can be included in this category and is manifested as various symptoms such as headache, cognitive disorder, and gait disorder of subacute course, causing confusion with degenerative diseases.

Conclusion

Compared to ischemic strokes, concepts and classification of hemorrhagic strokes have not been clearly understood, because of relatively low incidence of hemorrhagic stroke and lack of interest.

In terms of studying and practicing the hemorrhagic stroke, there is a need for a clear classification based on the exact concept of disease and the pathophysiology. I hope that suggested classifications in this chapter would help to resolve these issues.

References

1. Flint AC, Roebken A, Singh V. Primary intraventricular hemorrhage: yield of diagnostic angiography and clinical outcome. Neurocrit Care. 2008;8:330–6.
2. Macellari F, Paciaroni M, Agnelli G, et al. Neuroimaging in intracerebral hemorrhage. Stroke. 2014;45:903–8.
3. Qureshi AI, Tuhrim S, Broderick JP, et al. Spontaneous intracerebral hemorrhage. N Engl J Med. 2001;344:1450–60.
4. van Asch CJ, Luitse MJ, Rinkel GJ, et al. Incidence, case fatality, and functional outcome of intracerebral haemorrhage over time, according to age, sex, and ethnic origin: a systematic review and meta-analysis. Lancet Neurol. 2010;9:167–76.
5. Krishnamurthi RV, Moran AE, Forouzanfar MH, et al. Global burden of diseases, injuries, and risk factors 2010 study stroke expert group. The global burden of hemorrhagic stroke: a summary of findings from the GBD 2010 study. Glob Heart. 2014;9:101–6.
6. De Rooij NK, Linn FH, van der Plas JA, et al. Incidence of subarachnoid haemorrhage: a systematic review with emphasis on region, age, gender and time trends. J Neurol Neurosurg Psychiatry. 2007;78:1365–72.
7. Hop JW, Rinkel GJ, Algra A, et al. Case-fatality rates and functional outcome after subarachnoid hemorrhage: a systematic review. Stroke. 1997;28:660–4.
8. Pantoni L. Cerebral small vessel disease: from pathogenesis and clinical characteristics to therapeutic challenges. Lancet Neurol. 2010;9:689–701.

Risk Factors for Hemorrhagic Stroke

2

Alessandro Biffi

2.1 Risk Factors for Intracerebral Hemorrhage

2.1.1 Pathophysiology and Risk Factors for Primary Intracerebral Hemorrhage

Intracerebral hemorrhage (ICH) is the acute manifestation of a chronic progressive disease of the cerebral vessels [1]. The underlying vessel disease can be a mass, vascular malformation or other macroscopic abnormalities. However, for patients over the age of 55 years, the overwhelming majority of ICH cases occur in the presence of cerebral small vessel disease [2]. A number of pathology correlates have been identified, including (1) prominent degeneration of the arteriolar media and smooth muscles and (2) fibrinoid necrosis of the subendothelium with micro-aneurysms and focal dilatations. ICH is routinely classified according to the region of the brain in which it occurs: the thalamus, basal ganglia, brain stem, cerebellum ("deep" or "non-lobar" ICH), or at the junction of the cortical gray matter and subcortical white matter ("lobar" ICH). Pathological studies demonstrate that ICH location frequently correlates with different underlying small vessel diseases. Arteriolosclerosis leads to non-lobar ICH due to rupture of vessels damaged by long-standing, uncontrolled hypertension. Lobar ICH is more often associated with cerebral amyloid angiopathy (CAA), a degenerative disorder characterized by deposition of β-amyloid at capillaries, arterioles, and small- and medium-sized arteries in the cerebral cortex, leptomeninges, and cerebellum [3]. CAA is associated with sporadic ICH, preferentially lobar in location and affecting elderly individuals. From an epidemiological standpoint, CAA-related ICH is associated with higher risk of recurrence than non-lobar, hypertensive ICH [4]. This section will present risk factors for ICH and existing evidence supporting their role in increasing ICH risk, as also summarized in Fig. 2.1.

2.1.2 Family History and Genetic Risk Factors

From a genetic epidemiological standpoint, ICH syndromes can be characterized as either (1) familial, with an easily identifiable hereditary transmission pattern within families with multiple affected individuals, or (2) sporadic, with no overt evidence of familial inheritance [5].

2.1.2.1 Familial ICH

Multiple familial ICH syndromes, manifesting only in selected families with highly consistent phenotypes and a clear autosomal dominant

A. Biffi
Divisions of Stroke, Memory Disorders and Behavioral Neurology, Department of Neurology, Massachusetts General Hospital and Harvard Medical School, Boston, MA, USA
e-mail: abiffi@mgh.harvard.edu

S.-H. Lee (ed.), *Stroke Revisited: Hemorrhagic Stroke*, Stroke Revisited,
https://doi.org/10.1007/978-981-10-1427-7_2

		Strength of available evidence		
		Strong	**Moderate**	**Weak**
Effect size	**Substantial** (>100% risk modification)	Family history Race / ethnicity *APOE* gene Age Hypertension Alcohol consumption Oral anticoagulation	Sympathomimetic drugs	
	Modest (50–99% risk modification)	Body mass index Antiplatelet agents	Cholesterol levels Sleep apnea	Statin use Chronic kidney disease Migraine headache Lifestyle / Activity
	Minimal (<50% risk modification)	SSRI antidepressants	*1q22* locus *COL4A1* gene *COL4A2* gene	Sex / Gender

Fig. 2.1 Risk factors for intracerebral hemorrhage (ICH). Risk factors for ICH are presented and classified based on effect size (see figure for description) and strength of available, published evidence. Evidence strength defined as follows: Weak: evidence from a single study or conflicting results from multiple studies. Moderate: evidence from multiple studies, with one conflicting study at most. Strong: evidence from multiple studies and/or meta-analysis, without substantial conflicting findings and/or heterogeneity upon meta-analytical pooling. *SSRI* selective serotonin reuptake inhibitors

inheritance pattern, have been described [3, 5]. These syndromes usually reflect an underlying familial CAA disorder [3]. Familial forms of CAA (Table 2.1) generally present with more severe clinical manifestations than sporadic CAA and are almost always characterized by earlier age of onset, more severe clinical course, and earlier age of death [3]. Unlike sporadic CAA and CAA-ICH, these familial forms are very rare in the general population; indeed, they present only in selected families and usually are transmitted as autosomal dominant disorders. From a clinical perspective, both sporadic and familial CAA are often responsible for substantial cognitive impairment, but ICH is not a consistent feature of all familial forms (see Table 2.1). Of note, different individuals with the same mutation may present with substantially different clinical phenotypes (pleiotropy). For example, one kindred with the Iowa mutation (substitution of asparagine for aspartate at position 23) had a history of recurrent ICH; in another kindred, individuals presented with dementia and leukoaraiosis, but not ICH. These findings suggest that additional genetic factors likely modify the strong effect of this mutation (and other familial CAA mutations), although it does not appear that the *APOE* gene (see Sect. 2.1.2.2) is such a factor [6].

2.1.2.2 Sporadic ICH

Despite the existence of numerous familial ICH syndromes, the vast majority of ICH in the general population occurs as a sporadic event, unaccompanied by an easily identifiable strong family history. However, modern genetic epidemiology tools clarified that genetic risk factors play a substantial role in determining the risk for sporadic ICH. Investigators within the International Stroke Genetics Consortium (ISGC) estimated ICH risk heritability at 44% (standard error, 11%) in the first study to address this question [7]. While the precision of such estimates is limited by the small sample sizes available, thus far, these results

Table 2.1 Familial CAA syndromes

Amyloid peptide	Precursor protein	Chrom	Disease	Notes	CAA-ICH
Aβ	APP	21	CAA related to familial AD	Associated with presenilin-1, presenilin-2, and APP mutations	+
Aβ	APP	21	CAA in down syndrome	Lobar ICH has been reported in some cases	+/–
Aβ	APP	21	CAA in APP duplication	CAA pathology prominent Increased risk of lobar hemorrhage Also causes early-onset autosomal dominant familial AD	+
Aβ	APP	21	Hereditary cerebral hemorrhage with amyloidosis: Dutch type	Described in two large families from the Netherlands Age at onset: 50 years Lobar hemorrhages, focal neurological deficits, dementia, and leukoencephalopathy	+
Aβ	APP	21	Hereditary cerebral hemorrhage with amyloidosis: Italian type	Described in three Italian families Age at onset: 50 years Lobar hemorrhages and dementia	+
Aβ	APP	21	Hereditary cerebral hemorrhage with amyloidosis: Flemish type	Described in a Dutch family (discovered in Belgium, therefore called "Flemish") and a British family Age at onset: 45 years Progressive AD-like dementia, in some patients associated with a lobar hemorrhage	+/–
Aβ	APP	21	Hereditary cerebral hemorrhage with amyloidosis: Iowa type	Described in a Iowa family and a Spanish family Age at onset: 50–66 years Memory impairment, expressive language deficit, personality changes, myoclonic jerks, short-step gait No clinically manifest ICH (family from Iowa) or lobar hemorrhages (family from Spain)	+/–
Aβ	APP	21	Hereditary cerebral hemorrhage with amyloidosis: Piedmont type	Described in one family from piedmont (Italy) Age at onset: 50–70 years Recurrent lobar hemorrhages, cognitive decline	+
Aβ	APP	21	Hereditary cerebral hemorrhage with amyloidosis: Arctic (Icelandic) type	Described in one family from northern Sweden Age at onset: ~ 60 years Progressive cognitive decline (no strokes)	–
ACys	Cystatin C	20	Hereditary cerebral hemorrhage with amyloidosis: Icelandic type	Described in nine subfamilies in Iceland Causes systemic amyloidosis Age at onset: 20–30 years Recurrent lobar hemorrhages	+

(continued)

Table 2.1 (continued)

Amyloid peptide	Precursor protein	Chrom	Disease	Notes	CAA-ICH
ATTR	Transthyretin	18	Meningovascular amyloidosis	Causes systemic amyloidosis Polyneuropathy is the main clinical symptom Rarer findings: Ataxia, spasticity, and dementia	In some families (rare)
AGel	Gelsolin	9	Familial amyloidosis Finnish type	Causes systemic amyloidosis Progressive corneal lattice dystrophy, cranial and peripheral neuropathy, cutaneous amyloidosis	–
PrPSc	Prion protein	20	Gerstmann-Sträussler-Scheinker syndrome	Described in one family Progressive cognitive decline	–
ABri	ABri precursor protein	13	Familial British dementia	Described in four families Age at onset: 45–50 years Progressive dementia, cerebellar ataxia, and spastic tetraparesis	–
ADan	ABri precursor protein	13	Familial Danish dementia	Described in one family from Denmark Age at onset: 30 years Cataracts, deafness, progressive ataxia, dementia (previously known as "heredopatia ophtalmo-Oto-encephalica")	–

AD Alzheimer's Disease, *CAA* cerebral Amyloid Angiopathy, *Chrom* Chromosome provide compelling evidence for a substantial contribution of genetic variation to risk of sporadic ICH.

For sporadic lobar ICH, the ε2 and ε4 alleles of the apolipoprotein E (*APOE*) gene play a primary role in determining genetic risk. Indeed, in the population-based Greater Cincinnati/Northern Kentucky Study, the risk factor accounting for the largest proportion of cases of lobar ICH was possession of the APOE ε2 or ε4 allele, resulting in a population-attributable risk of 29% [6]. A multicenter meta-analysis published in 2010 and including more than 2000 ICH cases and more than 4000 controls definitively showed an association between APOE genotype and lobar ICH risk [8]. Of note, the association was also extended to individuals of African-American ancestry. A number of additional loci have been investigated for association with sporadic CAA-ICH. A variant within the CR1 gene previously associated with AD risk and pathology burden, single-nucleotide polymorphism (SNP) rs6656401, was found to be associated with both CAA-ICH risk and vascular amyloid burden [9]. Multiple variants within the translocase of outer mitochondrial membrane 40 (*TOMM40*) gene, lying in close proximity to the *APOE* locus, were associated with amyloid plaque and vascular burden, but not with CAA-ICH risk [10]. A consistent trend toward an association between CAA pathology and rs1800470 in the transforming growth factor-β1 (*TGF-β1*) gene was reported by two studies (total of 449 participants) [11, 12]. However, none of these associations have been independently confirmed by multicenter large lobar/CAA-ICH studies to date.

As for non-lobar ICH risk, it is generally assumed to be less influenced by genetic risk factors than lobar, CAA-related ICH. However, results from the population-based Greater Cincinnati/Northern Kentucky Stroke Study suggest that a large proportion of the population-attributable risk for deep ICH (about 20%) remains unexplained by known risk factors (including hypertension, which accounts for roughly 50% of the risk) [13]. These findings were confirmed by an ISGC collaborative study utilizing multicenter data [7]. These findings suggested that genetic risk loci for deep ICH exist. This hypothesis was recently confirmed by findings from the ICH genome-wide associations study (GWAS) conducted by the ISGC [14]. This study included (1) a discovery phase comprised of a case cohort of 1545 individuals (664 lobar and 881 non-lobar cases) and a control cohort of 1481 individuals and (2) a replication phase comprising a case cohort of 1681 individuals (484 lobar and 1194 non-lobar cases) and a control cohort of 2261 individuals. The investigators identified and replicated an association between deep ICH risk and genetic variant rs2984613 at the 1q22 locus. The 1q22 locus contains a number of genes, with *PMF1* and *SLC25A44* being of highest interest for further biological dissection. *PMF1* codes for polyamine-modulated factor 1, a nuclear protein regulated by polyamines required for normal chromosome alignment and kinetochore formation during mitosis. *SLC25A44* encodes solute carrier family 25-member 44, a member of the SLC25 family of mitochondrial carrier proteins. Of note, multiple variants at 1q22 associated with deep ICH risk were subsequently associated with cerebral white matter lesion burden, providing independent evidence of a biological role in cerebral small vessel disease [15, 16].

Previously published evidence suggested that *APOE* ε4 might also increase risk of deep ICH, albeit with a significantly smaller effect size when compared to the effect on lobar (CAA-related) ICH [8]. This finding suggests that multiple, beta-amyloid-independent mechanisms could underlie the impact of *APOE* on ICH, both lobar and deep. A subsequent analysis of the risk of ICH recurrence found that APOE ε(epsilon)4 carriers were at elevated risk of deep ICH recurrence (hazard ratio 1.31; 95% confidence interval 1.02–2.69) [17]. Low-density lipoprotein (LDL) cholesterol was found to modulate part of the effect of *APOE* on deep ICH risk, further supporting the hypothesis that *APOE* influences ICH risk by both beta-amyloid-dependent and independent mechanisms.

2.1.2.3 COL4A1-/COL4A2-Related Intracerebral Hemorrhage

The *COL4A1* and *COL4A2* genes are located in tandem on chromosome 13q34 and encode the collagen chains α1(IV) and α2(IV), which constitute a major component of the vascular basement membrane. Rare mutations within the *COL4A1* gene on chromosome 13q34 (encoding the alpha1 chain of type IV collagen) gene have been associated with autosomal dominant syndromes manifesting variably with perinatal intracerebral hemorrhage (ICH) with consequent porencephaly, adult-onset ICH (all anatomical locations), small foci of chronic blood products in normal (or near normal) brain tissue known as microbleeds, lacunar strokes, and leukoaraiosis (white matter damage). Most disease-causing mutations in this setting are missense variants involving a highly conserved hydrophobic glycine residue, which results in inhibition of heterotrimer deposition into the vascular basement membrane and altered structural properties. When imaged with electron microscopy, the basement membrane is uneven, with inconsistent density and focal disruptions [18]. Ultimately, these changes lead to increased fragility of vessel walls and ICH. Of note, *COL4A1* appears to play a major role in determining cerebral vessel tolerance to minor head trauma, as surgical delivery of mouse pups bearing a mutated *COL4A1* allele can prevent the severe perinatal cerebral hemorrhages that occur in spontaneous live births [19]. In humans, impaired responses to even mild trauma may include variable clinical manifestations such as subclinical microbleeds, subarachnoid hemorrhage, and devastating ICH.

A number of studies have explored potential associations between genetic variation at *COL4A1* and sporadic ICH. Rare, non-synonymous variants in *COL4A1* were identified in sporadic ICH cases, but not controls. Furthermore, these mutations impaired *COL4A1* secretion in striking similarity to mutations causing familial syndromes [20]. Previous studies had suggested that genetic variation within *COL4A2* (which is structurally and functionally associated with *COL4A1*) was also associated with sporadic ICH risk [21]. More recently, a multi-consortium effort uncovered evidence of association between common genetic variants at the *COL4A1/COL4A2* locus and a number of phenotype associated with cerebral small vessel disease. An intronic variant at *COL4A2* was found to be associated with deep ICH, lacunar ischemic stroke, and white matter disease severity among stroke patients [22]. Taken together, these findings strongly support a role for collagen IV deposition and function in sporadic ICH and other manifestations of cerebral small vessel disease.

2.1.3 Race and Ethnicity

A number of studies have identified disparities in ICH incidence based on self-reported race/ethnic background. Seminal observations in Greater Cincinnati metropolitan area in the United States demonstrated that black (i.e., African-American) individuals had 1.4 times the risk of intracerebral hemorrhage. Of note, among those age of 75 or younger, the risk of intracerebral hemorrhage among blacks was 2.3 times that of whites (95% confidence interval, 1.5–3.6), whereas the risk among those 75 or older was one fourth that of whites (95% confidence interval, 0.1–0.8). These observations suggested differential effects on race/ethnicity on ICH risk based on underlying etiology, as hypertensive hemorrhages are more common among younger individuals compared to amyloid-related hemorrhages [23]. A follow-up epidemiological study conducted in the same metropolitan area confirmed higher ICH incidence rates for blacks (48.9/100,000 persons) vs. whites (26.6/100,000 persons). Annual incidence rates per 100,000 black individuals in lobar, deep cerebral, brain stem, and cerebellar locations were 15.2, 25.7, 5.1, and 2.9, respectively. Annual incidence rates per 100,000 whites in the same locations were 9.4, 13.0, 1.3, and 2.9. As expected, the greatest excess risk for ICH among black individuals (compared with whites) was found among young- to middle-aged (35–54 years) persons with brain stem (RR, 9.8; 95%

CI, 4.2–23.0) and deep cerebral (RR, 4.5; 3.0–6.8) hemorrhage [24]. In another population-based study conducted in Northern Manhattan (USA), compared with whites, ICH relative risk was found to be higher for blacks for all ICH locations (3.8, 95% confidence interval 2.2–8.9), deep ICH (4.8, 95% confidence interval 2.3–21.1), and lobar ICH (2.8, 95% confidence interval 1.2–14.4). For Hispanics, the relative risk of ICH was higher for all ICH locations (2.6, 95% confidence interval 1.4–6.1) and deep ICH (3.7, 95% confidence interval 1.7–16.5), but not lobar ICH (1.4, 95% confidence interval 0.4–7.4) [25]. These findings strongly imply racial/ethnic differences in the role of chronic hypertension in determining risk of lobar ICH, especially non-lobar ICH. More recently, investigators in the United States launched and completed the ethnic/racial variations of intracerebral hemorrhage (ERICH) study, aimed at recruiting a large sample of ICH cases of white, black, and Hispanic racial/ethnic background (1000 participants in each category), with matched ICH-free controls [26]. Results from the ERICH study clarified that both treated and untreated hypertension exert a larger effect as ICH risk factors among blacks and Hispanics (compared to whites), regardless of ICH location [27]. Several reports have also clarified that individuals of Asian ancestry are at highest risk for ICH, accounting for the fact that ICH accounts for ~ 10% of strokes in Europe and Northern America but up to 18—24% of all strokes in Korea and Japan [28–30]. A systematic review of all published evidence in 2010 confirmed most aforementioned observations, identifying ICH incidence per 100,000 person-years of 24.2 (95% confidence interval 20.9–28.0) in white people, 22.9 (95% confidence interval 14.8–35.6) in black people, 19.6 (95% confidence interval 15.7–24.5) in Hispanic people, and 51.8 (95% confidence interval 38.8–69.3) in Asian people. It is likely that observed differences in ICH incidence based on race/ethnicity are deeply linked to biological, socioeconomic, and geographical disparities in hypertension risk and management.

2.1.4 Sexual Differences in ICH Risk

A number of observational studies conducted in different populations reported higher ICH incidence among men compared to women. An initial systematic review and meta-analysis of available evidence in 2003 found the crude relative ratio for sex effects (male vs. female) on ICH incidence was 3.73 (95% confidence interval 3.28–4.25) [31]. However, in a later meta-analysis of published evidence conducted in 2010 including 8145 patients with ICH incidence was not found to be significantly lower in women than in men (overall incidence ratio 0.85, 95% confidence interval 0.61–1.18) [32]. It is likely that disparities in ICH risk between sexes may reflect differential impact of other established risk factors (e.g., age at time of ICH, hypertension incidence and severity, alcohol consumption). However, primary biological effects related to genetic, hormonal, or metabolic differences cannot be ruled out, and additional studies will be required to advance our understanding of the impact of sex on ICH risk.

2.1.5 Hypertension

Among modifiable risk factors, hypertension is arguably the most important for development of spontaneous ICH [33]. While estimates vary, most studies suggest at least a doubling in risk for ICH associated with hypertension. As expected based on known ICH pathophysiology, the contribution of elevated blood pressure to ICH risk is greater for non-lobar ICH than for lobar ICH [34]. In a meta-analysis that pooled data from 28 studies, hypertension was twice as common in patients with deep ICH as in patients with lobar ICH (odds ratio (OR) 2.1, 95% confidence interval 1.82–2.42) [35]. More recently, however, hypertension has been implicated in recurrence risk for both lobar and non-lobar ICH, with comparable effect sizes [4]. A number of pitfalls exist in our current understanding of the association between ICH risk and hypertension. No study to date has identified specific blood pressure measures and their relationship to ICH risk. The role of blood pressure variability, while explored in stroke at large and ischemic stroke in particular, has not been the topic of dedicated investigations as it pertains to ICH risk [36]. As mentioned above, racial/ethnic and geographical differences in hypertension risk, diagnosis, and management are likely to account at least in part for differences in ICH incidence across the world.

2.1.6 Advancing Age

Advancing age has been consistently reported as a risk factor for ICH, with a systematic review of existing evidence being compiled in 2003 [31]. In this report the author attempted a meta-analysis of 14 case-control and 11 cohort studies of ICH. In cohort studies, the crude relative risk in ICH incidence for age (per every 10-year increase) was estimated at 1.97 (95% confidence interval 1.79–2.16). A more recent inpatient database study from the Netherlands estimated ICH incidences (per 100,000 individuals) of 5.9 among those age 35–54 years, 37.2 among those age 55–74 years, and 176.3 among those age 75–94 years old in 2010 [37]. A subsequent systematic meta-analysis published in 2010 confirmed the association between advancing age and increasing ICH incidence; using the age group 45–54 years as reference, incidence ratios increased from 0.10 (95% confidence interval 0.06–0.14) for people aged less than 45 years to 9.6 (95% confidence interval 6.6–13.9) for people older than 85 years. These findings likely reflect the chronic nature of cerebral small vessel disease underlying most cases of ICH, especially among those age 55 years and above. The slow but constant accumulation of small vessel abnormalities (due to either chronic hypertension or CAA) is likely to steadily increase risk for ICH over time, resulting in higher risk with advancing age. Furthermore, it is likely that advancing age also reflects increasing degree of hypertension severity and/or treatment resistance, in itself major risk factors for ICH [38].

2.1.7 Alcohol Consumption

A previously mentioned systematic review found an association between alcohol consumption and ICH incidence: among participants enrolled in case-control studies, the crude odds ratio for high alcohol intake (which was defined in a very variable manner across studies) was 3.36 (95% confidence interval 2.21–5.12) [31]. These findings were confirmed in a more recent systematic review and meta-analysis, which found high alcohol consumption (>2–4 drinks/day) to be associated with a modestly increased risk for both ICH and subarachnoid hemorrhage. Furthermore, the relative risk for heavy drinking (>4 drinks/day) was 1.67 (95% confidence interval 1.25–2.23) [39]. More recently, the ERICH study investigators conducted a more systematic case-control study of alcohol consumption and ICH risk. Patterns of alcohol consumption were categorized as none, rare (<1 drink per month), moderate (≥1 drink per month and ≤2 drinks per day), intermediate (>2 drinks per day and <5 drinks per day), and heavy (≥5 drinks per day). The investigators demonstrated an ordinal trend for alcohol consumption increasing ICH risk, ranging from rare use (odds ratio 0.57 compared to none) to moderate (odds ratio 0.65), to intermediate (odds ratio 0.82), and finally to heavy alcohol consumption (odds ratio 1.77). In subgroup analyses rare and moderate alcohol consumption were jointly associated with decreased risk of both lobar and non-lobar ICH. Heavy alcohol consumption was specifically and robustly associated with increased non-lobar ICH risk (odds ratio 2.04), with the effects being even more detrimental among black and Hispanic participants. The underlying pathophysiology linking high alcohol intake with increased ICH risk remains only partially understood. Most hypotheses revolved around regular and/or sizable alcohol consumption resulting in increased blood pressure (especially systolic blood pressure) and coagulation cascade abnormalities [40, 41].

2.1.8 Low Cholesterol and Statin Use

A number of studies reported an inverse relationship between total and/or LDL-cholesterol and ICH risk, with individuals showing low levels being at highest risk [42–46]. These and similar findings were compiled in a meta-analysis in 2013, including 23 studies with 7960 hemorrhagic strokes (including both ICH and subarachnoid hemorrhage) [47]. In a dose-response analysis, the summary relative risk of hemorrhagic stroke for 1 mmol/L increment of total cholesterol was 0.85 (95% confidence interval 0.80–0.91), for high-density lipoprotein cholesterol was 1.11 (95% confidence interval 0.99–1.25), and for low-density lipoprotein cholesterol was 0.90 (95% confidence interval 0.77–1.05). The pooled relative risk for intracerebral hemorrhage was 1.17 (95% CI, 1.02–1.35) for high-density lipoprotein cholesterol. Of note, in at least one study association between cholesterol levels and ICH incidence was stronger for non-lobar/hypertensive ICH than lobar hemorrhage [45]. Also of note, in a recent systematic review and meta-analysis relationships between cholesterol levels and risk of hemorrhagic stroke (including both ICH and subarachnoid hemorrhage) differed between East Asian and non-East Asian populations [48]. In terms of ICH risk, East Asians displayed no significant difference between high and low total cholesterol (relative risk =1.30, 95% confidence interval, 0.89–1.90), whereas among non-East Asians, low total cholesterol conferred higher ICH risk (relative risk = 1.70, 95% confidence interval 1.08–2.67). With respect to subarachnoid hemorrhage risk, among East Asians low total cholesterol conferred higher risk (relative risk = 1.48, 95% confidence interval 1.10–2.08), whereas non-East Asians displayed no significant difference in risk based on total cholesterol levels.

In light of the aforementioned results, a number of studies sought to identify potential associations between statin use (with associated lipid-lowering effects) and increased risk of primary ICH. However, a meta-analysis of data derived from 31 randomized controlled trials failed to identify associations between active statin therapy and significant increase in ICH risk (odds ratio 1.08; 95% confidence interval 0.88–1.32) [49]. Specifically, ICH risk was not related to the degree of low-density lipoprotein reduction or achieved low-density lipoprotein cholesterol. However, in a more recent meta-analysis of seven randomized clinical trials (involving 31,099 interventions subjects and 31,105 placebo subjects), high-dose statin therapy (defined as atorvastatin 80 mg, simvastatin 80 mg, pravastatin 40 mg, or rosuvastatin 20 mg per day) was associated with a significant increase in ICH risk (relative risk 1.53, 95% confidence interval 1.16–2.01) [50]. Because of these contradictory results and of the limited understanding of the biological mechanisms linking cholesterol levels, statin use and ICH risk optimal decision-making in regard to cholesterol treatment for ICH survivors remain controversial. Ultimately, additional studies will be required to clarify whether statin use is safe in patients with history of, or at high risk for, ICH.

2.1.9 Chronic Kidney Disease

Chronic kidney disease (CKD) was found to be a risk factor for ICH in a population-based study and cohort study including 4937 participants [51]. A number of limitations to this study were noted, chiefly including low number of hemorrhagic stroke events (n = 88) and joint analysis of ICH and subarachnoid hemorrhage as outcomes. A number of biological hypotheses may account for these findings, including (1) platelet dysfunction and bleeding propensity in individuals with chronic kidney disease and (2) chronic kidney disease which may represent a marker/analogue phenomenon to hypertensive cerebrovascular small vessel disease, the major mechanism accounting for ICH risk (and especially for non-lobar, hypertensive ICH). Supporting the latter theory is one study's findings associating CKD with a greater presence and number of cerebral microbleeds among patients with ICH [52]. Interestingly, these findings were also replicated in neurologically healthy adults, suggesting that chronic kidney and cerebral small vessel disease may be concomitantly present from the initial, subclinical stages [53]. Future studies will be required to clarify whether early diagnosis and/or treatment of chronic kidney disease may modify the natural history of cerebral small vessel disease and prevent ICH events.

2.1.10 Body Mass Index

Extremes of body mass index (BMI) are associated with increased incidence of ICH in several published studies [23]. In one case-control study including 384 ICH cases, low BMI (<18.5 kg/m^2) and very high BMI (>30.0 kg/m^2) were associated with deep ICH risk (odds ratio 1.76 and 1.75, respectively, both $p < 0.05$). However, no association effect was found for lobar ICH. These findings suggest that biological effects related to extremes of weight primarily impact the hypertensive subtype of cerebral small vessel disease. Proposed biological mechanisms accounting for these findings include low cholesterol levels (for low BMI) and increased hypertension incidence and severity as part of the metabolic syndrome complex (for high BMI), though additional studies will be required for further clarification.

2.1.11 Medication and Recreational Drugs Increasing ICH Risk

2.1.11.1 Selective Serotonin Reuptake Inhibitors

Selective serotonin reuptake inhibitors (SSRIs) have been associated with bleeding risk in general, as well as with intracranial hemorrhage, and specifically with intracerebral hemorrhage. In a meta-analysis of all published evidence, ICH was associated with SSRI exposure in both unadjusted (relative risk 1.68, 95% confidence interval 1.46–1.91) and adjusted (relative risk 1.42, 95% confidence interval 1.23–1.65) analyses. Of note, in a subset of five studies (three of intracranial hemorrhage and one each reporting hemorrhagic stroke and intracerebral hemorrhage), SSRI exposure in combination with oral anticoagulants was associated with an increased risk of bleeding compared with oral anticoagulants alone (RR 1.56, 95% CI 1.33–1.83). These findings are presumed to be related to known effects of SSRIs on platelet aggregation and thrombogenicity [54].

2.1.11.2 Statins

The existing evidence on the relationship between statin use and ICH risk has been summarized above. Briefly, a meta-analysis of data derived from 31 randomized controlled trials failed to identify associations between active statin therapy and significant increase in ICH risk [48]. However, in a more recent meta-analysis of seven randomized clinical trials, high-dose statin therapy was associated with a significant increase in ICH risk (relative risk 1.53, 95% confidence interval 1.16–2.01) [50].

2.1.11.3 Sympathomimetic Drugs

Associations have been reported between ICH and sympathomimetic drugs such as cocaine, heroin, amphetamine, and ephedrine, particularly in young patients [55]. The biological mechanisms accounting for cocaine-induced stroke in general (and ICH in particular) remain unclear. A number of contributing factors likely to be involved include vasospasm, cerebral vasculitis, enhanced platelet aggregation, cardioembolism, and hypertensive surges associated with altered cerebral autoregulation [56]. Of note, several studies have reported frequent angiographic abnormalities (up to 40%) in young patients diagnosed with ICH in the setting of cocaine use. Arteriography is therefore recommended as part of the evaluation of most young patients with non-traumatic ICH [57].

2.1.11.4 Anticoagulation Agents

Oral anticoagulation with warfarin (and other vitamin-K antagonists [VKA]) has been found to increase ICH risk by two- to fivefold, depending upon the intensity of anticoagulation [58]. As a result, VKA anticoagulation is estimated to account for approximately 5% of all non-traumatic ICH events in the United States annually. Of note, warfarin-associated ICH incidence was reported on the rise in the 1990s in the United States due to the increasing use of warfarin in older adult patients [59]. Multiple studies reported that combining warfarin with aspirin results in doubling of ICH risk, compared with similar intensity warfarin anticoagulation alone, thus resulting in an overall five- to tenfold increase in risk compared to no antithrombotic treatment at all [60]. ICH risk has been found to be lower among patients with non-valvular atrial fibrillation taking new oral anticoagulants (i.e., dabigatran, rivaroxaban, and apixaban), even when compared with well-controlled warfarin. Indeed, these agents have demonstrated increase in ICH risk comparable to aspirin monotherapy [61]. Combining new oral anticoagulation agents with aspirin increases the risk of ICH approximately twofold in published studies, while combination of new oral anticoagulants and dual antiplatelet therapy (i.e., aspirin plus clopidogrel) increases the risk of ICH an additional two- to threefold. It is important to remember that, in terms of absolute risk, ICH incidence rates remain relatively low even among those using anticoagulation agents. In most published studies, spontaneous ICH rates average 0.15% per year. Among those anticoagulated with warfarin (goal INR 2.0–3.0), ICH increases to 0.3–0.8% per year. Among patients taking new oral anticoagulation agents, ICH rates range from 0.2 to 0.8% per year. In the ATLAS-2 trial, rivaroxaban in addition to dual antiplatelet therapy (aspirin plus clopidogrel) at doses of 2.5 or 5 mg twice daily resulted in increase in yearly ICH incidence 0.2–0.4% and 0.6%, respectively [61]. These relatively small absolute increases in ICH risk are generally offset by much larger reductions in ischemic stroke events attributable to oral anticoagulation. However, absolute increase in ICH is substantially higher among certain ICH patient populations (especially those diagnosed with CAA), thus warranting a personalized approach to oral anticoagulation initiation and/or resumption [62].

2.1.11.5 Antiplatelet Agents

Antiplatelet agents (mainly aspirin and clopidogrel) were found to carry a small absolute increased risk of primary ICH based on meta-analysis of randomized controlled trial data [63]. In a subsequent review, ICH risk associated with aspirin use (for primary and secondary prevention of coronary heart disease) to be 0.2 events per 1000 patient years [64]. Existing evidence estimates dual antiplatelet therapy (aspirin plus clopidogrel) to increase ICH risk by approximately twofold compared with aspirin alone (0.4 vs. 0.2%) [65]. Of note, use of non-steroid anti-inflammatory drugs (NSAIDs) does not appear to increase ICH risk in published studies [61].

2.1.12 Other ICH Risk Factors

2.1.12.1 Sleep Apnea

Sleep apnea has been associated with increased risk for stroke in general, and hemorrhagic stroke in particular, with the bulk of available data pertaining to ICH [66]. These associations are most likely based on the known hemodynamic alterations associated with sleep apnea (especially obstructive sleep apnea), resulting in increased hypertension [67]. Published evidence suggests that obstructive sleep apnea is associated with increased likelihood of observing cerebral microbleeds on MRI, an established marker of cerebral small vessel disease, and associated with increased ICH risk [68].

2.1.12.2 Migraine and ICH Risk

A number of studies initially raised the possibility of migraine headache being associated with increased ICH risk [69]. In a meta-analysis of 8 studies (4 case-control and 4 cohort studies) involving a total of 1600 hemorrhagic strokes, the effect estimate of hemorrhagic stroke in subjects with any migraine versus control subjects was 1.48 (95% confidence interval 1.16–1.88) [70]. However, this study was limited by at least modest statistical heterogeneity in its results, as well as by the lack of specification of hemorrhagic stroke subtype (ICH vs. subarachnoid hemorrhage). However, in a more recent study involving 1797 incident cases of intracerebral hemorrhage (ICH) and 1340 of subarachnoid hemorrhage (SAH), the odds ratio of ICH among migraine patients was 1.2 (95% confidence interval 0.9–1.5) and of SAH was 1.2 (95% confidence interval 0.9–1.5) [71]. Additional studies will be required to clarify whether migraine is associated with sporadic hemorrhagic stroke subtypes (if any).

2.1.12.3 Lifestyle and Activity

A number of lifestyle, activity, and occupational factors have been associated with increased hemorrhagic stroke and/or ICH risk. In a nationwide matched case-control study conducted in Korea including 940 cases of incident hemorrhagic stroke cases (498 ICH cases and 442 subarachnoid hemorrhage cases), blue-collar workers (compared to white collar workers) had a higher risk for hemorrhagic stroke (odds ratio 1.33, 95% confidence interval, 1.06–1.66). Longer working hours were also associated with increased risk of hemorrhagic stroke. Exposure to ≥8 h/week of strenuous activity was also associated with hemorrhagic stroke risk (odds ratio 1.61, 95% confidence interval 1.26–2.05), when compared with no strenuous activity. It is likely that these findings may reflect differences in hypertension severity based on duration/intensity of work-related activities.

2.2 Risk Factors for Subarachnoid Hemorrhage

2.2.1 Pathophysiology and Risk Factors for Subarachnoid Hemorrhage

Approximately 10–15% of all strokes are hemorrhagic in nature, with subarachnoid hemorrhage (SAH) and ICH each accounting for 5–10% each. Despite recent improvement in therapeutic and supportive care strategies, SAH remains one of the most fatal forms of stroke. Survivors are also commonly affected by cognitive impairment, mood disorders, fatigue, and sleep disturbances [72]. In approximately 85% of SAH cases, the underlying etiology is rupture of saccular intracranial aneurysms. Other causes of SAH that will not be reviewed here include trauma, arteriovenous malformations/fistulae, several vasculitides, intracranial arterial dissections, and subarachnoid extension of intraparenchymal bleeding. It is worth clarifying that risk factors for aneurysm formation, rupture of an unruptured aneurysm, and aneurysmal subarachnoid hemorrhage largely overlap. Studies of SAH risk factors to date resulted in oftentimes conflicting evidence, likely reflecting bias in the studies and/or incomplete understanding of the biological mechanisms underlying aneurysms' formation and rupture. This section will be present risk factors for SAH and existing evidence supporting their role in increasing SAH risk, as summarized in Fig. 2.2.

2.2.2 Family History and Genetic Risk Factors

2.2.2.1 Family History of SAH and/or Intracranial Aneurysms

In regard to genetic contribution, SAH cases due to aneurysmal rupture can be classified as either sporadic (with no report family history) or familial (one of more family members affected). Familial clustering studies identified a threshold of two (or more) first-degree relatives with SAH as conferring the highest degree of risk [73, 74]. Family history of SAH (defined as two first-degree relatives with SAH) is associated with increased personal risk and accounts for 11% of all SAH events [75]. Overall, SAH risk is two- to sevenfold increased among first-degree relatives of SAH patients than in the general population. First- and second-degree relatives of patient diagnosed with SAH or an unruptured intracranial aneurysm also have a greater risk of an unruptured IA (8.7–13.9%), compared with the general population (1%). However, risk for SAH due to aneurysmal rupture among second-degree relatives of SAH patients is similar to the general population.

		Strength of available evidence		
		Strong	**Moderate**	**Weak**
Effect size	**Substantial** (>100% risk modification)	Family history Cigarette smoking Age Hypertension Sympathomimetic drugs Alcohol consumption		Geographical variations
	Modest (50–99% risk modification)		Cholesterol levels Short-term aspirin use	Race / Ethnicity Body mass index Statin use Diabetes mellitus
	Minimal (<50% risk modification)	Multiple genetic loci	Recent physical exertion	Regular physical exercise

Fig. 2.2 Risk factors for subarachnoid hemorrhage (SAH). Risk factors for SAH are presented and classified based on effect size (see figure for description) and strength of available, published evidence. Evidence strength defined as follows: Weak: evidence from a single study or conflicting results from multiple studies. Moderate: evidence from multiple studies, with one conflicting study at most. Strong: evidence from multiple studies and/or meta-analysis, without substantial conflicting findings and/or heterogeneity upon meta-analytical pooling

2.2.2.2 Genetic Association Studies of SAH and/or Intracranial Aneurysms

Because environmental and modifiable risk factors play a substantial role in determining SAH risk, it is possible that familial co-exposure may be falsely attributed to genetic influences on SAH risk. Identification of specific gene variants and loci affecting SAH risk is therefore a necessary logical step in clarifying the genetic architecture of this disorder. Candidate gene association studies of SAH and/or intracranial aneurysms identified numerous potential risk variants. However, these studies have been historically limited by small sample sizes and lack of consistent replication of reported findings. GWAS conducted in the last decade provided an opportunity for more robust, unbiased survey of the entire genome for associations with traits of interest. A recent meta-analysis pooled results from 61 studies (both candidate genetic studies and GWAS), including 32,887 cases of SAH/intracranial aneurysms and 83,683 controls data from [76]. A total of 11 risk variants located in eight genetic loci of interest were found to be consistently associated with intracranial aneurysms, including 9p21 (rs1333040 and rs10757278), 8q11 (variants rs9298506 and rs10958409), 4q31.23 (rs6841581), 9p21.3 (rs2891168), 2q33 (rs1429412 and rs700651), 7q13 (rs4628172), 12q22 (rs6538595), and 20p20.1 (rs1132274). Several genes of interest corresponding to these findings may shed additional light on the pathophysiology of SAH/aneurysm formation. SNP rs1333040 (chromosome 9p21.3) is located in the cyclin-dependent kinase inhibitor 2B (CDKN2B) antisense gene locus, which is associated with a wide spectrum of arterial disorders (including coronary artery disease and abdominal aortic aneurysms). These findings raise the possibility of shared common biological processes underlying several common cardiovascular conditions;

unfortunately the exact function of the CDKN2B gene is not fully understood [72]. SNP rs10757278 on chromosome 9p21.3 is located in a noncoding RNA region called ANRIL (antisense noncoding RNA in the INK4 locus), whose function remains unclear. However, prior functional studies suggest a relationship with expression of the CDKN2B and CDKN2A genes, involved in cell cycle signaling [77]. Two SNPs on chromosome 8q (rs10958409 and rs9298506) surround the SOX17 gene, which plays an important role in generation and maintenance of stem cells of endothelial and hematopoietic lineages, crucial in the formation and maintenance of vascular endothelium. SNP rs6841581 is located on chromosome 4q31.23, coding for the endothelin receptor type A (EDNRA) gene, a G-protein-coupled receptor for endothelins. The EDNRA gene protein product is thought to modulate vasoconstriction and vasodilatation after hemodynamic insult, therefore likely impacting aneurysm formation risk. SNPs rs1429412 and rs700651 are located at 2q33 and flank both the BOLL gene (involved in germ cell development) and the phospholipase C–like 1 gene (involved in intracellular cascade reactions with abolished phospholipase C activity). SNP rs4628172 on chromosome 7 is located within the TMEM195 gene, which encodes transmembrane proteins, possibly involved in fatty acid biosynthesis and iron binding.

2.2.3 Race/Ethnic and Geographical Differences in SAH Risk

The overall incidence of SAH in population-based studies (including out-of-hospital deaths) has been estimated at 9.1/100,000 people per year, with 95% confidence interval of 8.8–9.5 [78]. However, substantial regional variations in incidence have been reported. In the United States, the incidence is reportedly between 10 and 15/100,000. Much lower rates have been reported in China (2/100,000) and in South and Central America (4/100,000), while higher rates are reported in Finland and Japan (19 to 23/100,000). It is currently widely debated whether these variations reflect the true underlying differences based on racial/ethnic/geographic factors, as opposed to differences in case ascertainment and capture across different studies. In one US study including 107 SAH patients, the overall age-adjusted risk ratio in Mexican-Americans compared with non-Hispanic whites was 1.67 (95% confidence interval 1.13–2.47) [79]. These findings are in contrast with low overall SAH incidence rates in South and Central America, likely pointing to a complex interplay of genetic, cultural, and geographic factors in determining any association of race/ethnicity with SAH risk.

2.2.4 Advancing Age

Multiple studies have shown increasing SAH incidence with age. In a systematic review and meta-analysis, the existing calculated SAH incidence for average age 35 years was 8.6/100,000 (95% confidence interval 8.0–9.2). For every year of increase in mean age, SAH incidence was found to be 1.06 times higher (95% confidence interval 1.05–1.07) [78]. Among age categories, SAH incidence ranged from 2.0/100,000 (95% confidence interval 1.6–2.6), for those aged <25 years, to 31.3/100,000 (95% confidence interval 24.6–39.8) among those age > 85 years. Overall these findings likely reflect prolonged exposures to other established SAH risk factors (smoking, hypertension, alcohol consumption) among older individuals. It is worth noting that the aforementioned systematic review found that at younger ages (<45 years), SAH incidence was slightly higher in men, whereas in the fifth decade and beyond, SAH incidence was markedly higher in women. These findings point to hormonal effects and related changes later in life as crucial factors in the association between age and SAH risk among women.

2.2.5 Sexual Differences in SAH Risk

As mentioned above, SAH incidence is approximately 1.6 times higher in women than in men, but this difference becomes evident only after the fifth decade [78]. Estrogen and, less commonly, progesterone, have been postulated to have protective effects and thus to contribute to the increased SAH incidence in postmenopausal women. However, a recent meta-analysis showed that while these hormones might affect SAH risk, existing data are conflicting [80]. Among participants in 18 studies, the combined adjusted odds ratios for SAH were 1.31 (95% confidence interval 1.05–1.64) for current use of combined oral contraceptives, 0.90 (95% confidence interval 0.74–1.09) for ever combined oral contraceptive use, 0.86 (95% confidence interval 0.69–1.08) for current use of hormone replacement therapy, 0.74 (95% confidence interval 0.54–1.00) for ever use of HRT, and 1.29 (95% confidence interval) for postmenopausal women. Similarly, while prior studies reported associations between SAH risk and parity or age at menarche, this systematic review found results to be heterogeneous. Additional studies are therefore required to more definitively ascertain how hormonal levels and their changes over time directly impact SAH risk.

2.2.6 Cigarette Smoking

Cigarette smoking appears to be the most powerful modifiable risk factor for SAH [81]. In published longitudinal and case-control studies, the reported relative risks associated with smoking are of 2.0 and above. Most studies demonstrated a dose-dependent effect of cigarette smoking on SAH risk, with heavy smokers being at higher risk than lighter smokers. Individuals who stop smoking were shown to have decreasing SAH over time, with benefits less evident for prior heavy smokers [81]. In one cohort study, smoking was found to be a stronger SAH risk factor in women than men [82]. Similarly, in another study hypertension and smoking history interacted to increase risk above the level expected from the sum of the two independent effects [83]. A number of putative biological mechanisms have been postulated to account for the association between smoking and SAH risk [84]. Smoking has been found to promote increase in blood levels of proteases (such as elastase) and to influence their activity, thus potentially contributing to vessel wall damage. Smoking also leads to elevated fibrinogen blood levels, potentially resulting in increased blood viscosity and increased hemodynamic stress. Additionally, transient blood pressure elevations have been documented for hours after smoking, likely due to nicotine-induced catecholamine release leading to increased hemodynamic stress. Finally, smoking has been shown to exert antiestrogenic effects, thus likely nullifying the previously discussed beneficial effects of estrogens on SAH risk.

2.2.7 Hypertension

Hypertension has been associated with an increased SAH risk in multiple studies, with relative risk ratios ranging from 2.0 to 3.4 [84]. Hypertension is thought to impact risk for aneurysm formation and rupture by (1) causing increased endothelial damage; (2) leading to ischemic occlusion of the arterial vasa vasorum; (3) altering biosynthesis of elastin and collagen; (4) causing indirect vessel wall damage by affecting endothelial production of several molecules, including matrix metalloproteinase-13 and NO; and (5) causing direct mechanical damage by increasing hemodynamic stress on the vessel wall of cerebral arteries [84]. As previously mentioned for hypertension and ICH risk, our understanding of the association between SAH risk and hypertension remains incomplete. Existing evidence has failed to uncover specific blood pressure measures/treatment goal specifically associated with increased SAH risk. The role of blood pressure variability (if any) in determining SAH risk remains poorly understood and is the topic of limited investigative efforts. Finally racial/ethnic and geographical variations in hypertension epidemiology likely account, at least in part, for previously presented regional differences in SAH incidence worldwide.

2.2.8 Alcohol Consumption

The relationship between alcohol consumption and increased SAH risk has been the topic of multiple studies [84]. SAH risk has been shown to increase for weekly consumption of ~120–150 g of alcohol, with increasing amounts of alcohol elevating risk in a dose-dependent fashion. Published studies report relative risk ratios ranging from 2.1 to 4.7. However, light-to-moderate alcohol consumption (~100 g/week or less) has been inversely associated with SAH risk in some studies, suggesting a potential protective effect. Of note, most studies have reported higher relative risk for SAH in women vs. men for identical amounts of alcohol consumed [84]. The protective effect of light-to-moderate drinking could be related to beneficial antioxidant and anti-inflammatory effects reducing vessel wall damage. Conversely, heavy alcohol consumption is associated with increased oxidative stress, as well as with increased blood pressure, hematocrit, plasma osmolarity, and fibrinogen levels in blood – overall resulting in increased hemodynamic stress [41].

2.2.9 Other SAH Risk Factors

2.2.9.1 Sympathomimetic Drugs

As for hemorrhagic stroke in general, sympathomimetic drugs (chiefly cocaine) have been associated with an increased SAH risk, with reported relative risk indicating an increase in risk above tenfold among cocaine users [84]. As previously mentioned, cocaine use is associated with vasospasm (by promoting intracellular calcium release from the sarcoplasmic reticulum in cerebral vascular smooth muscle cells), impaired cerebral autoregulation, and systemic elevation in blood pressure. In case-control studies, phenylpropanolamine present in appetite suppressants (and possibly certain cold remedies) was associated with increased risk for hemorrhagic stroke (including both intracerebral hemorrhage and subarachnoid hemorrhage) among women [85]. Similarly, caffeine-containing medications have also been associated with increased SAH risk in isolated reports [86].

2.2.9.2 Low Cholesterol and Statin Use

As previously mentioned (see Sect. 2.1.8), elevated cholesterol is inversely associated with risk for hemorrhagic stroke, including SAH [47]. Of note, in comparison with ICH, studies associating cholesterol levels with SAH risk have been less consistent. As previously mentioned, a recent systematic review and meta-analysis found differential associations between cholesterol levels and risk of SAH vs. ICH among East Asian vs. non-East Asian populations [48]. Multiple studies failed to report associations between SAH risk and statin exposure [72].

2.2.9.3 Diabetes Mellitus

Diabetes mellitus was associated with a reduced risk of SAH in one review [87]. These findings are in contrast with established evidence linking insulin resistance with endothelial dysfunction, inflammation, and oxidative stress [84]. However, these findings were statistically significant only in case-control studies upon systematic review. The authors of the review themselves suggested conclude that the association between diabetes and reduced SAH risk may reflect bias related to either (1) increased competing mortality caused by diseases other than SAH or (2) better control of other SAH risk factors (especially hypertension and smoking) among diabetic patients.

2.2.9.4 Physical Exercise

A systematic review of SAH risk factors found that one longitudinal study demonstrated a weak, nonsignificant protective effect of regular rigorous physical activity in men only [87]. However, two case-control studies showed an opposite, detrimental effect of regular rigorous physical activity on SAH risk. Additional studies will be required to clarify the effect on long-term physical activity on SAH risk. A number of studies in the literature have also focused on the role of vigorous exertion (including sports and intercourse) on immediate risk of aneurysmal rupture. A systematic review found that 19% of SAH events occurred during or within 2 h of moderate or heavy exercise (odds ratio 2.7, 95% confidence interval 1.6–4.6 for comparison with no or light exercise) [72]. However, the absolute number of exertion-related cases was deemed to be low (population-attributable risk of 7.9%).

2.2.9.5 Body Mass Index

Low BMI was associated with an ~ 70% decrease in SAH risk in a longitudinal study, but it was associated with increased risk (although not statistically significant) in two case-control studies [87]. A more recent report from Japan found evidence of a J-shaped association between SAH risk and body mass index, with both very low and very high values increasing risk [88].

2.2.9.6 Antiplatelet Agents and Oral Anticoagulants

Although very limited data is currently available, oral anticoagulation is generally considered to increase risk for SAH [72]. On the contrary, several studies suggested that the use of low-dose aspirin may reduce SAH risk. However, in a recent meta-analysis including seven studies, no significant association was found between aspirin use (of any duration or frequency) and SAH risk (odds ratio 1.00; 95% confidence interval 0.81–1.24) [89]. The authors of this meta-analysis uncovered a significant association between short-term use of aspirin (<3 months) and increased SAH risk (odds ratio 1.61; 95% confidence interval 1.20–2.18), but not for longer use. Additional studies are needed to quantify the increase in SAH risk conferred by antiplatelet agents and anticoagulants, especially newer anticoagulation agents.

References

1. Qureshi AI, Tuhrim S, Broderick JP, et al. Spontaneous intracerebral hemorrhage. N Engl J Med. 2001;344:1450–60.
2. Pantoni L. Cerebral small vessel disease: from pathogenesis and clinical characteristics to therapeutic challenges. Lancet Neurol. 2010;9:689–701.
3. Biffi A, Greenberg SM. Cerebral amyloid angiopathy: a systematic review. J Clin Neurol. 2011;7:1–9.
4. Biffi A, Anderson C, Battey TW, et al. Association between blood pressure control and risk of recurrent intracerebral hemorrhage. JAMA. 2015;314(9):904–12.
5. Rost NS, Greenberg SM, Rosand J. The genetic architecture of intracerebral hemorrhage. Stroke. 2008;39:2166–73.
6. Woo D, Sekar P, Chakraborty R, et al. Genetic epidemiology of intracerebral hemorrhage. J Stroke Cerebrovasc. 2005;14:239–43.
7. Devan WJ, Falcone GJ, Anderson CD, et al. Heritability estimates identify a substantial genetic contribution to risk and outcome of intracerebral hemorrhage. Stroke. 2013;44:1578–83.
8. Biffi A, Sonni A, Anderson CD, et al. Variants at APOE influence risk of deep and lobar intracerebral hemorrhage. Ann Neurol. 2010;68:934–43.
9. Biffi A, Shulman JM, Jagiella JM, et al. Genetic variation at CR1 increases risk of cerebral amyloid angiopathy. Neurology. 2012;78:334–41.
10. Valant V, Keenan B, Anderson C, et al. TOMM40 in cerebral amyloid angiopathy related intracerebral hemorrhage: comparative genetic analysis with Alzheimer's disease. Transl Stroke Res. 2012;3(Suppl 1):S102–12.
11. Hamaguchi T, Okino S, Sodeyama N, et al. Association of a polymorphism of the transforming growth factor-{beta}1 gene with cerebral amyloid angiopathy. J Neurol Neurosur Ps. 2005;76:696–9.
12. Peila R, Yucesoy B, White LR, et al. A TGF-beta1 polymorphism association with dementia and neuropathologies: the HAAS. Neurobiol Aging. 2007;28:1367–73.
13. Woo D, Broderick JP. Spontaneous intracerebral hemorrhage: epidemiology and clinical presentation. Neurosurg Clin N Am. 2002;13:265–79.
14. Woo D, Falcone GJ, Devan WJ, et al. Meta-analysis of genome-wide association studies identifies 1q22 as a susceptibility locus for intracerebral hemorrhage. Am J Hum Genet. 2014;94:511–21.
15. Fornage M, Debette S, Bis JC, et al. Genome-wide association studies of cerebral white matter lesion burden: the CHARGE consortium. Ann Neurol. 2011;69:928–39.
16. Verhaaren BF, Debette S, Bis JC, et al. Multiethnic genome-wide association study of cerebral white matter hyperintensities on MRI. Circ Cardiovasc Genet. 2015;8:398–409.
17. Raffeld MR, Biffi A, Battey TW, et al. APOE epsilon4 and lipid levels affect risk of recurrent nonlobar intracerebral hemorrhage. Neurology. 2015;85:349–56.
18. Volonghi I, Pezzini A, Del Zotto E, et al. Role of COL4A1 in basement-membrane integrity and cerebral small-vessel disease. The COL4A1 stroke syndrome. Curr Med Chem. 2010;17:1317–24.
19. Gould DB, Phalan FC, Van Mil SE, et al. Role of COL4A1 in small-vessel disease and hemorrhagic stroke. N Engl J Med. 2006;354:1489–96.
20. Weng YC, Sonni A, Labelle-Dumais C, et al. COL4A1 mutations in patients with sporadic late-onset intracerebral hemorrhage. Ann Neurol. 2012;71:470–7.

21. Jeanne M, Labelle-Dumais C, Jorgensen J, et al. COL4A2 mutations impair COL4A1 and COL4A2 secretion and cause hemorrhagic stroke. Am J Hum Genet. 2012;90:91–101.
22. Rannikmae K, Davies G, Thomson PA, et al. Common variation in COL4A1/COL4A2 is associated with sporadic cerebral small vessel disease. Neurology. 2015;84:918–26.
23. Poon MT, Bell SM, Al-Shahi Salman R. Epidemiology of intracerebral haemorrhage. Front Neurol Neurosci. 2015;37:1–12.
24. Flaherty ML, Woo D, Haverbusch M, et al. Racial variations in location and risk of intracerebral hemorrhage. Stroke. 2005;36:934–7.
25. Labovitz DL, Halim A, Boden-Albala B, et al. The incidence of deep and lobar intracerebral hemorrhage in whites, blacks, and Hispanics. Neurology. 2005;65:518–22.
26. Woo D, Rosand J, Kidwell C, et al. The ethnic/racial variations of intracerebral hemorrhage (ERICH) study protocol. Stroke. 2013;44:e120–5.
27. Walsh KB, Woo D, Sekar P, et al. Untreated hypertension: a powerful risk factor for lobar and nonlobar intracerebral hemorrhage in whites, blacks, and hispanics. Circulation. 2016;134:1444–52.
28. Hong KS, Bang OY, Kang DW, et al. Stroke statistics in Korea: part I. Epidemiology and risk factors: a report from the Korean stroke society and clinical research center for stroke. J Stroke. 2013;15:2–20.
29. Toyoda K. Epidemiology and registry studies of stroke in Japan. J Stroke. 2013;15:21–6.
30. Benjamin EJ, Blaha MJ, Chiuve SE et al. Heart disease and stroke statistics-2017 update: a report from the American Heart Association. Circulation. 2017; 135:00–00.
31. Ariesen MJ, Claus SP, Rinkel GJE, et al. Risk factors for intracerebral hemorrhage in the general population: a systematic review. Stroke. 2003;34:2060–5.
32. Van Asch CJ, Luitse MJ, Rinkel GJ, et al. Incidence, case fatality, and functional outcome of intracerebral haemorrhage over time, according to age, sex, and ethnic origin: a systematic review and meta-analysis. Lancet Neurol. 2010;9:167–76.
33. Zia E, Pessah-Rasmussen H, Khan FA, et al. Risk factors for primary intracerebral hemorrhage: a population-based nested case-control study. Cerebrovasc Dis. 2006;21:18–25.
34. Martini SR, Flaherty ML, Brown WM, et al. Risk factors for intracerebral hemorrhage differ according to hemorrhage location. Neurology. 2012;79:2275–82.
35. Jackson CA, Sudlow CLM. Is hypertension a more frequent risk factor for deep than for lobar supratentorial intracerebral haemorrhage? J Neurol Neurosurg. 2006;77:1244–52.
36. Rothwell PM, Howard SC, Dolan E, et al. Effects of beta blockers and calcium-channel blockers on within-individual variability in blood pressure and risk of stroke. Lancet Neurol. 2010;9:469–80.
37. Jolink WM, Klijn CJ, Brouwers PJ, et al. Time trends in incidence, case fatality, and mortality of intracerebral hemorrhage. Neurology. 2015;85:1318–24.
38. Lionakis N, Mendrinos D, Sanidas E, et al. Hypertension in the elderly. World J Cardiol. 2012;4:135–47.
39. Larsson SC, Wallin A, Wolk A, et al. Differing association of alcohol consumption with different stroke types: a systematic review and meta-analysis. BMC Med. 2016;14:178.
40. Xin X, He J, Frontini MG, et al. Effects of alcohol reduction on blood pressure: a meta-analysis of randomized controlled trials. Hypertension. 2001;38:1112–7.
41. Gorelick PB, Kelly MA. Alcohol as a risk factor for stroke. Heart Dis Stroke. 1992;1:255–8.
42. Thrift AG, Mcneil JJ, Forbes A, et al. Risk factors for cerebral hemorrhage in the era of well-controlled hypertension. Melbourne risk factor study (MERFS) group. Stroke. 1996;27:2020–5.
43. Giroud M, Creisson E, Fayolle H, et al. Risk factors for primary cerebral hemorrhage: a population-based study—the stroke registry of Dijon. Neuroepidemiology. 1995;14:20–6.
44. Iribarren C, Jacobs DR, Sadler M, et al. Low total serum cholesterol and intracerebral hemorrhagic stroke: is the association confined to elderly men? Stroke. 1996;27:1993–8.
45. Segal AZ, Chiu RI, Eggleston-Sexton PM, et al. Low cholesterol as a risk factor for primary intracerebral hemorrhage: a case-control study. Neuroepidemiology. 1999;18:185–93.
46. Yano K, Reed DM, Maclean CJ. Serum cholesterol and hemorrhagic stroke in the Honolulu heart program. Stroke. 1989;20:1460–5.
47. Wang X, Dong Y, Qi X, et al. Cholesterol levels and risk of hemorrhagic stroke: a systematic review and meta-analysis. Stroke. 2013;44:1833–9.
48. Xie L, Wu W, Chen J, et al. Cholesterol levels and hemorrhagic stroke risk in east Asian versus non-east Asian populations: a systematic review and meta-analysis. Neurologist. 2017;22:107–15.
49. Mckinney JS, Kostis WJ. Statin therapy and the risk of intracerebral hemorrhage: a meta-analysis of 31 randomized controlled trials. Stroke. 2012;43:2149–56.
50. Pandit AK, Kumar P, Kumar A, et al. High-dose statin therapy and risk of intracerebral hemorrhage: a meta-analysis. Acta Neurol Scand. 2016;134:22–8.
51. Bos MJ, Koudstaal PJ, Hofman A, et al. Decreased glomerular filtration rate is a risk factor for hemorrhagic but not for ischemic stroke: the Rotterdam study. Stroke. 2007;38:3127–32.
52. Ovbiagele B, Wing JJ, Menon RS, et al. Association of chronic kidney disease with cerebral microbleeds in patients with primary intracerebral hemorrhage. Stroke. 2013;44:2409–13.
53. Kim SH, Shin DW, Yun JM, et al. Kidney dysfunction and cerebral microbleeds in neurologically healthy adults. PLoS One. 2017;12:e0172210.
54. Hoirisch-Clapauch S, Nardi AE, Gris JC, et al. Are the antiplatelet and profibrinolytic properties of selective serotonin-reuptake inhibitors relevant to their brain effects? Thromb Res. 2014;134:11–6.

55. Pozzi M, Roccatagliata D, Sterzi R. Drug abuse and intracranial hemorrhage. Neurol Sci. 2008;29(Suppl 2):S269–70.
56. Treadwell SD, Robinson TG. Cocaine use and stroke. Postgrad Med J. 2007;83:389–94.
57. Mcevoy AW, Kitchen ND, Thomas DG. Intracerebral haemorrhage and drug abuse in young adults. Brit J Neurosurg. 2000;14:449–54.
58. Rosand J, Eckman MH, Knudsen KA, et al. The effect of warfarin and intensity of anticoagulation on outcome of intracerebral hemorrhage. Arch Intern Med. 2004;164:880–4.
59. Flaherty ML, Haverbusch M, Sekar P, et al. The increasing burden of anticoagulant-associated intracerebral hemorrhage. Stroke. 2006;37:623.
60. Shireman TI, Howard PA, Kresowik TF, et al. Combined anticoagulant-antiplatelet use and major bleeding events in elderly atrial fibrillation patients. Stroke. 2004;35:2362–7.
61. An SJ, Kim TJ, Yoon BW. Epidemiology, risk factors, and clinical features of intracerebral hemorrhage: an update. J Stroke. 2017;19:3–10.
62. Charidimou A, Shoamanesh A, Al-Shahi Salman R, et al. Cerebral amyloid angiopathy, cerebral microbleeds and implications for anticoagulation decisions: the need for a balanced approach. Int J Stroke. 2018;13:117–20.
63. Hart RG, Pearce LA, Aguilar MI. Meta-analysis: antithrombotic therapy to prevent stroke in patients who have nonvalvular atrial fibrillation. Ann Intern Med. 2007;146:857–67.
64. Gorelick PB. Combining aspirin with oral anticoagulant therapy: is this a safe and effective practice in patients with atrial fibrillation? Stroke. 2007;38:1652–4.
65. Investigators A, Connolly SJ, Pogue J, et al. Effect of clopidogrel added to aspirin in patients with atrial fibrillation. N Engl J Med. 2009;360:2066–78.
66. Covassin N, Somers VK. Sleep apnea, hypertension, and hemorrhagic stroke-deja vu all over again. J Am Soc Hypertens. 2016;10:197–200.
67. Floras JS. Hypertension and sleep apnea. Can J Cardiol. 2015;31:889–97.
68. Koo DL, Kim JY, Lim JS, et al. Cerebral microbleeds on MRI in patients with obstructive sleep apnea. J Clin Sleep Med. 2017;13:65–72.
69. Sacco S, Ricci S, Carolei A. Migraine and vascular diseases: a review of the evidence and potential implications for management. Cephalalgia. 2012;32:785–95.
70. Sacco S, Ornello R, Ripa P, et al. Migraine and hemorrhagic stroke: a meta-analysis. Stroke. 2013;44:3032–8.
71. Gaist D, Gonzalez-Perez A, Ashina M, et al. Migraine and risk of hemorrhagic stroke: a study based on data from general practice. J Headache Pain. 2014;15:74.
72. Macdonald RL, Schweizer TA. Spontaneous subarachnoid haemorrhage. Lancet. 2017;389:655–66.
73. Broderick JP, Brown RD Jr, Sauerbeck L, et al. Greater rupture risk for familial as compared to sporadic unruptured intracranial aneurysms. Stroke. 2009;40:1952–7.
74. Broderick JP, Sauerbeck LR, Foroud T, et al. Familial intracranial aneurysm (FIA) study protocol. BMC Med Genet. 2005;6(17)
75. Ruigrok YM, Buskens E, Rinkel GJ. Attributable risk of common and rare determinants of subarachnoid hemorrhage. Stroke. 2001;32:1173–5.
76. Alg VS, Sofat R, Houlden H, et al. Genetic risk factors for intracranial aneurysms: a meta-analysis in more than 116,000 individuals. Neurology. 2013;80:2154–65.
77. Yasuno K, Bilguvar K, Bijlenga P, et al. Genome-wide association study of intracranial aneurysm identifies three new risk loci. Nat Genet. 2010;42:420–5.
78. De Rooij NK, Linn FH, Van Der Plas JA, et al. Incidence of subarachnoid haemorrhage: a systematic review with emphasis on region, age, gender and time trends. J Neurol Neurosurg. 2007;78:1365–72.
79. Eden SV, Meurer WJ, Sanchez BN, et al. Gender and ethnic differences in subarachnoid hemorrhage. Neurology. 2008;71:731–5.
80. Algra AM, Klijn CJ, Helmerhorst FM, et al. Female risk factors for subarachnoid hemorrhage: a systematic review. Neurology. 2012;79:1230–6.
81. Kim CK, Kim BJ, Ryu WS, et al. Impact of smoking cessation on the risk of subarachnoid haemorrhage: a nationwide multicentre case control study. J Neurol Neurosurg. 2012;83:1100–3.
82. Lindekleiv H, Sandvei MS, Njolstad I, et al. Sex differences in risk factors for aneurysmal subarachnoid hemorrhage: a cohort study. Neurology. 2011;76:637–43.
83. Lindekleiv H, Sandvei MS, Romundstad PR, et al. Joint effect of modifiable risk factors on the risk of aneurysmal subarachnoid hemorrhage: a cohort study. Stroke. 2012;43:1885–9.
84. Andreasen TH, Bartek J Jr, Andresen M, et al. Modifiable risk factors for aneurysmal subarachnoid hemorrhage. Stroke. 2013;44:3607–12.
85. Yoon BW, Bae HJ, Hong KS, et al. Phenylpropanolamine contained in cold remedies and risk of hemorrhagic stroke. Neurology. 2007;68:146–9.
86. Lee SM, Choi NK, Lee BC, et al. Caffeine-containing medicines increase the risk of hemorrhagic stroke. Stroke. 2013;44:2139–43.
87. Feigin VL, Rinkel GJ, Lawes CM, et al. Risk factors for subarachnoid hemorrhage: an updated systematic review of epidemiological studies. Stroke. 2005;36:2773–80.
88. Kawate N, Kayaba K, Hara M, et al. Body mass index and incidence of subarachnoid hemorrhage in Japanese community residents: the Jichi medical school cohort study. J Stroke Cerebrovasc. 2017;26:1683–8.
89. Phan K, Moore JM, Griessenauer CJ, et al. Aspirin and risk of subarachnoid hemorrhage: systematic review and meta-analysis. Stroke. 2017;48:1210–7.

3 Pathophysiology of Primary Intracerebral Hemorrhage: Insights into Cerebral Small Vessel Disease

Marco Pasi and Anand Viswanathan

3.1 Introduction

Spontaneous intracerebral, non-traumatic intracerebral hemorrhage (ICH) results from rupture and bleeding of small arteries and arterioles into the brain resulting in the formation of a parenchymal hematoma [1, 2]. Depending on the underlying cause, ICH may be classified as primary or secondary. Secondary causes of ICH include vascular malformations, brain tumors with hemorrhage, a variety of bleeding disorders, infection-associated bleeding, or inflammatory disorders [3]. This chapter will focus on primary ICH which accounts for 77–88% of ICH cases and results from sporadic aged-related cerebral small vessel disease [1, 3–7].

The term small vessel disease is generally used to describe all the diseases that affect the small arteries, arterioles, and capillaries that are located in the brain parenchyma or in the leptomeningeal vessels [8–11]. While recent investigational work has suggested that it may be possible to visualize pathologies in these small arteries with 7 Tesla MRI [12, 13], standard neuroimaging used in clinical practice does yet not allow the direct visualization of these vessels. Thus, the term small vessel disease as it is currently used does not describe the vessel pathology per se but rather encompasses all the consequences of small vessel pathology on brain parenchymal tissue [14].

The two main forms of sporadic small vessel disease which are strongly associated with ICH are hypertensive small vessel disease and cerebral amyloid angiopathy (CAA; Table 3.1). The location of ICH is suggestive of the dominant underlying microangiopathy [1, 15, 16]. Pathologic evaluation of serial sections of hematoma tissue has shown that degenerative vessel wall changes related to long-term hypertension are responsible of the rupture of deep perforating arteries, thus manifesting as hemorrhagic hypertensive small vessel disease [1, 17, 18]. The rupture of these deep arteries with a diameter between 50 and 400 μm is the main mechanism underlying putaminal, caudate, thalamic, and pontine ICHs [1, 19]. Similarly, extensive amyloid deposition in the medium-sized arteries of the cerebral cortex and overlying leptomeninges may also lead to vasculopathic changes [20, 21]. The breakdown of disrupted amyloid-laden vessel walls appears to be the substrate for lobar CAA-related ICH [21–23].

This chapter discusses ICH related to these two common forms of sporadic cerebral small vessel disease, highlighting the pathophysiology related to small- and medium-sized artery rupture. We additionally discuss the different MRI

M. Pasi · A. Viswanathan (✉)
Hemorrhagic Stroke Research Program, Department of Neurology, Massachusetts General Hospital Stroke Research Center, Harvard Medical School, Boston, MA, USA
e-mail: aviswanathan1@partners.org

S.-H. Lee (ed.), *Stroke Revisited: Hemorrhagic Stroke*, Stroke Revisited,
https://doi.org/10.1007/978-981-10-1427-7_3

Table 3.1 Neuropathological, clinical, and neuroimaging characteristics of hypertensive small vessel disease and cerebral amyloid angiopathy-related ICH

Characteristics	Hypertensive small vessel disease-related ICH	Cerebral amyloid angiopathy-related ICH
Small vessel pathology	Arteriolosclerosis [57], lypohialinosis [1, 53], fibrinoid necrosis [50, 55], in absence of cerebral amyloid angiopathy	Amyloid-β deposition and associated vasculopathy in cortical and leptomeningeal vessels [20, 22, 23]
Risk factors	Hypertension [1, 24, 28, 29] and vascular risk factors [28, 35]	Age, apolipoprotein E ε4 and ε2 [21–23, 79–81]
Location ICH	Typically deep: Putamen [41], caudatus [19, 41], thalamus [42], pons [17]; cerebellum (deep area) [17]	Lobar (cortical-subcortical) [7, 22, 23], less common cerebellum (superficial area) [83]
Cerebral microbleeds	Predominantly deep [87, 98–100], with or without lobar [87]	Strictly lobar [15, 71]
Cortical superficial siderosis	Rare [104]	Very common in symptomatic CAA [68–70, 103]
White matter hyperintensities	No predilection for a specific brain region, peri-basal ganglia pattern [93]	Posterior predominance [92], white matter spots [93]
Enlarged perivascular spaces	Basal ganglia [93, 109, 110]	Centrum semiovale [93, 109, 110]
Lacunes	Usually in the basal ganglia or deep white matter [1, 90]. Further evidence is needed	Reported to be located in lobar area in one study [90]. Further evidence is needed
DWI-positive lesions	Not a preferential distribution, reported to be less common than in lobar ICH [113]. Further evidence is needed	Reports to be present in 15% of patients, not preferential distribution [113]. Further evidence is needed

ICH intracerebral hemorrhage, *DWI* diffusion-weighted imaging

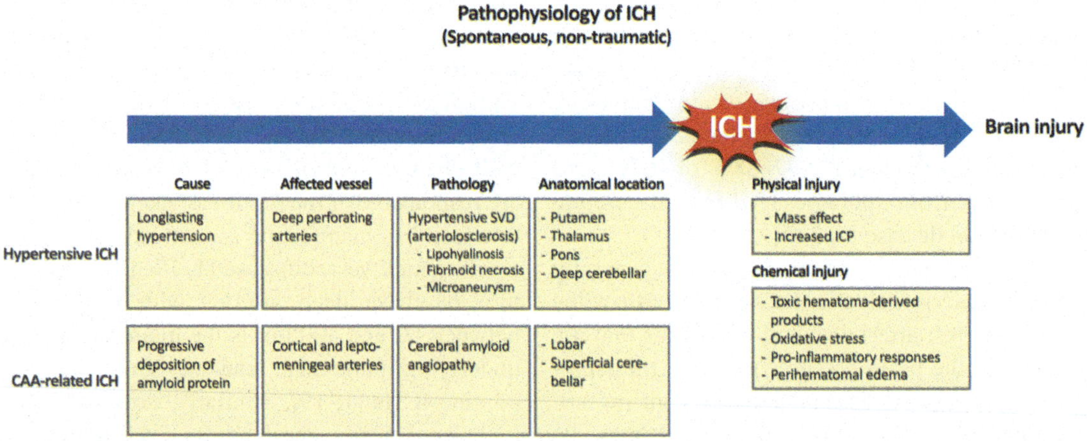

Fig. 3.1 Pathophysiology of intracerebral hemorrhage (ICH). *ICH* intracerebral hemorrhage, *SVD* small vessel disease, *CAA* cerebral amyloid angiopathy

manifestations encountered in ICH patients, specifically focusing on the location and patterns suggestive of a specific type of underlying small vessel disease. In the second part of the chapter, dynamic processes related to hematoma evolution and mechanism of primary and secondary brain injury will also be explored. Conceptual diagram of pathophysiology of ICH is described in Fig. 3.1.

3.2 Pathophysiology of Hypertensive Intracerebral Hemorrhage

Hypertensive ICH most commonly occurs in the basal ganglia, thalamus, and brainstem and less commonly in the cerebellum (Fig. 3.2) [1]. When ICH occurs in those regions, a history of hypertension has been reported with a frequency

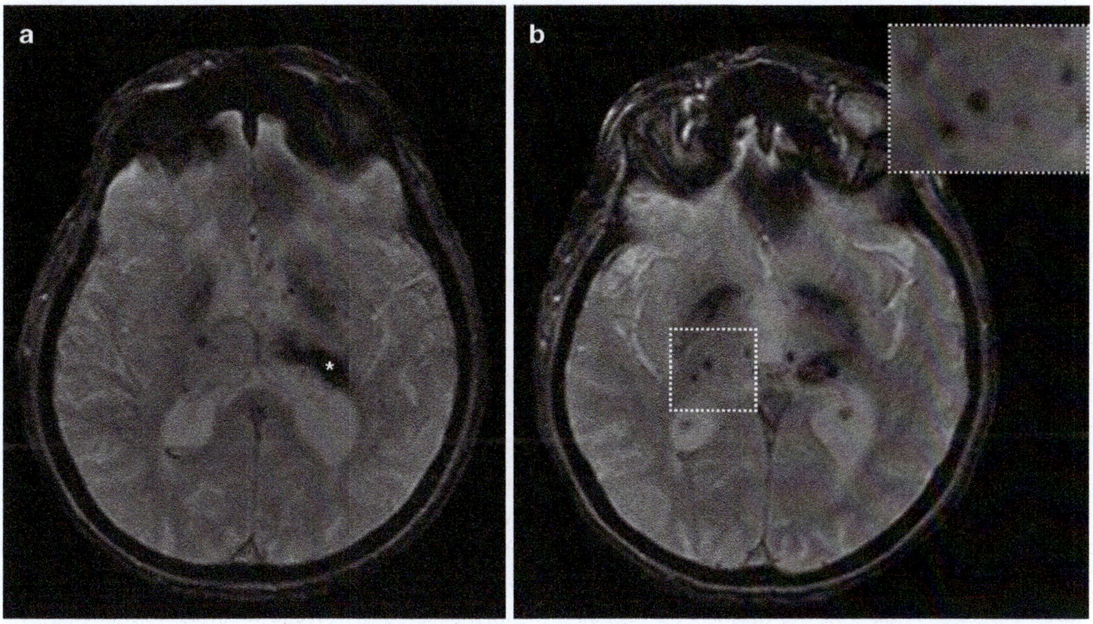

Fig. 3.2 Hypertensive small vessel disease-related intracerebral hemorrhage. T2*-gradient echo MRI sequences in a patient with hypertensive small vessel disease-related intracerebral hemorrhage. Panel **a** shows a left thalamic hematoma (*star*). The same patient showed strictly deep located cerebral microbleeds (**b**, *inset*) without any lobar cerebral microbleeds

that ranges from 50 to 86% [24–26]. In the majority of studies, history of hypertension was more prevalent in patients with deep than in those with lobar primary ICH [27–29]. In contrast with these results, a population-based study performed in Greater Cincinnati found that in 188 ICH cases, hypertension was equally prevalent in both lobar and deep ICH (67% and 73%, respectively) without significant differences in prevalence between different age groups [30]. Hypertension and poor blood pressure control seem also a risk factor of future ICH, irrespective of the location of the hematoma [31–34]. The PROGRESS trial showed beneficial effects of antihypertensive treatment in reducing the risk of ICH with a 76% relative risk reduction in comparison with the placebo-treated group at 4 years follow-up [31]. As hypertension is a multisystem disease, studies have suggested that pathology in other organs may also be concurrently found in patients with ICH. Autopsy studies have shown that left ventricular hypertrophy is a common finding in ICH patients [29]. Furthermore, population-based study participants with electrocardiographic left ventricular hypertrophy carry a higher risk of ICH than those without (hazard ratio [HR]: 1.7, 95% confidence interval [CI]: 0.77–3.7) in Cardiovascular Health Study (HR 2.8, 95% CI: 1.2–6.4 in the Atherosclerosis Risk in Communities Study) [35]. Similarly, renal dysfunction is a frequent comorbidity in patients with spontaneous ICH [36–38]. One major hypothesis for this association is the coexistence of small vessel microangiopathies in the brain and kidney [39]. Both are low-resistance end organs which are exposed to high-volume blood flow throughout the cardiac cycle [39]. Furthermore, there are similarities between the microvascular systems of the kidney and the brain [40]. Recently, in 97 primary ICH patients, it has been shown that renal dysfunction (estimated glomerular filtration rate [eGFR] <60 mL/min/1.73 m^2) was present in 12% of the patients [37]. Similar rates were reported in the Intensive Blood Pressure Reduction in Acute Cerebral Hemorrhage Trial (INTERACT 2). In this trial, 280 (11%) of the recruited patients had moderately/severely decreased eGFR [38]. In the population-based Rotterdam Study, renal dysfunction was a strong risk factor for hemorrhagic, but not ischemic stroke [36]. However, more studies are needed to specifically evaluate the prevalence and effects on outcomes of end-organ damage in large primary ICH cohorts. The examination of different expressions of end-organ damage in ICH subtypes (e.g., deep versus lobar ICH) is also required.

3.2.1 Pathologic Mechanisms Associated with Hypertensive Intracerebral Hemorrhage

Deep hypertensive ICH occurs in areas supplied by perforating deep arteries that arise from the large cerebral vessels in the brain (Fig. 3.2) [1]. The putamen is consistently reported as the most common location for brain hematoma (35–50% of all ICH cases) [41–43], followed by thalamus (10–15%) [42–45], and then pons (5–12%) [17, 42, 43]. Putaminal ICH results from the rupture of a lateral branch of the striate arteries whose diameter ranges between 200 and 400 μm [41]. Though relatively uncommon, rupture of distal segments of the lateral striate arteries can lead to caudate hematomas [19, 41]. Based on their location, thalamic hematomas may originate from the rupture of four groups of arteries: (1) anterior thalamic group artery rupture results in anterior thalamic hematomas (6% of all thalamic ICH), (2) tuberothalamic artery rupture results in posteromedial thalamic hematomas (14% of all thalamic ICH), (3) thalamoperforating artery rupture results in posterolateral thalamic hematoma (44% of all thalamic ICH), and (4) posterior choroidal artery rupture results in dorsal thalamic hematomas (18% of all thalamic ICH) [44]. Pontine hemorrhages are usually caused by bleeding of small paramedian basilar perforating arteries [17]. The result is a medially located hematoma that predominantly involves the basis pontis [17]. Less frequently, the hematoma may be located in the tegmentum when a distal segments of long circumferential branches of the basilar artery are the source of the bleeding [46].

Previous findings suggest that perforator arteries are more directly exposed to the effects of high blood pressure because of the lack of gradual decrease in vessel caliber as in other areas of the cerebrovascular circulation [47]. Thus, longstanding hypertension appears to cause a series of degenerative pathologic changes that eventually weakens these deep perforators [1, 18, 48]. The mechanism of actual bleeding is presumably related to rupture of these fragile vessels – while several detailed neuropathologic studies have examined this question, it has been difficult to prove pathologically [1, 48–50]. The first pathological reports described "miliary aneurysms" as the main vasculopathic changes related to deep hypertensive ICH [51]. These lesions were initially believed to be true dilation of the arterial wall; however, it was only with the availability of more precise histologic techniques that pathologists could show that miliary aneurysms were "false aneurysms" that are made of masses of blood outside the vessel wall [52]. At that time, the rupture of the vessel and the formation of the hematoma was believed to be secondary to an intimal lesion that could either extend to the media and adventitia or led to the formation of a dissecting aneurysm [52]. Later work that combined postmortem angiography and histology found that miliary aneurysms were present in almost all hypertensive ICH patients (15/16 patients) and were located mainly in the basal ganglia, internal capsule, and thalamus [19, 48]. Even if the presence of microaneuryms in hypertensive patients with ICH are common, a causal role in causing ICH has never been firmly established. Fisher, using serial sections of blocks of tissue containing the hemorrhage, found that in putaminal hemorrhages, primary arterial bleeding sites occurred along multiple secondary sites of bleedings. Microaneurysms in the immediate relation of the hematoma were not reported, whereas degenerative arteriole changes called "lipohyalinosis" were a very common abnormality in the walls of small arteries harboring the bleeding sites [1]. In conclusion, based on Fisher's studies, hypertensive ICH most likely results from the rupture of one or two lipohyalinotic arteries, followed by a second rupture at the periphery of the enlarging hematoma in a "avalanche fashion" [1, 2]. The bleeding sites appear as round collections of platelets combined with and surrounded by concentric lamellae of fibrin, so-called bleeding globes or fibrin globes [1]. Fibrin or bleeding globes at the primary and secondary sites are histologically identical, except that the fibrin globes are larger. Histologically, the bulk of the hematoma is formed by a compact mass of red blood cells, and the bleeding sites are characteristically found at its periphery [1].

Pathologically, lipohyalinosis is a term that describes a destructive vascular process with deposition of hyaline and fat-laden macrophages in the wall of the penetrating arteries [1, 53]. These degenerative arterial changes are also suggested to cause lacunar infarcts, a subgroup of ischemic stroke that is associated hypertension and diabetes (Fig. 3.3) [53]. Thus, lipohyalinosis affecting deep perforating arteries can either led to vessel rupture (mechanism of hematoma formation) or occlusion (mechanism of lacunar infarction). It is unclear as to what factors predispose lipohyalinotic vessels toward rupture versus occlusion [54]. Another small vessel disease pathologic feature that has been related to blood leakage and ICH is fibrinoid necrosis [50, 55]. Fibrinoid necrosis appears in small arteries and arterioles of the brain, kidneys, and other organs, predominantly in patients with uncontrolled hypertension. Fibrinoid material deposits segmentally and commonly occupy a portion of the vessel. Electron microscopic and immunohistochemical studies show that they consist of exudated plasma protein and necrotic smooth muscle cells with a staining pattern reminiscent of fibrin. Fibrinoid necrosis has been related to aneurysmal dilatation of weakened small and medium arteries with subsequent leakage of blood components [50].

The above pathologic processes have been related to hypertension and grouped under different terms in the literature including "hypertensive arteriopathy," hypertensive microangiopathy, arteriolosclerosis, age-related or vascular risk factor-related small vessel disease, or degenerative microangiopathy [1, 56, 57]. Throughout this chapter, we have employed the term hypertensive small vessel disease in relationship to ICH. While hypertension has traditionally been regarded as the cardinal risk factor for primary deep ICH, not all patients have hypertension [25, 58]. Thus, the use of the term hypertensive small vessel disease, especially in ICH patients, is to some extent an oversimplification. On the other hand, "normotensive" primary

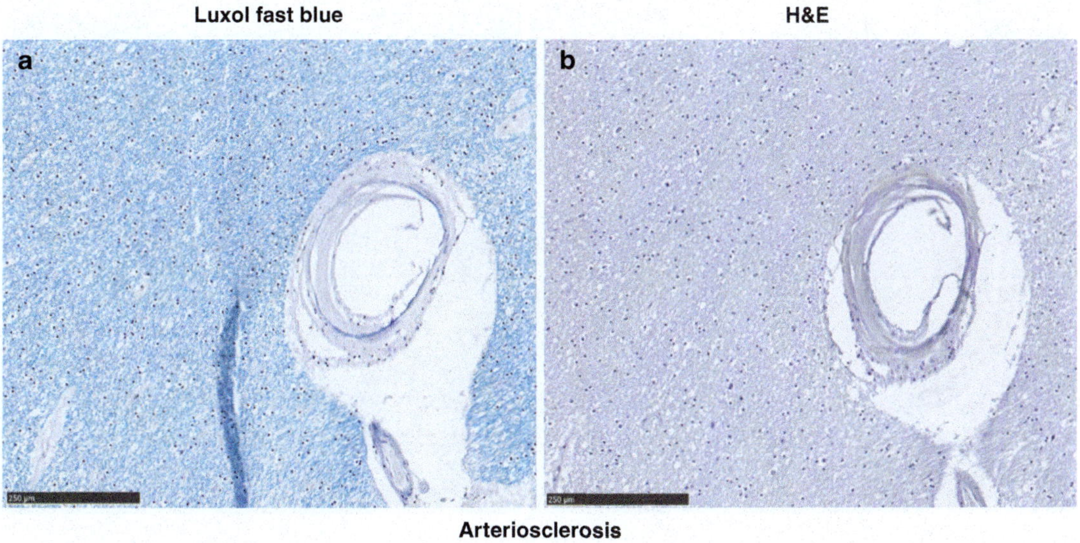

Fig. 3.3 Hypertensive-related small vessel changes. A vessel in the deep white matter with arteriolosclerosis on a Luxol fast blue and hematoxylin-stained section (**a**). The adjacent section show negative immunohistochemistry for amyloid β (**b**)

ICH patients may have had mild undetected degrees of hypertension. There is evidence to suggest that isolated blood pressure measurement obtained in the office setting may have limitations in detecting subclinical hypertensive disease [59]. Hypertension is a multisystem disease that may result in systemic damage even before it is clinically recognized [60]. Some data suggest that the identification of arteriolar disease may precede the diagnosis of hypertension based on office measurements [60]. Nonetheless, the overall body of evidence suggest that hypertension and age remain the most important risk factors for primary deep hemorrhage [25, 32].

3.3 Pathophysiology of Cerebral Amyloid Angiopathy Intracerebral Hemorrhage

Cerebral amyloid angiopathy is a common microangiopathy in the elderly defined pathologically by the progressive deposition of amyloid protein in the walls of cortical and leptomeningeal small arteries, arterioles, and less often capillaries of the brain [11, 16, 20, 22]. The term CAA describes a heterogeneous group of biochemically and genetically diverse system disorders [61–65]. In this chapter, the use of the term CAA refers to the sporadic form of this specific microangiopathy associated with symptomatic hemorrhagic stroke. CAA is a major cause of lobar symptomatic ICH (Fig. 3.4) [20] and an important contributor to vascular cognitive impairment [66, 67]. One of the first attempts to clarify the relationship between CAA and lobar ICH was made by Okazaki and colleagues in 1979 [7]. The authors analyzed 23 consecutive cases of moderate-to-severe CAA from autopsies and found that history of multiple lobar hemorrhages was very common in these patients. CAA is now recognized as a key contributor of cortical-subcortical (lobar) ICH especially in posterior regions, where the pathology appears most severe [22, 23, 68]. In pathologic series, CAA appears to account for a substantial proportion of all

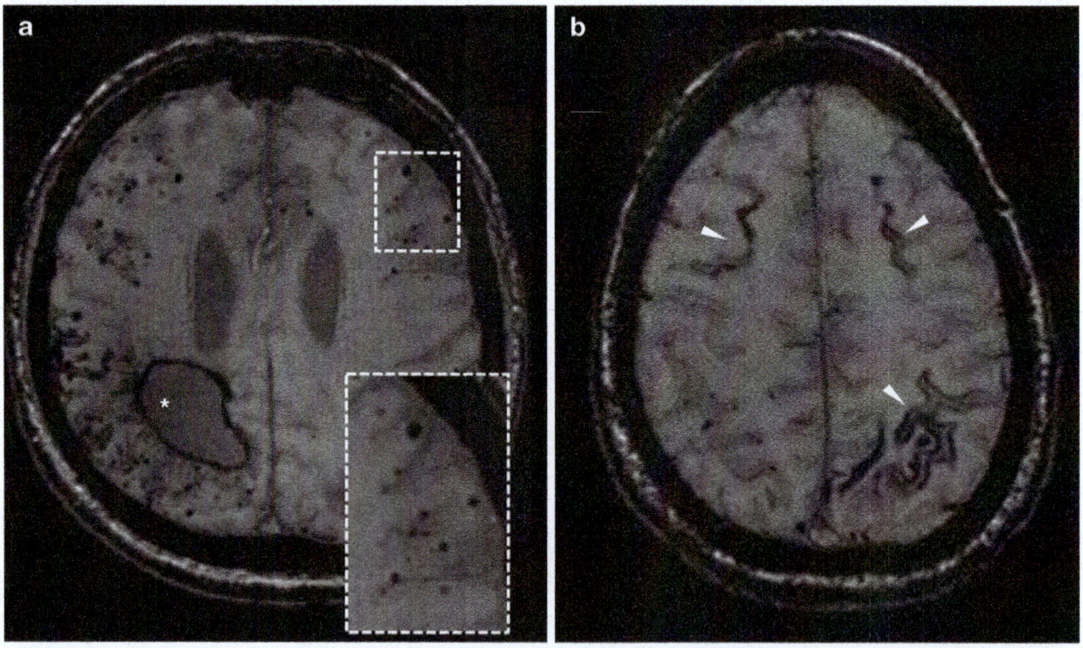

Fig. 3.4 Cerebral amyloid angiopathy-related intracerebral hemorrhage. Panel A shows an axial slice from susceptibility-weighted imaging (SWI) MRI in a patient with cerebral amyloid angiopathy (CAA). Right lobar hematoma (*) with strictly lobar cerebral microbleeds (*inset*). Panel B (susceptibility-weighted imaging (SWI) sequence) shows a different CAA patient with disseminated cortical superficial siderosis (*arrowheads*)

spontaneous lobar ICH in elderly patients. In one study, among 39 cases of lobar ICH, CAA was present in 29 cases, with an overall prevalence of 74% [15]. In patients with previous lobar ICH, the risk of recurrent hemorrhage appears to be approximately 10% per year [69]. Some CAA patients appear to harbor a more severe form of the disease and experience recurrent ICH weeks or months after their initial hemorrhage [70]. This appears to be related to the presence of sulcal bleeding events, termed cortical superficial siderosis (Fig. 3.4; cSS) [70, 71]. The modified Boston criteria can be used to determine the likely etiology of ICH for relatively high specificity by using clinical data, imaging signs, and, if available, histopathologic findings. More recently, it has been shown that these criteria have high positive predictive value for the diagnosis of CAA even in the absence of lobar ICH (Fig. 3.4) [72, 73].

3.3.1 Pathologic Mechanisms Associated with Cerebral Amyloid Angiopathy-Related Intracerebral Hemorrhage

The lobar predominance of CAA-related ICH is a driven amyloid deposition in the cortical and leptomeningeal vessels (and less commonly the cerebellum). The brainstem and deep hemispheric structures are generally spared [20, 22, 23]. The frequent involvement of posterior areas, especially the occipital lobe, is not well understood. It has been hypothesized that greater tortuosity of occipital small arteries may impair perivascular drainage [74]. Beta-amyloid deposition usually starts in the abluminal portion of the tunica media, often surrounding smooth muscle cells. It then involves the adventitia subsequently infiltrating all layers of the vessel with associated loss of smooth muscle cells. In the later stages, the architecture of the vessel is severely disrupted, and microaneurysm formation, fibrinoid necrosis, and "double barreling'" may be present (Fig. 3.5) [20, 23, 75, 76]. One postmortem histopathologic study, which compared CAA patients with and without symptomatic lobar ICH, found that patients with ICH had a severe degree of vascular amyloid deposition with foci of vessel wall fragmentation and the presence of fibrinoid necrosis [20]. However, a more recent study with pathologic data has shown that patients with CAA-related ICH have a similar vascular β-amyloid burden and severity compared to those patients with CAA who did not have a symptomatic ICH [77]. It is possible that biological pathways distinct from those involved in amyloid vascular accumulation play a role in determining clinical expression in patients with CAA. Indeed, clinical, genetic, and serological factors have been proposed as contributors to CAA-related ICH. The presence and combination of different apolipoprotein E (ApoE) alleles are the best established genetic risk factor for sporadic CAA development [62, 78]. ApoE ε4 and ε2 have been associated with an increased risk of CAA-related lobar ICH. These alleles have also been associated with hematoma expansion, worse clinical outcome, and risk of recurrence after ICH [79, 80]. ApoE ε4 appears to be involved in β-amyloid deposition, while ApoE ε2 appears to promote vasculopathic changes in amyloid-laden vessels, leading to rupture [21, 81–83].

The role of hypertension as a predisposing factor in CAA-related ICH is not fully defined and remains an area of active research. In pathological series of CAA-ICH patients, the estimate prevalence of hypertension is in the range of 32–58%, generally lower than other ICH population [25, 76, 84]. However, recent data suggest inadequate BP control during follow-up is associated with a higher risk of both lobar (HR: 3.53, CI: 1.65–7.54) and non-lobar (HR: 4.23, CI: 1.02–17.52) ICH recurrences [32].

3.4 Pathophysiology of Cerebellar and Mixed Intracerebral Hemorrhage

Spontaneous (non-traumatic and not due to vascular malformations) cerebellar ICH has been mainly reported secondary to hypertension, but in some cases, cerebellar ICH can be related to CAA [17, 85]. In cerebellar ICH, the hematoma

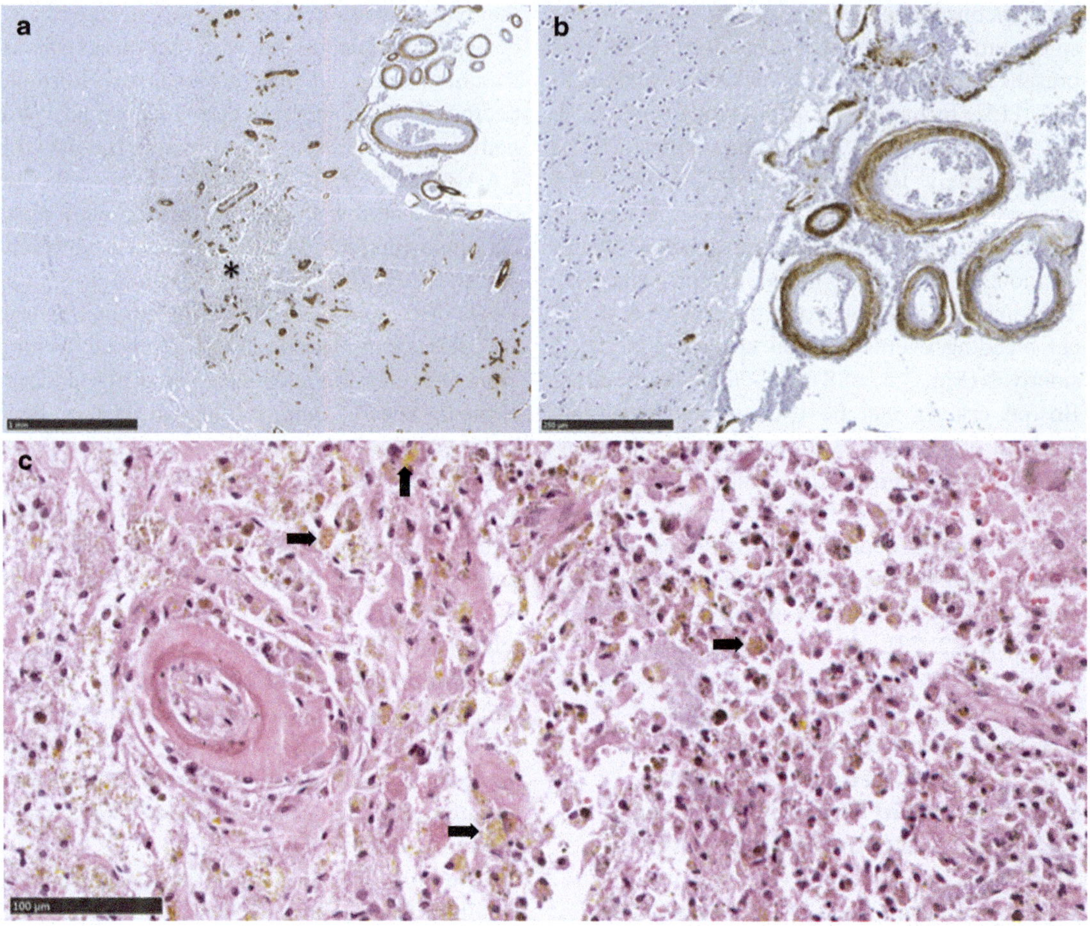

Fig. 3.5 Cerebral amyloid angiopathy-related vessel changes. An example of moderate-to-severe cerebral amyloid angiopathy and an old hemorrhage (*) on a section that underwent immunohistochemistry against amyloid β (**a**). Both cortical and leptomeningeal vessels show widespread circumferential amyloid β deposition (**b**). An adjacent hematoxylin and eosin-stained section shows multiple hemosiderin deposits within the hemorrhagic area (**c**, *arrows*)

is generally located in or close to one of the dentate nuclei (termed the deep cerebellar location; see Fig. 3.6, Panel A) [17, 86]. By contrast, in a subgroup of cases, hematoma location can be restricted to the cerebellar cortex and vermis (termed superficial cerebellar location) [85]. Interestingly, data based on autopsy series suggest that when the primary cerebellar bleed is located in the deep cerebellar gray nuclei and white matter, the underlying etiology is more likely to be related to hypertension [17, 85, 86]. In line with these pathologic findings, we recently reported in an MRI-based study that patients with deep cerebellar hematoma frequently had hypertension (65%), whereas in superficial cerebellar ICH, hypertension was much less common (12%) [87]. Additionally, patients with superficial cerebellar ICH were more frequently found to have strictly lobar cerebral microbleeds, a marker of CAA [15, 73, 87]. The artery commonly implicated as the source of bleeding in deep cerebellar ICH is a large branch of the superior cerebellar artery and is the major blood supply to the dentate nucleus. In a minority of individuals, this artery may arise from the anterior inferior or posterior inferior cerebellar arteries [17]. In superficial cerebellar ICH, penetrating pial arteries arising appear to be the source of bleeding [85].

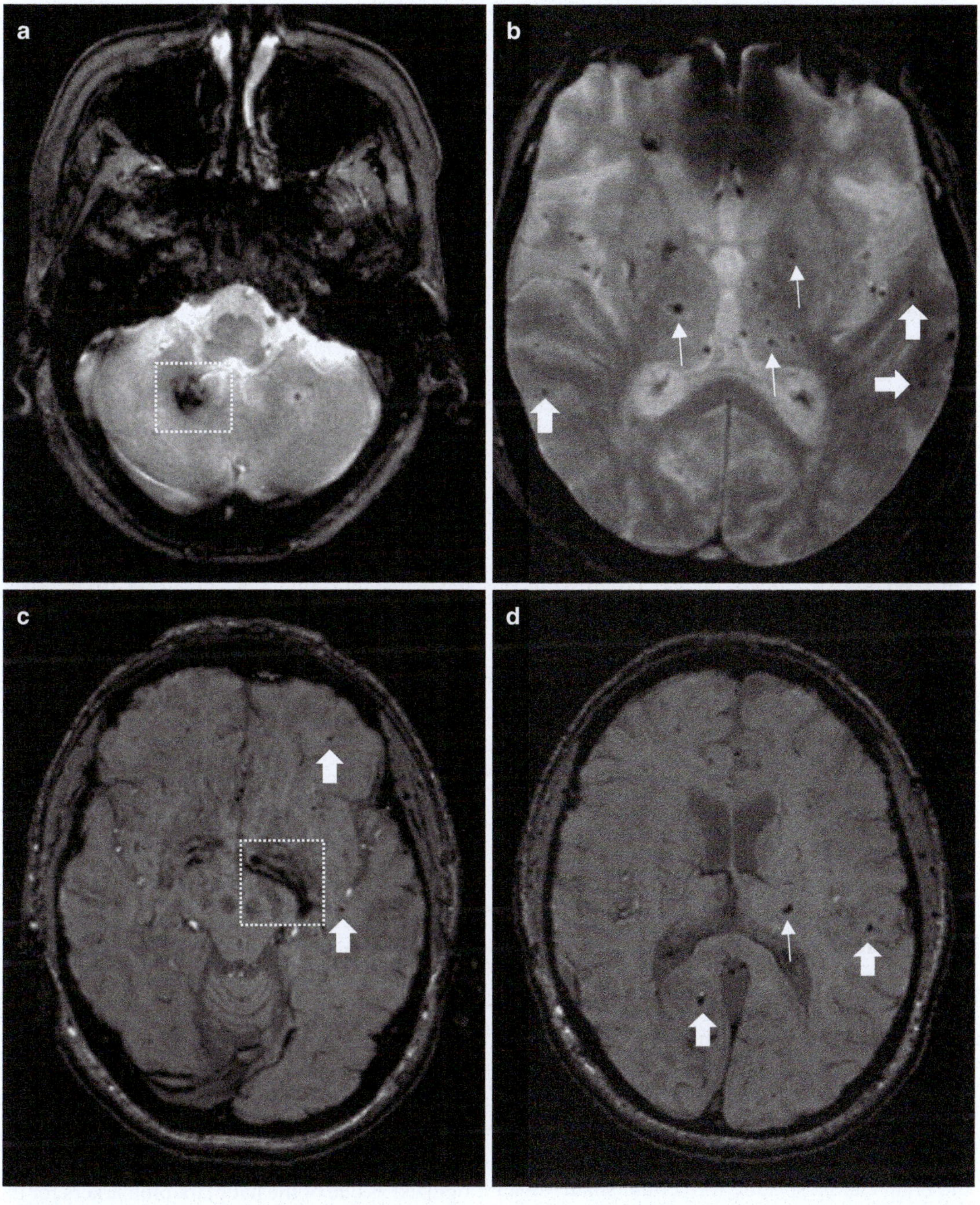

Fig. 3.6 Cerebellar intracerebral hemorrhage and mixed intracerebral hemorrhage. Panels A and B show T2*-gradient echo MRI sequences in a patient with cerebellar hemorrhage. Right deep cerebellar hematoma (**a**, *dotted square box*) with mixed distribution of supratentorial cerebral microbleeds (CMB) (**b**, *thick arrows* show lobar CMBs; *thin arrows* show deep CMBs). Panels C and D show susceptibility-weighted imaging (SWI) sequences in a patient with a mixed distribution of hemorrhages (mixed ICH). Deep hematoma is indicated in the dotted square box (**c**). Thick arrows mark lobar CMBs and thin arrows mark deep CMB (**d**)

In clinical practice one commonly encounters patients with hemorrhages (microbleeds or ICH) in both lobar and deep brain regions (mixed ICH patients; Fig. 3.6, Panels C and D). The pathologic processes underlying mixed ICH have not been fully elucidated. It is likely that mixed ICH represents a severe vasculopathy caused by risk factors such as hypertension and diabetes [88, 89]. Indeed, patients with mixed ICH appear to have a vascular risk factor profile similar to those with hypertensive-related ICH [89]. Larger pathologic and epidemiologic studies are required to more fully address this question. Alternatively, patients with hemorrhages in lobar and deep areas may harbor both CAA and hypertensive small vessel diseases [88, 90]. A recent study using in vivo brain amyloid imaging suggested that vascular amyloid and hypertensive small vessel disease might have synergistic effects on the progression of lobar cerebral microbleeds [91]. Patients with mixed ICH appear to have a lower ICH recurrence rate (5.1% per year) compared to patients with CAA-related ICH (10.4% per year) and a higher recurrence rate compared to those with HTN-ICH (1.6% per year) [89].

3.5 The Use of MRI in Evaluation of Small Vessel Disease-Related Intracerebral Hemorrhage

The broad availability of MRI has proved to be extremely useful as a noninvasive tool for the evaluation of small vessel disease-related brain damage in patients with ICH. MRI markers of small vessel disease occur frequently in patients with ICH, and their topographical distribution in the brain can be specific for certain small vessel pathologies [88, 92–95]. MRI markers of small vessel disease in ICH can be divided into hemorrhagic markers (cerebral microbleeds and cSS) and non-hemorrhagic markers (white matter hyperintensities, enlarged perivascular spaces, diffusion-weighted-positive [DWI] lesions, and lacunes).

3.5.1 Cerebral Microbleeds

Cerebral microbleeds are defined small areas of signal void with associated blooming appreciable on T2*-gradient echo/SWI (susceptibility-weighted imaging) (Fig. 3.2, Panel B; Fig. 3.4, Panel A) [96]. Various cut-off points in size have been used to classify cerebral microbleeds, but because of the blooming effect that depends on the MRI field strength and sequence, an absolute size criterion is not recommended (the majority fall within the range of 5–10 mm in size) [96, 97]. Pathologically, these signal abnormalities correlate with hemosiderin-laden macrophages in perivascular tissue, consistent with vascular leakage of blood cells [90, 98]. However, recent studies using ex vivo MRI have been suggested that a subset of visualized microbleeds may be due to other vascular pathologies that may have different pathophysiologic mechanisms [98]. In the context of CAA, it had been hypothesized that vessel fragility and rupture occur at site of Aβ deposition in the walls of cortical vessels. However, recent work may suggest that microbleeds occur in proximity to cortical vessels with relatively low, not high, Aβ burden [99]. Further research regarding the mechanisms of bleeding are required.

Cerebral microbleeds are most commonly located in the cortico-subcortical junction, deep gray or white matter in the cerebral hemispheres, brainstem, or cerebellum [96, 100]. As discussed above, cerebral microbleeds located in strictly lobar regions are strongly predictive of advanced CAA pathology (Fig. 3.4, panel A) [15, 73], while cerebral microbleeds in deep areas appear most commonly to be associated with hypertensive small vessel disease [88, 90, 101]. Strictly lobar microbleeds detected on MRI are now recognized as one of the hallmark biomarkers for the presence of advanced CAA and are useful for the diagnosis of CAA in patients with and without ICH [15, 73]. Detailed pathologic validation studies that correlate the presence of deep cerebral microbleeds (Fig. 3.2, Panel B) and hypertensive small vessel disease have not been performed. However, both population-based

vessel trigger secondary ruptures from surrounding vessels [1, 2]. Individuals with high numbers of cerebral microbleeds may be protected from secondary rupture after an initial ICH due to the nature of their vessel walls.

In contrast to the immediate primary injury related to hematoma formation, secondary injury of ICH may result from the potentiation of parallel cascades resulting in activation of microglia and astrocytes, perihematomal edema, and neuronal death [125, 129, 140–144].

Perihematomal tissue is exposed to extravasated blood components including red blood cells, leukocytes, and plasma protein activating the surrounding microglia and astrocytes [125, 141, 143, 145]. Activated microglia are believed to have neuroprotective properties by clearing the hematoma and debris [146]. However, preclinical studies have also shown that activated microglia and astrocytes release inflammatory cytokines, reactive oxygen species, and proteases promoting blood-brain barrier damage and contributing to secondary injury damage [125, 141, 143, 145].

Perihematomal edema appears within hours secondary to clot retraction and release of plasma proteins into the surrounding white matter [131, 147–151]. Later, delayed thrombin formation may contribute directly to neural toxicity or indirectly through damage to the blood-brain barrier with subsequent worsening of vasogenic edema [125, 140, 152]. After 3–7 days, peak perihematomal edema occurs and corresponds with the lysis of red blood cells [153–155]. Red blood lysis may occur up to 7 days after ICH and is usually secondary to the complement cascade [155]. Heme degradation products – carbon monoxide, biliverdin, and iron – are believed to contribute to oxidative stress, edema formation, and neuronal death contributing to secondary injury after ICH [125, 131, 144, 147, 155]. It has also been reported that high plasma levels of proinflammatory molecules, such as glutamate, cytokines, and adhesion molecules, within 24 h of ICH onset are correlated with the magnitude of the subsequent perihematomal brain edema [127, 150, 156, 157].

The role of cerebral ischemia in ICH-related brain injury remains unclear. Large hematomas cause increased intracranial pressure and may consequently reduce cerebral blood flow [123]. Additionally, if the tissue supplied by the ruptured vessel has insufficient collateral supply, the blood flow in the perihematomal region may decrease [131]. However, clinical and animal studies have not found levels of blood flow decreases in the perihematomal regions sufficient to cause ischemic damage [158, 159]. In line with this evidence, decreased perfusion in the perihematomal zone seems related mainly to decreased tissue metabolic demand in the setting of ICH without falling below a perfusion threshold to trigger ischemic damage [160].

Conclusions

Primary ICH results from the rupture of a small- and medium-sized deep perforators or cortical arteries. Age-associated sporadic cerebral small vessel disease is the main cause of primary ICH. The two major forms of small vessel disease are hypertensive small vessel disease and CAA. The identification of the microangiopathy underlying ICH is clinically relevant, as hypertensive small vessel disease and CAA have different risks of recurrence [69]. Hematoma location can be strongly suggestive of the etiology of ICH. Deep supratentorial ICH and pontine hematomas are mainly secondary to hypertensive small vessel disease, while lobar ICHs are commonly associated with CAA. MRI small vessel disease markers can additionally be used to better classify underlying pathology. Future work should begin to focus on the histopathological lesions in patients with ICH and aim to validate neuroimaging biomarkers with pathologic data [98, 161].

References

1. Fisher CM. Pathological observations in hypertensive cerebral hemorrhage. J Neuropathol Exp Neurol. 1971;30:536–50.
2. Fisher CM. Hypertensive cerebral hemorrhage. Demonstration of the source of bleeding. J Neuropathol Exp Neurol. 2003;62:104–7.

3. Qureshi AI, Tuhrim S, Broderick JP, et al. Spontaneous intracerebral hemorrhage. N Engl J Med. 2001;344:1450–60.
4. Foulkes MA, Wolf PA, Price TR, et al. The stroke data bank: design, methods, and baseline characteristics. Stroke. 1988;19:547–54.
5. Mohr JP, Caplan LR, Melski JW, et al. The Harvard cooperative stroke registry: a prospective registry. Neurology. 1978;28:754–62.
6. Béjot Y, Cordonnier C, el al DJ. Intracerebral haemorrhage profiles are changing: results from the Dijon population-based study. Brain. 2013;136:658–64.
7. Okazaki H, Reagan TJ, Campbell RJ. Clinicopathologic studies of primary cerebral amyloid angiopathy. Mayo Clin Proc. 1979;54:22–31.
8. Greenberg SM. Small Vessels, big problems. N Engl J Med. 2006;354:1451–3.
9. Pantoni L. Cerebral small vessel disease: from pathogenesis and clinical characteristics to therapeutic challenges. Lancet Neurol. 2010;9:689–701.
10. Wardlaw JM, Smith C, Dichgans M. Mechanisms of sporadic cerebral small vessel disease: insights from neuroimaging. Lancet Neurol. 2013;12:483–97.
11. Charidimou A, Boulouis G, Gurol ME, et al. Emerging concepts in sporadic cerebral amyloid angiopathy. Brain. 2017;140:1829–50.
12. Bouvy WH, Geurts LJ, Kuijf HJ, et al. Assessment of blood flow velocity and pulsatility in cerebral perforating arteries with 7-T quantitative flow MRI. NMR Biomed. 2016;29:1295–304.
13. van Veluw SJ, Zwanenburg JJM, Hendrikse J, et al. High resolution imaging of cerebral small vessel disease with 7 T MRI. Acta Neurochir Suppl. 2014;119:125–30.
14. Wardlaw JM, Smith EE, Biessels GJ, et al. Neuroimaging standards for research into small vessel disease and its contribution to ageing and neurodegeneration. Lancet Neurol. 2013;12:822–38.
15. Knudsen KA, Rosand J, Karluk D, et al. Clinical diagnosis of cerebral amyloid angiopathy: validation of the Boston criteria. Neurology. 2001;56:537–9.
16. Viswanathan A, Greenberg SM. Cerebral amyloid angiopathy in the elderly. Ann Neurol. 2011;70:871–80.
17. Dinsdale HB. Spontaneous hemorrhage in the posterior fossa: a study of primary cerebellar and pontine hemorrhages with observations on their pathogenesis. Arch Neurol. 1964;10:200–17.
18. Takebayashi S, Kaneko M. Electron microscopic studies of ruptured arteries in hypertensive intracerebral hemorrhage. Stroke. 1983;14:28–36.
19. Russell RWR. Observations on intracerebral aneurysms. Brain. 1963;86:425–42.
20. Vonsattel JPG, Myers RH, Tessa Hedley-Whyte E, et al. Cerebral amyloid angiopathy without and with cerebral hemorrhages: a comparative histological study. Ann Neurol. 1991;30:637–49.
21. McCarron MO, Nicoll JA, Stewart J, et al. The apolipoprotein E epsilon2 allele and the pathological features in cerebral amyloid angiopathy-related hemorrhage. J Neuropathol Exp Neurol. 1999;58:711–8.
22. Gilbert JJ, Vinters HV. Cerebral amyloid angiopathy: incidence and complications in the aging brain. I. Cerebral hemorrhage. Stroke. 1983;14:915–23.
23. Vinters HV, Gilbert JJ. Cerebral amyloid angiopathy: incidence and complications in the aging brain. II. The distribution of amyloid vascular changes. Stroke. 1983;14:924–8.
24. Brott T, Thalinger K, Hertzberg V. Hypertension as a risk factor for spontaneous intracerebral hemorrhage. Stroke. 1986;17:1078–83.
25. Woo D, Sauerbeck LR, Kissela BM, et al. Genetic and environmental risk factors for intracerebral hemorrhage: preliminary results of a population-based study. Stroke. 2002;33:1190–6.
26. Viswanathan A, Rakich SM, Engel C, et al. Antiplatelet use after intracerebral hemorrhage. Neurology. 2006;66:206–9.
27. Jackson CA, Sudlow CLM. Is hypertension a more frequent risk factor for deep than for lobar supratentorial intracerebral haemorrhage? J Neurol Neurosurg Psychiatry. 2006;77:1244–52.
28. Massaro AR, Sacco RL, Mohr JP, et al. Clinical discriminators of lobar and deep hemorrhages: the stroke data Bank. Neurology. 1991;41:1881–5.
29. Bahemuka M. Primary intracerebral hemorrhage and heart weight: a clinicopathologic case-control review of 218 patients. Stroke. 1987;18:531–6.
30. Broderick J, Brott T, Tomsick T, et al. Lobar hemorrhage in the elderly. The undiminishing importance of hypertension. Stroke. 1993;24:49–51.
31. PROGRESS Collaborative Group. Randomised trial of a perindopril-based blood-pressure-lowering regimen among 6105 individuals with previous stroke or transient ischaemic attack. Lancet. 2001;358:1033–41.
32. Biffi A, Anderson CD, Battey TWK, et al. Association between blood pressure control and risk of recurrent intracerebral hemorrhage. JAMA. 2015;314:904–12.
33. Arima H, Anderson C, Omae T, et al. Degree of blood pressure reduction and recurrent stroke: the PROGRESS trial. J Neurol Neurosurg Ps. 2014;85:1284–5.
34. Arima H, Tzourio C, Anderson C, et al. Effects of perindopril-based lowering of blood pressure on intracerebral hemorrhage related to amyloid angiopathy: the PROGRESS trial. Stroke. 2010;41:394–6.
35. Folsom AR, Yatsuya H, Psaty BM, et al. Carotid intima-media thickness, electrocardiographic left ventricular hypertrophy, and incidence of intracerebral hemorrhage. Stroke. 2011;42:3075–9.
36. Bos MJ, Koudstaal PJ, Hofman A, et al. Decreased glomerular filtration rate is a risk factor for hemorrhagic but not for ischemic stroke: the Rotterdam study. Stroke. 2007;38:3127–32.
37. Laible M, Horstmann S, Möhlenbruch M, et al. Renal dysfunction is associated with deep cerebral microbleeds but not white matter hyperintensities

in patients with acute intracerebral hemorrhage. J Neurol. 2015;262:2312–22.
38. Zheng D, Sato S, Arima H, et al. Estimated GFR and the effect of intensive blood pressure lowering after acute intracerebral hemorrhage. Am J Kidney Dis. 2016;68:94–102.
39. O'Rourke MF, Safar ME. Relationship between aortic stiffening and microvascular disease in brain and kidney: cause and logic of therapy. Hypertension. 2005;46:200–4.
40. Ikram MA, Vernooij MW, Hofman A, et al. Kidney function is related to cerebral small vessel disease. Stroke. 2008;39:55–61.
41. Hier DB, Davis KR, Richardson EP, et al. Hypertensive putaminal hemorrhage. Ann Neurol. 1977;1:152–9.
42. Mutlu N, Berry RG, Alpers BJ. Massive cerebral hemorrhage: clinical and pathological correlations. Arch Neurol. 1963;8:644–61.
43. Freytag E. Fatal hypertensive intracerebral haematomas: a survey of the pathological anatomy of 393 cases. J Neurol Neurosurg Ps. 1968;31:616–20.
44. Chung CS, Caplan LR, Han W, et al. Thalamic haemorrhage. Brain J Neurol. 1996;119:1873–86.
45. Walshe TM, Davis KR, Fisher CM. Thalamic hemorrhage: a computed tomographic-clinical correlation. Neurology. 1977;27:217–22.
46. Caplan LR, Goodwin JA. Lateral segmental brainstem hemorrhages. Neurology. 1982;32:252–60.
47. Garcia JH, Ho KL. Pathology of hypertensive arteriopathy. Neurosurg Clin N Am. 1992;3:497–507.
48. Cole FM, Yates PO. Pseudo-aneurysms in relationship to massive cerebral haemorrhage. J Neurol Neurosurg Ps. 1967;30:61–6.
49. Cole FM, Yates P. Intracerebral microaneurysms and small cerebrovascular lesions. Brain. 1967;90:759–68.
50. Rosenblum WI. Miliary aneurysms and "Fibrinoid" degeneration of cerebral blood vessels. Hum Pathol. 1977;8:133–9.
51. Charcot JM, Bouchard C. Nouvelles recherches sur la pathogénie de l'hémorragie cérébrale. Arch Physiol Norm Pathol. 1868;1:110.
52. Ellis AG. The pathogenesis of spontaneous cerebral hemorrhage. Proc Pathol Soc. 1909;12:197.
53. Fisher CM. The arterial lesions underlying lacunes. Acta Neuropathol. 1968;12:1–15.
54. Alistair DG. Hypertensive cerebral small vessel disease and stroke. Brain Pathol. 2002;12:358–70.
55. Ogata J, Fujishima M, Tamaki K, et al. Vascular changes underlying cerebral lesions in stroke-pronc spontaneously hypertensive rats. A serial section study. Acta Neuropathol. 1981;54:183–8.
56. Charidimou A, Pantoni L, Love S. The concept of sporadic cerebral small vessel disease: a road map on key definitions and current concepts. Int J Stroke. 2016;11:6–18.
57. Deramecourt V, Slade JY, Oakley AE, et al. Staging and natural history of cerebrovascular pathology in dementia. Neurology. 2012;78:1043–50.
58. Lammie GA, Brannan F, Slattery J, et al. Nonhypertensive cerebral small-vessel disease: an autopsy study. Stroke. 1997;28:2222–9.
59. Hara A, Tanaka K, Ohkubo T, et al. Ambulatory versus home versus clinic blood pressure: the association with subclinical cerebrovascular diseases: the Ohasama study. Hypertension. 2012;59:22–8.
60. Wong TY, Klein R, Sharrett AR, et al. Retinal arteriolar diameter and risk for hypertension. Ann Intern Med. 2004;140:248.
61. Biffi A, Greenberg SM. Cerebral amyloid angiopathy: a systematic review. J Clin Neurol. 2011;7:1–9.
62. Rannikmäe K, Kalaria RN, Greenberg SM, et al. APOE associations with severe CAA-associated vasculopathic changes: collaborative meta-analysis. J Neurol Neurosurg Ps. 2014;85:300–5.
63. Reinvang I, Espeseth T, Westlye LT. APOE-related biomarker profiles in non-pathological aging and early phases of Alzheimer's disease. Neurosci Biobehav Rev. 2013;37:1322–35.
64. Zhang-Nunes SX, Maat-Schieman MLC, Duinen SG, et al. The cerebral β-amyloid angiopathies: hereditary and sporadic. Brain Pathol. 2006;16:30–9.
65. Charidimou A, Blacker D, Viswanathan A. Context is everything: from cardiovascular disease to cerebral microbleeds. Int J Stroke. 2018;13:6–10.
66. Moulin S, Labreuche J, Bombois S, et al. Dementia risk after spontaneous intracerebral haemorrhage: a prospective cohort study. Lancet Neurol. 2016;15:820–9.
67. Xiong L, Boulouis G, Charidimou A, et al. Dementia incidence and predictors in cerebral amyloid angiopathy patients without intracerebral hemorrhage. J Cereb Blood Flow Metab. 2018;38:241–9.
68. Rosand J, Muzikansky A, Kumar A, et al. Spatial clustering of hemorrhages in probable cerebral amyloid angiopathy. Ann Neurol. 2005;58:459–62.
69. Biffi A, Halpin A, Towfighi A, et al. Aspirin and recurrent intracerebral hemorrhage in cerebral amyloid angiopathy. Neurology. 2010;75:693–8.
70. Roongpiboonsopit D, Charidimou A, William CM, et al. Cortical superficial siderosis predicts early recurrent lobar hemorrhage. Neurology. 2016;87:1863–70.
71. Charidimou A, Boulouis G, Roongpiboonsopit D, et al. Cortical superficial siderosis multifocality in cerebral amyloid angiopathy a prospective study. Neurology. 2017;89:2128–35.
72. Linn J, Halpin A, Demaerel P, et al. Prevalence of superficial siderosis in patients with cerebral amyloid angiopathy. Neurology. 2010;74:1346–50.
73. Martinez-Ramirez S, Romero J-R, Shoamanesh A, et al. Diagnostic value of lobar microbleeds in individuals without intracerebral hemorrhage. Alzheimers Dement. 2015;11:1480–8.
74. Attems J, Jellinger K, Thal DR, et al. Review: sporadic cerebral amyloid angiopathy. Neuropathol Appl Neurobiol. 2011;37:75–93.

75. Revesz T, Holton JL, Lashley T, et al. Sporadic and familial cerebral amyloid angiopathies. Brain Pathol. 2002;12:343–57.
76. Vinters HV. Cerebral amyloid angiopathy. A critical review. Stroke. 1987;18:311–24.
77. Charidimou A, Martinez-Ramirez S, Shoamanesh A, et al. Cerebral amyloid angiopathy with and without hemorrhage evidence for different disease phenotypes. Neurology. 2015;84:1206–12.
78. Verghese PB, Castellano JM, Holtzman DM. Apolipoprotein E in Alzheimer's disease and other neurological disorders. Lancet Neurol. 2011;10:241–52.
79. Biffi A, Anderson CD, Jagiella JM, et al. APOE genotype and extent of bleeding and outcome in lobar intracerebral haemorrhage: a genetic association study. Lancet Neurol. 2011;10:702–9.
80. O'Donnell HC, Rosand J, Knudsen KA, et al. Apolipoprotein E genotype and the risk of recurrent lobar intracerebral hemorrhage. N Engl J Med. 2000;342:240–5.
81. Schmechel DE, Saunders AM, Strittmatter WJ, et al. Increased amyloid beta-peptide deposition in cerebral cortex as a consequence of apolipoprotein E genotype in late-onset Alzheimer disease. Proc Natl Acad Sci USA. 1993;90:9649–53.
82. Greenberg SM, Vonsattel JP, Segal AZ, et al. Association of apolipoprotein E epsilon2 and vasculopathy in cerebral amyloid angiopathy. Neurology. 1998;50:961–5.
83. Greenberg SM, William Rebeck G, Vonsattel JPG, et al. Apolipoprotein E ϵ4 and cerebral hemorrhage associated with amyloid angiopathy. Ann Neurol. 1995;38:254–9.
84. Charidimou A, Martinez-Ramirez S, Reijmer YD, et al. Total magnetic resonance imaging burden of small vessel disease in cerebral amyloid angiopathy: an imaging-pathologic study of concept validation. JAMA Neurol. 2016;73:994–1001.
85. Itoh Y, Yamada M, Hayakawa M, et al. Cerebral amyloid angiopathy: a significant cause of cerebellar as well as lobar cerebral hemorrhage in the elderly. J Neurol Sci. 1993;116:135–41.
86. Fisher CM, Picard EH, Polak A, et al. Acute hypertensive cerebellar hemorrhage: diagnosis and surgical treatment. J Nerv Ment Dis. 1965;140:38–57.
87. Pasi M, Marini S, Morotti A, et al. Cerebellar hematoma location: implications for the underlying microangiopathy. Stroke. 2018;49:207–10.
88. Smith EE, Nandigam KRN, Chen Y-W, et al. MRI markers of small vessel disease in lobar and deep hemispheric intracerebral hemorrhage. Stroke. 2010;41:1933–8.
89. Pasi M, Charidimou A, Boulouis G et al (2018) Mixed-location cerebral hemorrhage/microbleeds: underlying microangiopathy and recurrence risk. Neurology 9;90:e119-e126.
90. Fazekas F, Kleinert R, Roob G, et al. Histopathologic analysis of foci of signal loss on gradient-echo T2*-weighted MR images in patients with spontaneous intracerebral hemorrhage: evidence of microangiopathy-related microbleeds. Am J Neuroradiol. 1999;20:637–42.
91. Kim YJ, Kim HJ, Park J-H, et al. Synergistic effects of longitudinal amyloid and vascular changes on lobar microbleeds. Neurology. 2016;87:1575–82.
92. Pasi M, Boulouis G, Fotiadis P, et al. Distribution of lacunes in cerebral amyloid angiopathy and hypertensive small vessel disease. Neurology. 2017;88:2162–8.
93. Charidimou A, Boulouis G, Haley K, et al. White matter hyperintensity patterns in cerebral amyloid angiopathy and hypertensive arteriopathy. Neurology. 2016:10–1212.
94. Thanprasertsuk S, Martinez-Ramirez S, Pontes-Neto OM, et al. Posterior white matter disease distribution as a predictor of amyloid angiopathy. Neurology. 2014;83:794–800.
95. Charidimou A, Boulouis G, Pasi M, et al. MRI-visible perivascular spaces in cerebral amyloid angiopathy and hypertensive arteriopathy. Neurology. 2017;88:1157–64.
96. Greenberg SM, Vernooij MW, Cordonnier C, et al. Cerebral microbleeds: a guide to detection and interpretation. Lancet Neurol. 2009;8:165–74.
97. Greenberg SM, Nandigam RNK, Delgado P, et al. Microbleeds versus macrobleeds. Stroke. 2009;40:2382–6.
98. van Veluw SJ, Biessels GJ, Klijn CJM, et al. Heterogeneous histopathology of cortical microbleeds in cerebral amyloid angiopathy. Neurology. 2016;86:867–71.
99. van VSJ, Kuijf HJ, Charidimou A, et al. Reduced vascular amyloid burden at microhemorrhage sites in cerebral amyloid angiopathy. Acta Neuropathol. 2017;133:409–15.
100. Cordonnier C, Al-Shahi Salman R, Wardlaw J. Spontaneous brain microbleeds: systematic review, subgroup analyses and standards for study design and reporting. Brain. 2007;130:1988–2003.
101. Vernooij MW, van der LA, Ikram MA, et al. Prevalence and risk factors of cerebral microbleeds the Rotterdam scan study. Neurology. 2008;70:1208–14.
102. Banerjee G, Wahab KW, Gregoire SM, et al. Impaired renal function is related to deep and mixed, but not strictly lobar cerebral microbleeds in patients with ischaemic stroke and TIA. J Neurol. 2016;263:760–4.
103. Charidimou A, Linn J, Vernooij MW, et al. Cortical superficial siderosis: detection and clinical significance in cerebral amyloid angiopathy and related conditions. Brain. 2015;138:2126–39.
104. Charidimou A, Boulouis G, Xiong L, et al. Cortical superficial siderosis and first-ever cerebral hemorrhage in cerebral amyloid angiopathy. Neurology. 2017;88:1607–14.
105. Ni J, Auriel E, Jindal J, et al. The characteristics of superficial siderosis and convexity subarachnoid hemorrhage and clinical relevance in suspected

cerebral amyloid angiopathy. Cerebrovasc Dis. 2015;39:278–86.
106. Wollenweber FA, Baykara E, Zedde M, et al. Cortical superficial siderosis in different types of cerebral small vessel disease. Stroke. 2017;48:1404–7.
107. Charidimou A, Baron J-C, Werring DJ. Transient focal neurological episodes, cerebral amyloid angiopathy, and intracerebral hemorrhage risk: looking beyond TIAs. Int J Stroke. 2013;8:105–8.
108. van VSJ, Lauer A, Charidimou A, et al. Evolution of DWI lesions in cerebral amyloid angiopathy: evidence for ischemia. Neurology. 2017;89:2136–42.
109. Wardlaw JM, Valdés Hernández MC, Muñoz-Maniega S. What are white matter hyperintensities made of? Relevance to vascular cognitive impairment. J Am Heart Assoc. 2015;4:e001140.
110. Zhu Y-C, Chabriat H, Godin O, et al. Distribution of white matter hyperintensity in cerebral hemorrhage and healthy aging. J Neurol. 2012;259:530–6.
111. Charidimou A, Meegahage R, Fox Z, et al. Enlarged perivascular spaces as a marker of underlying arteriopathy in intracerebral haemorrhage: a multicentre MRI cohort study. J Neurol Neurosurg Ps. 2013;84:624–9.
112. Charidimou A, Hong YT, Jäger HR, et al. White matter perivascular spaces on magnetic resonance imaging: marker of cerebrovascular amyloid burden? Stroke. 2015;46:1707–9.
113. Keable A, Fenna K, Yuen HM, et al. Deposition of amyloid β in the walls of human leptomeningeal arteries in relation to perivascular drainage pathways in cerebral amyloid angiopathy. Biochim Biophys Acta. 2016;1862:1037–46.
114. Manousopoulou A, Gatherer M, Smith C, et al. Systems proteomic analysis reveals that clusterin and tissue inhibitor of metalloproteinases 3 increase in leptomeningeal arteries affected by cerebral amyloid angiopathy. Neuropathol Appl Neurobiol. 2017;43:492–504.
115. Kimberly WT, Gilson A, Rost NS, et al. Silent ischemic infarcts are associated with hemorrhage burden in cerebral amyloid angiopathy. Neurology. 2009;72:1230–5.
116. Prabhakaran S, Gupta R, Ouyang B, et al. Acute brain infarcts after spontaneous intracerebral hemorrhage: a diffusion-weighted imaging study. Stroke. 2010;41:89–94.
117. Gregoire SM, Charidimou A, Gadapa N, et al. Acute ischaemic brain lesions in intracerebral haemorrhage: multicentre cross-sectional magnetic resonance imaging study. Brain J Neurol. 2011;134:2376–86.
118. Menon RS, Burgess RE, Wing JJ, et al. Predictors of highly prevalent brain ischemia in intracerebral hemorrhage. Ann Neurol. 2012;71:199–205.
119. Auriel E, Gurol ME, Ayres A, et al. Characteristic distributions of intracerebral hemorrhage–associated diffusion-weighted lesions. Neurology. 2012;79:2335–41.
120. Kidwell CS, Rosand J, Norato G, et al. Ischemic lesions, blood pressure dysregulation, and poor outcomes in intracerebral hemorrhage. Neurology. 2017;88:782–8.
121. Fisher CM. Lacunes: small, deep cerebral infarcts. Neurology. 1998;50:841.
122. Martinez-Ramirez S, Pontes-Neto OM, Dumas AP, et al. Topography of dilated perivascular spaces in subjects from a memory clinic cohort. Neurology. 2013;80:1551–156.
123. Broderick JP, Brott TG, Duldner JE, et al. Volume of intracerebral hemorrhage. A powerful and easy-to-use predictor of 30-day mortality. Stroke. 1993;24:987–93.
124. Felberg RA, Grotta JC, Shirzadi AL, et al. Cell death in experimental intracerebral hemorrhage: the "black hole" model of hemorrhagic damage. Ann Neurol. 2002;51:517–24.
125. Wang J. Preclinical and clinical research on inflammation after intracerebral hemorrhage. Prog Neurobiol. 2010;92:463–77.
126. Tsunoda A, Mitsuoka H, Bandai H, et al. Intracranial cerebrospinal fluid measurement studies in suspected idiopathic normal pressure hydrocephalus, secondary normal pressure hydrocephalus, and brain atrophy. J Neurol Neurosurg Ps. 2002;73:552–5.
127. Castillo J, Dávalos A, Álvarez–Sabín J et al (2002) Molecular signatures of brain injury after intracerebral hemorrhage. Neurology 58:624–629.
128. Morotti A, Phuah C-L, Anderson CD, et al. Leukocyte count and intracerebral hemorrhage expansion. Stroke. 2016;47:1473–8.
129. Mayne M, Fotheringham J, Yan H-J, et al. Adenosine A2A receptor activation reduces proinflammatory events and decreases cell death following intracerebral hemorrhage. Ann Neurol. 2001;49:727–35.
130. Hernandez-Guillamon M, Martinez-Saez E, Delgado P, et al. MMP-2/MMP-9 plasma level and brain expression in cerebral amyloid angiopathy-associated hemorrhagic stroke. Brain Pathol. 2012;22:133–41.
131. Keep RF, Hua Y, Xi G. Intracerebral haemorrhage: mechanisms of injury and therapeutic targets. Lancet Neurol. 2012;11:720–31.
132. Brott T, Broderick J, Kothari R, et al. Early hemorrhage growth in patients with intracerebral hemorrhage. Stroke. 1997;28:1–5.
133. Goldstein JN, Fazen LE, Snider R, et al. Contrast extravasation on CT angiography predicts hematoma expansion in intracerebral hemorrhage. Neurology. 2007;68:889–94.
134. Demchuk AM, Dowlatshahi D, Rodriguez-Luna D, et al. Prediction of haematoma growth and outcome in patients with intracerebral haemorrhage using the CT-angiography spot sign (PREDICT): a prospective observational study. Lancet Neurol. 2012;11:307–14.
135. Boulouis G, Morotti A, Charidimou A, et al. Noncontrast computed tomography markers of intracerebral hemorrhage expansion. Stroke. 2017;48:1120–5.

136. Boulouis G, Morotti A, Brouwers HB, et al. Association between hypodensities detected by computed tomography and hematoma expansion in patients with intracerebral hemorrhage. JAMA Neurol. 2016;73:961–8.
137. Boulouis G, Morotti A, Brouwers HB, et al. Noncontrast computed tomography hypodensities predict poor outcome in intracerebral hemorrhage patients. Stroke. 2016;47:2511–6.
138. Boulouis G, van Etten ES, Charidimou A, et al. Association of key magnetic resonance imaging markers of cerebral small vessel disease with hematoma volume and expansion in patients with lobar and deep intracerebral hemorrhage. JAMA Neurol. 2016;73:1440.
139. Falcone GJ, Biffi A, Brouwers HB, et al. Predictors of hematoma volume in deep and lobar supratentorial intracerebral hemorrhage. JAMA Neurol. 2013;70:988–94.
140. Masada T, Hua Y, Xi G, et al. Attenuation of intracerebral hemorrhage and thrombin-induced brain edema by overexpression of interleukin-1 receptor antagonist. J Neurosurg. 2001;95:680–6.
141. Power C, Henry S, Del Bigio MR, et al. Intracerebral hemorrhage induces macrophage activation and matrix metalloproteinases. Ann Neurol. 2003;53:731–42.
142. Rynkowski MA, Kim GH, Garrett MC, et al. C3a receptor antagonist attenuates brain injury after intracerebral hemorrhage. J Cereb Blood Flow Metab. 2009;29:98–107.
143. Zhao X, Sun G, Zhang J, et al. Hematoma resolution as a target for intracerebral hemorrhage treatment: role for peroxisome proliferator-activated receptor γ in microglia/macrophages. Ann Neurol. 2007;61:352–62.
144. Wang J, Doré S. Heme oxygenase-1 exacerbates early brain injury after intracerebral haemorrhage. Brain. 2007;130:1643–52.
145. Taylor RA, Chang C-F, Goods BA, et al. TGF-β1 modulates microglial phenotype and promotes recovery after intracerebral hemorrhage. J Clin Invest. 2017;127:280–92.
146. Mantovani A, Biswas SK, Galdiero MR, et al. Macrophage plasticity and polarization in tissue repair and remodelling. J Pathol. 2013;229:176–85.
147. Wagner KR, Xi G, Hua Y, et al. Lobar intracerebral hemorrhage model in pigs: rapid edema development in perihematomal white matter. Stroke. 1996;27:490–7.
148. Xi G, Keep RF, Hoff JT. Erythrocytes and delayed brain edema formation following intracerebral hemorrhage in rats. J Neurosurg. 1998;89:991–6.
149. Abilleira S, Montaner J, Molina CA, et al. Metalloproteinase-9 concentration after spontaneous intracerebral hemorrhage. J Neurosurg. 2003;99:65–70.
150. Alvarez-Sabín J, Delgado P, Abilleira S, et al. Temporal profile of matrix metalloproteinases and their inhibitors after spontaneous intracerebral hemorrhage: relationship to clinical and radiological outcome. Stroke. 2004;35:1316–22.
151. Mehdiratta M, Kumar S, Hackney D, et al. Association between serum ferritin level and perihematoma edema volume in patients with spontaneous intracerebral hemorrhage. Stroke. 2008;39:1165–70.
152. Xue M, Hollenberg MD, Yong VW. Combination of thrombin and matrix metalloproteinase-9 exacerbates neurotoxicity in cell culture and intracerebral hemorrhage in mice. J Neurosci. 2006;26:10281–91.
153. Xi G, Keep RF, Hoff JT. Mechanisms of brain injury after intracerebral haemorrhage. Lancet Neurol. 2006;5:53–63.
154. Zazulia AR, Diringer MN, Derdeyn CP, et al. Progression of mass effect after intracerebral hemorrhage. Stroke. 1999;30:1167–73.
155. Wu J, Hua Y, Keep RF, et al. Iron and iron-handling proteins in the brain after intracerebral hemorrhage. Stroke. 2003;34:2964–9.
156. Silva Y, Leira R, Tejada J, et al. Molecular signatures of vascular injury are associated with early growth of intracerebral hemorrhage. Stroke. 2005;36:86–91.
157. Castellazzi M, Tamborino C, De Santis G, et al. Timing of serum active MMP-9 and MMP-2 levels in acute and subacute phases after spontaneous intracerebral hemorrhage. Acta Neurochir Suppl. 2010;106:137–40.
158. Herweh C, Jüttler E, Schellinger PD, et al. Evidence against a perihemorrhagic penumbra provided by perfusion computed tomography. Stroke. 2007;38:2941–7.
159. Qureshi AI, Wilson DA, Hanley DF, et al. No evidence for an ischemic penumbra in massive experimental intracerebral hemorrhage. Neurology. 1999;52:266–72.
160. Zazulia AR, Diringer MN, Videen TO, et al. Hypoperfusion without ischemia surrounding acute intracerebral hemorrhage. J Cereb Blood Flow Metab. 2001;21:804–10.
161. Veluw V, J S, Charidimou A, et al. Microbleed and microinfarct detection in amyloid angiopathy: a high-resolution MRI-histopathology study. Brain. 2016;139:3151–62.

Pathophysiology of Subarachnoid Hemorrhage

4

Sook Young Sim and Yong Sam Shin

4.1 Pathophysiology of Aneurysmal Subarachnoid Hemorrhage

Cerebral aneurysm is defined as a thin-walled outpouching of the cerebral artery. Its rupture leads to arterial bleeding into the subarachnoid space, so-called subarachnoid hemorrhage (SAH) [1]. Aneurysmal SAH accounts for up to 85–98% of spontaneous SAH and represents about 15% of all strokes [2–4]. SAH usually affects a relatively young age compared to other types of stroke, with a mean age of 50~55 at rupture; it also has a high fatality rate, leading to a high rate of years of potential life lost with major personal and socioeconomic impact [2–6].

4.1.1 Mechanism of Aneurysmal Genesis, Growth, and Rupture

Intracranial aneurysms are believed to be acquired lesions that occur with age. They arise mainly in arterial branching around the circle of Willis [3]. A number of different mechanisms have been proposed to explain aneurysm formation, growth, and rupture. The pathogenesis of a cerebral aneurysm is multifactorial and heterogeneous; nevertheless, it has been speculated that key factors involving aneurysmal formation can be summarized as vessel wall injury, inflammation, and subsequent maladaptive vascular remodeling under the influence of specific hemodynamic stress [1, 6–10]. Individual genetic susceptibility and medical risk factors also play an important role in this process [1, 7].

4.1.1.1 Vessel Wall Degradation and Vascular Remodeling

The vessel wall of cerebral arteries consists of adventitia, media, and intima, with endothelial lining. An internal elastic lamina separates the intima from the media and serves as an important component of structural support because the external elastic lamina is absent in intracranial arteries [1]. The media comprises smooth muscle cells and an extracellular matrix. Defects of the smooth muscle cell layer and the internal elastic lamina might be the most important pathologic factors in the development of cerebral aneurysms [7]. It is observed that the endothelium around the aneurysm wall is separated from the basement membrane, and there is no internal elastic lamina at the base of the aneurysm; there is only thin or fragmented internal elastic lamina in the periphery [7].

S. Y. Sim
Department of Neurosurgery, College of Medicine, Seoul Paik Hospital, Inje University, Seoul, South Korea

Y. S. Shin (✉)
Department of Neurosurgery, College of Medicine, Seoul St. Mary's Hospital, The Catholic University of Korea, Seoul, South Korea

S.-H. Lee (ed.), *Stroke Revisited: Hemorrhagic Stroke*, Stroke Revisited,
https://doi.org/10.1007/978-981-10-1427-7_4

It has been generally accepted that aneurysm formation might be initiated with disruption of the internal elastic lamina and loss of medial smooth muscle cells in response to various stimuli, including hemodynamic insult and genetic and environmental risk factors [7, 8]. It is observed that the aneurysmal wall exhibits the architectural disruption in media in which it has a disorganized vascular wall with the expression of vascular endothelial growth factor and basic fibroblast growth factor [9]. These findings indicate that arterial wall degradation and disruption of the normal vascular remodeling process are associated with aneurysm formation [7, 9].

It has been suggested that pathologic remodeling of the vascular wall is initiated by endothelial damage or hemodynamic oscillation [1, 8]. Inflammation of the vascular wall proceeds as endothelial cell swelling, fibrin accumulation, and cellular infiltration. Subsequent thickening of the intimal layer prevents the nutritional flow to the intimal and medial layers. This leads to the degradation of the internal elastic lamina and the extracellular matrix, both of which provide the elasticity and strength of the vessel wall in normal physiologic status [1]. Thus, this process ends with the formation of a partial defect in the affected vessel wall, which would allow vascular outpouching under hemodynamic stress in the future [1]. The synergistic effects of hemodynamic stress and vessel wall injury play an important role in aneurysm formation, growth, and rupture [1].

Degradation of the extracellular matrix of the vascular wall is partially mediated by toxins and proteolytic enzymes such as elastase [1]. It can also be induced by decreased activity of an inhibitory enzyme on the proteases, such as in α1-antitrypsin deficiency, leading to an imbalance between elastase and α1-antitrypsin (elastase inhibitor) [1]. Consequently, increased proteolytic activity and subsequent cytokine-mediated inflammation after vascular injury play a role in the degeneration of the structural component of the vessel wall [1]. Tumor necrosis factor-α (TNF-α) promotes infiltration of inflammatory cells into the vessels and damages the vascular structures [1]. It also inhibits endothelial repair and degrades structural components of the vessel wall, such as elastin and collagen [1].

4.1.1.2 Hemodynamic Stress

It has been suggested that the hemodynamic environment seems to play a fundamental role in the pathogenesis of cerebral aneurysms [1, 6, 8, 10]. Intracranial aneurysms frequently develop at specific locations, such as arterial bifurcations, where the hemodynamic stress tends to be high [8]. Recently, image-based computational fluid dynamics (CFD) has been implicated in the evaluation of hemodynamics in intracranial aneurysms, shedding light on the understanding of the peri-aneurysmal hemodynamic environment [6, 8, 10]. Wall shear stress (WSS), one of the most crucial parameters in fluid hemodynamics, is defined as a tangential frictional force of blood flow on the vessel lumen [6, 10]. It has been proposed that aberrant levels of WSS elicit endothelial cell-mediated destructive vascular remodeling, including pro-inflammatory reaction, matrix metalloproteinase (MMP) activation, and extracellular matrix degradation [8, 10]. However, it has been reported that both high and low WSS are correlated with aneurysmal growth and rupture across the CFD studies [6, 10]. These controversial results might be due to inconsistent parameter definitions, small data sets, and hemodynamic complexities around aneurysmal geometry [6, 10]. In a meta-analysis of CFD studies investigating the association of aneurysmal genesis with hemodynamic parameters, it was found that high WSS is strongly correlated with genesis of bifurcation aneurysms, whereas low WSS is correlated with side wall aneurysm [6]. One mechanism that might explain the association between WSS and aneurysm formation is that endothelium, which senses the tension in the blood vessels at the time of WSS elevation, dilates to lower the elevated WSS; if this phenomenon continues, the vessel wall may weaken [6]. Examinations of flow dynamics have also linked peri-aneurysmal hemodynamics to other indices, such as gradient oscillatory number (GON), aneurysm formation index (AFI), and the oscillatory shear index (OSI) [6, 10].

Anatomic geometry around the aneurysm, including aneurysmal size, location, and configuration, has long been regarded as one of the influencing factors for rupture risk [6]. A possible relationship between aneurysm diameter and the risk of rupture has been put forth [5, 11]. Arterial bifurcation apices are common sites for cerebral aneurysms. In animal studies, arterial bifurcation, or a branching site, has a specific pattern of vascular wall remodeling, such as hyperplasia; this forms an intimal pad at the bifurcation and adjacent destructive remodeling, including disruption of internal elastic lamina, loss of medial smooth muscle cells, reduced proliferation of smooth muscle cells, and loss of fibronectin resembling the initiation of an intracranial aneurysm [8]. A biomechanical study has demonstrated that an aneurysm ruptures when the ratio of the wall thickness to the radius of the aneurysm decreases [10]. It is assumed that aneurysmal geometry and its hemodynamic susceptibility play an important role in aneurysmal formation, growth, and rupture [6].

4.1.1.3 Individual Medical Risk Factors

The most commonly known modifiable risk factors for intracranial aneurysm are smoking, hypertension, and heavy alcohol consumption [1, 3, 7]. Cigarette smoking is the most consistent risk factor, being 3–10 times higher and dose-dependent [7]. Smoking has been known to increase the risk of aneurysm formation and rupture via release of cigarette toxins and carbon monoxide [1]. These chemicals precipitate an inflammatory reaction by increasing protease levels, reducing α1-antitrypsin activity, inducing oxidative stress, and increasing blood viscosity due to the elevated fibrinogen level [1, 7]. The consequent imbalance between proteases and antiproteases leads to increased proteolysis of connective tissue of the vessel wall and extracellular matrix surrounding the cerebral artery as well as disruption of the normal homeostatic mechanism involving vascular repair [7]. Smoking has also been associated with transient elevation of blood pressure and antiestrogenic effect [1].

Hypertension increases the risk of SAH approximately 2.8-fold in longitudinal studies and has a relative risk of 2.9 in population-based studies [7]. Elevation in blood pressure might cause an increase in vascular resistance of the vasa vasorum and result in ischemic necrosis and thinning of the medial layer [1]. It is also proposed that uncompensated blood flow resulting from hypercapnia-induced impairment of cerebral autoregulation and increased blood viscosity possibly contributes to hemodynamic stress on the vasculatures in the genesis of aneurysms, as WSS is known to be proportional to the blood viscosity and the velocity gradients [1]. In patients with intracranial aneurysm, there may be alteration of biochemical pathways associated with arterial homeostasis involving activation of nitric oxide (NO) in the endothelium, and its effects on smooth muscle cell relaxation through hyperpolarization via potassium channel activation may be altered. Prolonged impairment of arterial homeostasis results in excessive loss of vascular tone and endothelial injury [7].

Heavy alcohol consumption also increases the risk of aneurysmal SAH in a dose-dependent manner, with a relative risk of 2.8–4.7 [7]. It damages the endothelium by activation of TNF-α and NO-inducing oxidative stress [1]. Interestingly, a protective effect of light drinking against vessel inflammation has also been suggested in relation with increased high-density lipoprotein levels and decreased TNF-α activity [1]. Estrogens have beneficial effects on the integrity of vessel walls through strengthening collagen and lowering TNF-α activity [1]. However, a high dose of estrogen in oral contraceptive pills or hormone replacement therapy has been shown to mitigate this beneficial effect by elevation of blood pressure resulting from retention of sodium and body fluid [1].

4.1.1.4 Genetic Predisposition

Most intracranial aneurysms occur sporadically, but it is well known that family history is related to the occurrence of multiple and large cerebral aneurysms and development of SAH in about 10% of cases [3, 7]. Unfortunately, genetic research on aneurysms has been limited even in the era of remarkable advances in molecular biology and genetics. This is partly because molecular pathogenesis and pathobiological features associated with aneurysm genesis are poorly understood; thus it is difficult to select candidate markers for aneurysms [7]. Much of the effort to find genetic markers associated with aneurysms targets the structural abnormality in genetic syndromes with aneurysm phenotypes. Structural alterations in most genetic syndromes associated with cerebral aneurysm involve the extracellular matrix of connective tissue, as with polycystin in polycystic kidney disease, fibrillin-1 in Marfan's syndrome, and type III collagen in Ehlers-Danlos syndrome [7, 12]. Among the group of MMPs, which are endopeptidase with selective, specific activities against the extracellular matrix of basement membranes [7], type IV collagenase (MMP-9) has been suggested as an important component for aneurysm genesis since the functional polymorphic changes associated with it have been found in aneurysm [13]. Other candidate genes in familial intracranial aneurysm include endoglin (ENG) and α1-antitrypsin (SERPINA1) [14]. Several limitations of genome-wide linkage studies and advances in genetics research techniques enable genome-wide association studies to help identify genomic regions associated with cerebral aneurysm. A number of single-nucleotide polymorphisms (SNPs) have been identified on the SOX17, CDKN2A-CDKN2B, EDNRA, and PRDM6 genes that are presumably associated with intracranial aneurysm [14].

Despite the continual efforts to find genetic and molecular markers of cerebral aneurysms, the results are conflicting and unsatisfactory; this likely indicates that aneurysm genesis might be a multifactorial process with genetic heterogeneity [7, 15]. It is suggested that patients with a genetic predisposition, when exposed to a long-term environmental risk factor, may fail to undergo a normal arterial remodeling process because of their inability to maintain arterial homeostasis, leading to formation of an aneurysm [7] (Fig. 4.1).

4.1.1.5 Factors Relating to Aneurysmal Growth and Rupture

Generally, aneurysm growth during follow-up is considered to be a risk factor for aneurysmal rupture, as such an aneurysm is 10–30 times more likely to rupture compared with stable aneurysms [16, 17]. Meta-analyses of longitudinal observational studies, including follow-up with over 13,000 cases, showed that 9% of aneurysms were enlarged at follow-up. Risk factors for aneurysmal growth were age (older than 50 years), female gender, smoking history, cavernous carotid artery and basilar artery location, irregular shape, multiple aneurysm, and larger aneurysm size (≥10 mm) [16, 18]. It also revealed that growing aneurysms were associated with a higher rupture rate of 3.1%/year compared with 0.1%/year for stable aneurysms [16]. Aneurysms with daughter sacs or lobulations had a 14.7% growth rate per year, while the overall aneurysm growth rate was 2.5% per year [16].

Aneurysmal rupture might be affected by complex factors. Of these, a sudden increase in transmural arterial pressure (differences in intra-aneurysmal and cerebrospinal fluid [CSF] pressures) is one of the most important factors [3]. Physical activity, such as exercise, sexual intercourse, and physical straining, precedes SAH in about 20% of cases [3]. A number of risk factors might contribute to aneurysm rupture, including clinical factors such as female gender, hypertension, smoking, prior history of SAH, and family history and anatomic factors such as multiple aneurysm, larger aneurysm size, irregular shape, and posterior circulation location [19, 20]. A substantial portion of clinical and anatomical risk factors for aneurysm rupture overlaps with risk factors associated with aneurysm growth, with little to moderate heterogeneity between studies; this suggests that these two processes share similar pathogenesis [16, 18, 21].

4.1.2 Pathophysiology After Aneurysmal Subarachnoid Hemorrhage

A number of pathophysiologic phenomena occur in patients with aneurysmal SAH. These include aneurysmal rebleeding, hydrocephalus, delayed neurologic deterioration with or without cerebral vasospasm, and medical complications in cardiac, pulmonary, body fluid, and electrolyte systems. Along with the initial ictal

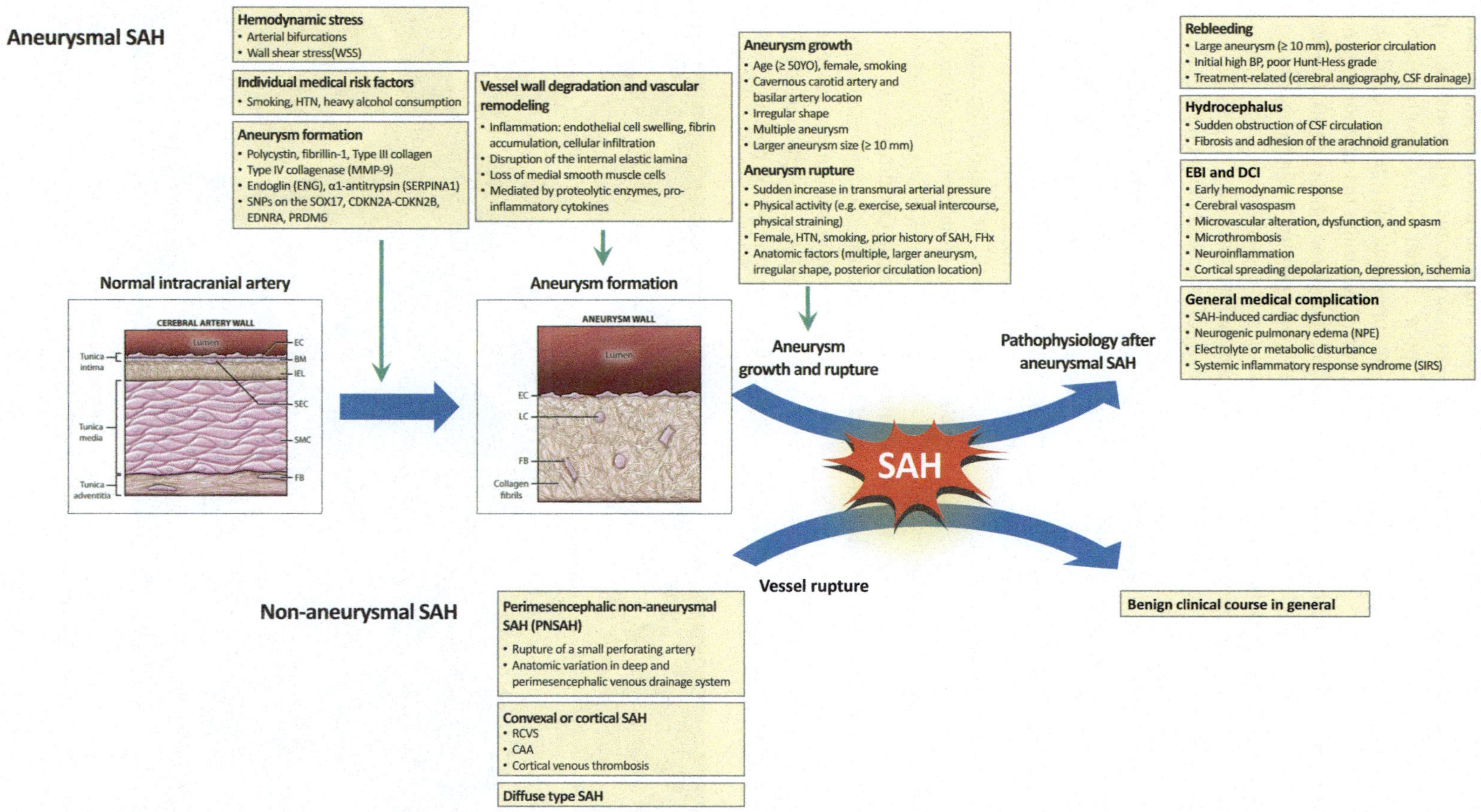

Fig. 4.1 Conceptual diagram of pathophysiology of subarachnoid hemorrhage (SAH). *HTN* hypertension, *SNP* single-nucleotide polymorphism, *FHx* family history, *BP* blood pressure, *CSF* cerebrospinal fluid, *EBI* early brain injury, *DCI* delayed cerebral ischemia, *RCVS* reversible cerebral vasoconstriction syndrome, *CAA* cerebral amyloid angiopathy, *EC* endothelial cells, *BM* basal membrane, *IEL* internal elastic lamina, *SEC* subendothelial cells, *SMC* smooth muscle cells, *FB* fibroblasts, *LC* lymphocytes. Illustrations of the structural composition of a cerebral artery wall and aneurysmal wall are reproduced by permission of Stroke [52]

injury, these complications significantly contribute to a poor clinical outcome in patients with aneurysmal SAH.

4.1.2.1 Rebleeding

Aneurysmal rebleeding before aneurysmal clipping or coiling in acute SAH is one of the leading causes of mortality with a mortality rate of 50–80%. Rebleeding occurs in approximately 8–28.4% of ruptured aneurysms, mostly during the first 24–72 h after the initial bleed (Fig. 4.2) [2, 3, 5, 15, 22]. Recent literature has clarified that aneurysmal rebleeding occurs more frequently in the earlier period than previously expected, with a peak incidence during the first 2–6 h [22, 23].

The underlying mechanism of rebleeding is not precisely defined but is thought to be complex and influenced by a variety of factors. It has been assumed that the fibrin net covering the rupture point at the initial status of rupture is very fragile and not able to withstand even small intra-aneurysmal pressure changes [24].

The current known risk factors for aneurysmal rebleeding include aneurysmal size and location; presence of intraventricular, subdural, and intracerebral hematoma; age; hypertension; hyperglycemia; poor initial clinical grade; multiple aneurysm; presence of sentinel headache; and coagulopathy, although the relationship between rebleeding and some of these risk factors is not consistent between the studies [15, 22].

Aneurysmal Factors

A number of studies, including clinical series, large prospective cohort studies, and the meta-analysis of risk factors for aneurysmal rebleeding, consistently revealed that larger aneurysms were at a higher risk for rebleeding, especially for an aneurysm larger than 10 mm [5, 11, 22]. The location of aneurysm is also implicated to be associated with the risk of rebleeding, mainly with aneurysms arising from posterior circulation [11].

Individual Systemic Condition and Predisposition

Initial elevated blood pressure at presentation is known to be associated with increased rebleeding rates [5, 22]. Systolic blood pressure higher than

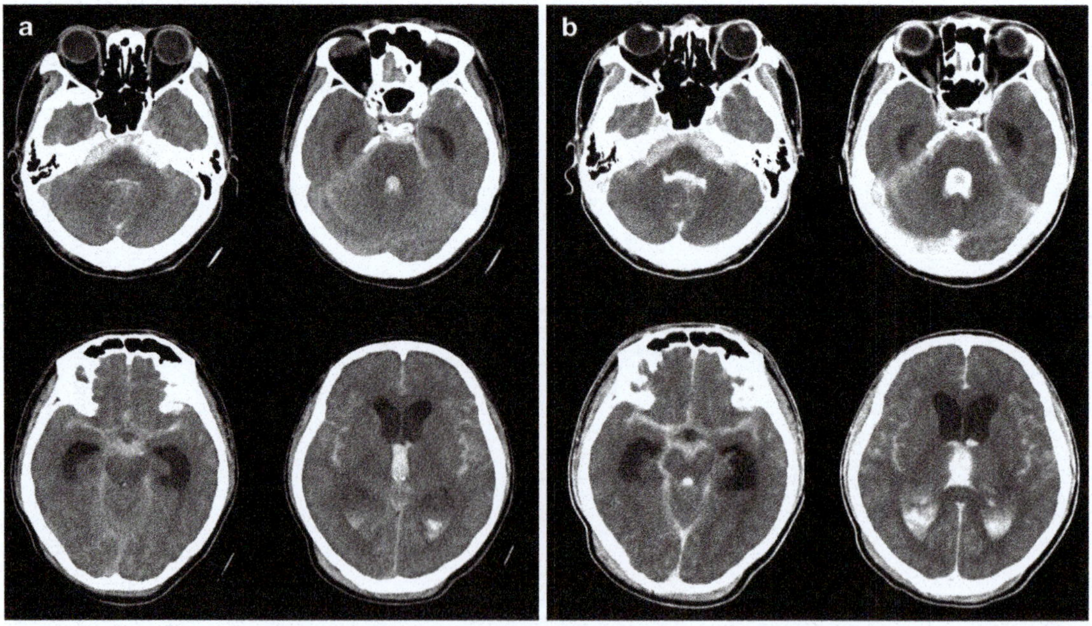

Fig. 4.2 (**a**) Initial brain computed tomography (CT) scan of a 42-year-old male with stuporous mental status shows subarachnoid hemorrhage in the Sylvian, basal, prepontine, cerebellopontine, and cerebellomedullary cistern. Intraventricular hemorrhage in the third, fourth, and lateral ventricles is also noted. (**b**) Follow-up images 2 h after the initial scan demonstrate a massive rebleeding, especially in the fourth ventricle. Hydrocephalus is more evident

160 mmHg and a poor Hunt-Hess grade are also statistically correlated with increased risk of rebleeding [22]. Advanced age has been proposed as an independent risk factor for aneurysmal rebleeding [22].

Fibrin degradation products (FDP) and D-dimer, markers of fibrinolysis, were found to be elevated in the acute stage of SAH. Tissue plasminogen activator (t-PA), which converts plasminogen to plasmin, is activated and released from endothelial cells by endothelial damage and fibrin deposition in the SAH-induced brain. Moreover, it has been reported that decreased activity of plasminogen activator inhibitor-1 (PAI-1), an endogenous inhibitor of t-PA, may be a reason for higher fibrinolytic activity even when t-PA is within the normal range [15]. These increased fibrinolytic activities may dissolve clots covering the aneurysmal rupture point and be associated with rebleeding [15]. There are several reports that reduced clot stability due to decreased platelet aggregation and factor XIII activity is found in patients with rebleeding. Factor XIII, activated by thrombin, is a factor that cross-links fibrin into polymer. It also binds α 2-antiplasmin to fibrin and produces a strong clot that is resistant to fibrinolysis. In summary, reduced clot stability and increased fibrinolytic activity may play important roles in rebleeding in the acute stage of SAH [15].

Treatment-Related Factors

Performance of cerebral angiography in the acute stage, especially within 6 h after SAH, increases the risk of rebleeding by 3.3–23.9% [15]. It has also been reported that CSF drainage before aneurysm closure increases the risk of rebleeding. It has been speculated that changes in the transmural pressure are related to this phenomenon [15, 25]. CSF drainage can increase the transmural pressure by reducing CSF pressure, while cerebral angiography may increase the transmural pressure by temporarily increasing the intra-aneurysmal pressure during the contrast injection. A short interval between CSF diversion and permanent aneurysmal repair might help reduce the risk of rebleeding in this situation [22]. Fibrinolytic therapy to reduce delayed cerebral ischemia in SAH is another risk factor for aneurysmal rebleeding for hospitalized patients [15].

4.1.2.2 Hydrocephalus

The incidence of hydrocephalus after SAH has been reported to be about 15–35% [26–28]. A blood clot in the subarachnoid space, if large, subsequently spills into the ventricles, impeding CSF resorption and circulation. Sudden obstruction of CSF circulation is considered an important contributor to acute development of hydrocephalus [27, 29]. It is known that about 1/5 of the total hydrocephalus occurs in the acute stage; this is most likely due to decreased CSF absorption into the venous sinus owing to the blood clot in the arachnoid granulation. The chronic, long-term, communicating hydrocephalus is secondary to the fibrosis and adhesion of the arachnoid granulation [26]. In addition to the mechanical obstruction of the CSF pathway and inflammatory processes, dysfunctional cerebral pulsation and brain compliance contribute to the development of hydrocephalus after SAH [28]. Ependymal cell desquamation and subependymal basal membrane destruction due to spasm of the choroidal artery and an increase in CSF production due to a series of inflammatory responses following SAH have also been suggested as underlying mechanisms in the development of hydrocephalus [26, 28, 30]. In an experimental study, it was noted that fluid-filled vesicles in the choroid plexus were more related with the SAH model; thus, the authors speculated that CSF secretion might be stimulated by the irritant receptor of glossopharyngeal and vagal nerve endings, which innervate the healthy choroidal plexus epithelium and arteries [30]. However, these suggestions should be further validated.

Patients with hydrocephalus are at greater risk of neurologic impairment and morbidity than those without hydrocephalus [27]. Acute hydrocephalus is more frequently developed in patients with a large clot burden, an episode of rebleeding, or a poor clinical grade on admission [26, 27]. Furthermore, it is observed that acute hydrocephalus reduces cerebral blood flow (CBF), especially in the vicinity of the ventricles, in addition to the direct mass effect [25].

The incidence of hydrocephalus requiring permanent CSF diversion has been reported in 8–63% of cases [27]. Risk factors for shunt-dependent hydrocephalus include presence of intraventricular hemorrhage, aneurysm of posterior circulation, diffuse and dense subarachnoid blood, hypertension, increased sympathetic activity, old age (≥60 years), and presence of in-hospital complications such as meningitis, pneumonia, vasospasm, and ischemic stroke [26, 27].

4.1.2.3 Early Brain Injury and Delayed Cerebral Ischemia After Subarachnoid Hemorrhage

At the onset of SAH, acute arterial bleeding from the cerebral aneurysm results in immediate increased intracranial pressure (ICP). Impaired CSF absorption and circulation lead to the development of acute hydrocephalus, promoting a further increase in ICP [29]. In addition, microvascular alterations, such as transient circulatory arrest, global cerebral ischemia, and reactive hyperemia, also occur along with brain edema and neuronal injury [2]. These initial pathophysiologic changes within the first 3 days are referred as an early brain injury (EBI) [2, 4, 29].

In addition to the initial injury, a complex of pathophysiologic processes occurs following SAH later, during the course of disease; this complex is commonly called delayed cerebral ischemia (DCI) or delayed ischemic neurological deficits (DIND) [2, 4, 31]. Delayed neurological deterioration after SAH typically appears 3–4 days after subarachnoid hemorrhage, reaching the highest incidence and severity at 6–8 days; most cases resolve within 2 weeks following ictus [2, 4, 32]. Interestingly, the observation of arterial narrowing following aneurysmal SAH during the same period of delayed-onset neurological deterioration has led to the assumption that cerebral vasospasm is a principal cause of this condition [2, 4, 29]. However, the presence of angiographic vasospasm is not always correlated with symptomatic DCI, and most clinical trials targeted at reducing vasospasm have failed to produce clinical improvement in DCI [4, 29, 31]. It has therefore been proposed that the pathophysiologic process involving DCI is not solely related to cerebral vasospasm; rather, a multifactorial process can be postulated [2, 4, 29].

The proposed mechanisms of DCI other than vasospasm of large arteries include microvascular alteration and dysfunction (microvascular spasm), microthrombosis, inflammation, and cortical spreading ischemia [2, 4, 29, 32]. It remains to be determined whether EBI might be a precondition for DCI or both EBI and DCI present as coinstantaneous processes in the development of early and delayed cerebral injury [2, 4]. Some events related to DCI may begin during the acute stage of SAH; they may have reciprocal influences and share common pathways with the process of EBI [4].

Early Hemodynamic Response After Subarachnoid Hemorrhage

Acute extravasation of blood from the ruptured aneurysm into the confined subarachnoid space causes abrupt elevation of ICP [2, 4]. The high level of ICP usually decreases within 10–15 minutes [2, 4]. In some cases, however, sustained elevation of ICP may follow due to the direct mass effect of the hemorrhage combined with the development of acute hydrocephalus [4]. If it exceeds the diastolic blood pressure, cerebral perfusion pressure (CPP) can be diminished [2, 4]. Early impairment of these hemodynamic parameters as an increase in ICP and a decrease in CPP results in the reduction of regional CBF; this leads to transient global arrest of intracranial circulation and manifests clinically as loss of consciousness [2, 4, 29].

The initial fall in CBF after SAH is accompanied by an impairment of cerebral autoregulation, reduced cerebral metabolic rate of oxygen, and the suppression of total electrocorticographic activity [4]. CBF autoregulation impairment affects both pressure autoregulation and chemoregulation [2, 4]. Disturbance in autoregulation is pronounced during the first 73 h after ictus and correlates with the severity of SAH [2, 4]. It may result from impaired endothelium-dependent control of vessel diameter [7]. In many studies, impaired CBF autoregulation precedes vasospasm, and the patients with cerebral autoregulatory dysfunction are at great risk of developing DIND [2]. Initial transient global or focal ischemia initiates a cascade of further pathophysiologic processes, such as early metabolic failure, ionic disturbance, and cerebral edema [2, 4, 29]. In animal and human studies, markers of brain ischemia are increased along with concentrations of the excitatory neurotransmitter glutamate [2, 29]. The neurovascular coupling of cortical activity and regional CBF contributes to further reduction of regional CBF, due to disruption of cortical signaling [4]. A noreflow phenomenon, the absence of vascular filling after a period of global cerebral ischemia, may occur despite restoration of cerebral flow in relation to persistent arteriolar vasoconstriction, mainly by pericyte constriction and subsequent capillary thrombosis [2, 4, 29]. It was recently proposed that initial hypoxia and inadequate distal perfusion also activate inflammatory pathways and the coagulation cascade [4, 29]. A large hemorrhagic clot burden, accompanying hydrocephalus, and secondary ischemia with progressive cerebral edema, if not corrected, could lead to a persistent, abnormally high level of ICP and cause a fatal brain herniation.

Cerebral Vasospasm

Since the first observation of arterial narrowing following SAH by Ecker and Riemenschneider in 1951 [33], cerebral vasospasm has been defined as consistent narrowing of cerebral arteries with arterial wall thickening [4]. It usually involves large cerebral arteries between 3 and 14 days and peaks at 1 week after hemorrhage (Fig. 4.3). Angiographic vasospasm can be observed in approximately 50%–70% of patients with SAH [4]. Among them, 20–30% of subjects

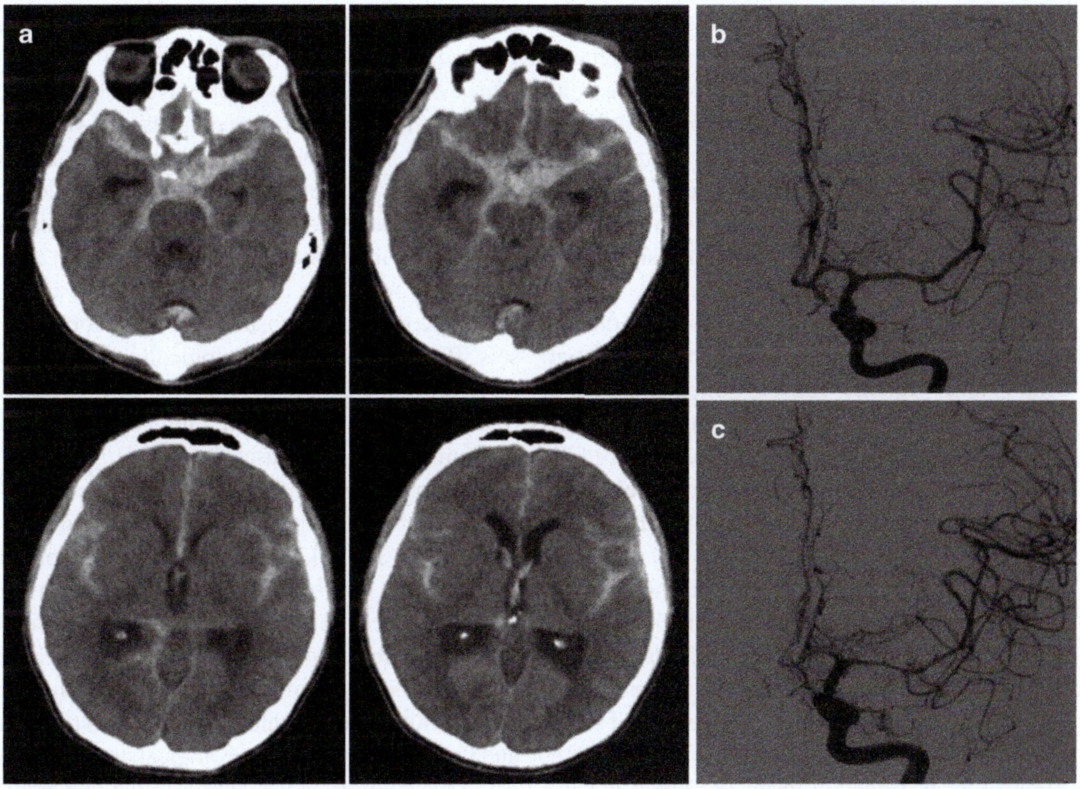

Fig. 4.3 (**a**) A 45-year-old male presents with sudden severe headache. Computed tomography (CT) scan shows acute subarachnoid hemorrhage. (**b**) Subsequent angiography reveals cerebral aneurysm arising at the left posterior communicating artery. The aneurysm was secured by coil embolization on the day of admission. (**c**) Follow-up angiography 7 days later shows diffuse narrowing of the vascular caliber in the proximal middle cerebral artery and anterior cerebral artery

develop delayed cerebral ischemia and infarction clinically [4, 32]. The amount of subarachnoid blood has been reported to correlate with the degree of vasospasm [34]. In addition to vasospasm of large arteries adjacent to the circle of Willis, vasoconstriction of small parenchymal vessels, referred as microvascular spasm, has been proposed to play a role in both EBI and DCI as well [4, 32]. Microvascular spasm occurs first in the early stage of SAH, followed by progressively larger vessel spasm in the delayed injury period [4].

The red blood cells that spill into the subarachnoid space break down and degrade over time, producing derivatives such as hemoglobin, methemoglobin, oxyhemoglobin, heme, and hemin [32]. Oxidized hemoglobin from lysis of the subarachnoid clot initiates complex pathophysiologic cascades in the early brain injury period [4, 32]. Free hemoglobin and hemin generate superoxide radicals, lipid peroxidation, bilirubin oxidation (BOX) products, endothelin-1, and the endogenous NO inhibitor; they peak at 3–8 days after SAH [2, 4, 29, 32]. Oxyhemoglobin also activates several pathways involving protein kinase C, Rho kinase, and Tyrosine kinase, promoting arteriolar smooth muscle contraction by increased Ca^{2+} influx via voltage-sensitive calcium channels [29].

Endothelial dysfunction is considered one of the factors in early vasoconstriction. Endothelial denudation, smooth muscle thickening, and impaired endothelial controls of vasomotor tone have been observed in vasospastic vessels [2]. Vasomotor tone is mainly controlled by releasing of spasmogens (such as endothelin-1 and 20-hydroxyeicosatetraenoic acid) and relaxant agents (such as NO, prostaglandin-I, and epoxyeicosatrienoic acid) from the endothelium [2, 7, 29]. Endothelin-1 is one of the most potent endogenous vasoconstrictors. It is produced mainly by endothelium as a consequence of stimulation by oxyhemoglobin, endothelial denudation, or ischemic insult [2, 29]. It is suggested that the early increase in endothelin-1 level as well as a decrease in NO activity promotes vascular constriction in delayed vasospasm in SAH [29].

Hemoglobin-induced oxidative stress also plays an important role in early and delayed brain injury [32]. Oxygen free radicals (ROS), such as superoxide anion, hydroxyl radical, hydrogen peroxide, NO, and peroxynitrite, are generated during oxidation of hemoglobin along with an increased NO synthase (NOS) activity, disrupted mitochondrial respiration, a hypoxic conversion of endothelial xanthine dehydrogenase to xanthine oxidase, lipid peroxidation, and upregulation of NADPH oxidase [2, 29]. As a result of oxidative stress, serial pathologic processes involving early and delayed brain injury occur; these include degradation of the vascular wall, disruption of the blood-brain barrier (BBB), vasoconstriction through releasing leukotriene C_4 and prostaglandin D_2 from the lipoxygenase and cyclooxygenase pathways, and apoptotic cell death [1, 2, 29]. Among these, alteration in cerebral NO level plays an important role in regulation of cerebral blood flow and smooth muscle cell proliferation [1]. A decrease in cerebral NO level immediately after SAH is due to a natural scavenging system, including hemoglobin, free radicals, and vascular neutrophils [2]. It then increases within 24 hours after SAH, recovering above the basal level, along with saturation of scavenging mechanisms combined with an increase in NOS activity [2]. A temporary reduction of cerebral NO level apparently accompanies constriction of cerebral vessels. If NO increases pathologically, it acts as a free radical itself in the form of peroxynitrite, resulting in NO-mediated cell injury of the endothelium and smooth muscle cell [1, 2].

Apoptosis of endothelial cells and necrosis of astrocytes by oxidative stress result in the disruption of the BBB [1, 2, 29, 32]. Activation of autophagy in neurons has been implicated in the pathogenesis of EBI. It has been demonstrated that serum levels of neuron-specific enolase, a marker of neuronal injury, and S100-B, a marker of glial injury, are elevated in poor-grade patients and those with delayed neurological deterioration [2]. Recent studies have demonstrated that apoptotic cell death is evoked via caspase-dependent intrinsic pathway (caspase-3, 8, and 9), activated by an increased intracellular calcium level in the early stage of SAH and an extrinsic death receptor pathway mediated by the TNF receptor in the late phase of SAH [2, 29].

Voltage-gated calcium channels are attributed to maintaining ionic gradients across the cell membrane. L-type Ca^{2+} channel has been shown to be strongly correlated with vasospasm in SAH, and dihydropyridine L-type Ca^{2+} channel antagonists are proved to be useful for the prevention of vasospasm and DCI in SAH [4]. Recently, the possible significance of impaired cellular calcium homeostasis through the R- and T-types has also been proposed in delayed cerebral ischemia [4]. The aberrant increase in intracellular calcium leads to vasoconstriction, release of glutamate, and activation of various molecules mediating cell death [2]. An increase in extracellular concentration of glutamate represents activation of the N-methyl-D-aspartate (NMDA) receptor with massive calcium influx; this consequently leads to cellular leakage and BBB disruption and is associated with the severity of initial brain injury [2].

Microvascular Alteration, Dysfunction, and Spasm

Regions of perfusion mismatch, in which perfusion deficit or infarction occurs without evidence of large vessel vasospasm, have been noticed in positron emission tomography (PET), magnetic resonance imaging (MRI), and computed tomography (CT) in the early brain injury period. Impaired neurovascular coupling, including neurons, astrocytes, and endothelium, results in a patchy microvascular constriction seen in the early phase following SAH, in approximately 70% of cerebral arterioles [4, 29]. This environmental change in microvasculature has been proposed as part of the fundamental background for an initiation of EBI and DCI. In addition to the direct vasospastic effect of oxygenated hemoglobin and its breakdown products, several other factors contribute to microvascular narrowing; these include swollen astrocytic end feet, constricted pericytes, and cerebral edema. Recently, the role of pericytes in the regulation of microcirculation has been emphasized based on its effect on the capillary microscopic distribution of blood, so-called capillary transit time heterogeneity (CTH) [4]. Prolonged constriction or thrombosis of cerebral arterioles after SAH may result in an impairment of cerebral autoregulation; this autoregulatory failure is more frequently associated with DCI than those with intact autoregulation [29].

Microthrombosis

When SAH occurs, the tissue factor is released from the damaged brain cells and endothelium to systemic circulation, which activates the coagulation cascade. The last step in the coagulation cascade is thrombin activation, which promotes fibrin and platelet aggregation on the damaged aneurysmal wall to prevent further bleeding [2, 15].

Platelet activation and aggregation appear in the early course of SAH, around 5 minutes after experimental SAH and 48 hours after clinical SAH [2, 29]. In an autopsy series, formation of microthrombi is seen as well, where platelet aggregates in intraparenchymal microvessels and within pial arterioles, with the exception of the parent vessel of the ruptured aneurysm or a vessel affecting vasospasm [2]. Interestingly, these microthrombi have been observed in a biphasic pattern, at 4 days and between 7 and 14 days after SAH [29]. In the clinical setting, microemboli can be observed using transcranial Doppler ultrasound in up to 30%–70% of the patients with SAH [4]. Antithrombin inhibits thrombin action by forming a thrombin-antithrombin (TAT) complex. This TAT complex is elevated in the acute state of SAH, especially in those with severe brain damage and rebleeding; this indicates that it is hypercoagulable in the early stage of SAH [15].

Formation of microthrombi is the result of a multifactorial process. Platelet activation and aggregation are initiated from the mechanical obstruction of vessel lumen and vasoconstriction via the release of serotonin, adenosine diphosphate (ADP), and platelet-derived growth factor (PDGF) [2, 29]. Denuded endothelium exposes collagen, von Willebrand factor, and thrombin, further activating platelets and the coagulation cascade [2, 29]. Platelet aggregates also release thromboxanes, which promote vasoconstriction in parenchymal and pial vasculatures [29].

Fibrinolytic activity is also impaired, leading to a vicious cycle of creating a procoagulable state [29]. Along with the procoagulable state and impaired fibrinolytic activity, the narrowing of the arteriole and capillary lumen by swollen astrocytic end feet and pericyte constriction also affects microvascular thrombosis [4].

Microthromboemboli may also originate from the site of the aneurysm rupture and move to parenchymal vessels [2]. A recent study indicates that microthrombi escape into the parenchyma from the lumen, where they originally form in the early stage of SAH [2]. The number of microthrombi seems to be correlated to the degree of SAH and vasoconstriction [2, 4].

Many experimental and clinical studies demonstrate that microthrombosis contributes to microvascular dysfunction and increases CTH. If continued, it initiates additional inflammatory processes and further aggravates brain injury, leading to destruction of major proteins of the vessel wall by releasing collagenases such as MMP-2 and 9 [2, 26, 29]. These may lead to irreversible ischemic degeneration in the surrounding neural structure. Indeed, microthrombosis has been associated with DCI, although not all patients with microthrombi develop permanent neurologic impairment [2, 4].

Neuroinflammation

A cascade of inflammatory reaction is initiated by erythrocyte breakdown products along with initial ischemia [32]. An increased concentration of inflammatory cytokines in the early period of SAH plays a critical role in the pathogenesis of both EBI and DCI [2, 4, 32]. Elevation of C-reactive protein (CRP), a highly sensitive inflammatory protein, along with systemic inflammatory response, including fever, leukocytosis, tachycardia, and tachypnea, is frequently observed in patients with acute stage SAH [2, 29, 35] and may be correlated with a poor clinical outcome [4].

CD68 (the activated microglial marker) and glial fibrillary acidic protein (GFAP, the specific marker of the astrocyte) are highly expressed in SAH, suggesting the microglia and the astrocyte are activated and involved in both the early and the delayed processes of SAH [4, 32]. Activation of microglia and astrocyte within the first several hours after SAH consequently upregulates endothelial expression of adhesion molecules, such as E-selectin, intercellular adhesion molecule-1 (ICAM-1), and vascular cell adhesion molecule-1 (VCAM-1), promoting parenchymal migration of the inflammatory cells such as macrophages and neutrophils [2, 4, 29, 32]. Further inflammatory cascades are preceded by pro-inflammatory cytokines, such as interleukin (IL)-1β, IL-6, TNF-α, and endothelin-1, released from recruited inflammatory cells [2, 4, 29, 35]. Activation of complementary and inflammatory pathways, such as a mitogen-activated protein kinase pathway, further exaggerates vasoconstriction, recruitment of inflammatory cells, increase in vascular permeability, BBB disruption, and neuronal cell death [2, 4, 29, 32, 35].

The role of the intracellular signaling pathways in inflammation has been studied [32]. Inhibition of inflammatory factors, such as toll-like receptor 4 or c-Jun N-terminal kinase, reduces the degree of vasospasm in animal studies [32]. The poly (ADP-ribose) polymerase pathway is activated in the smooth muscle and adventitia, promoting adhesion molecule expression and neutrophil recruitment [32]. The lectin-complement pathway has also been shown to be related with the degree of vasospasm [32]. Neuronal damage and apoptosis are demonstrated with increased intracerebral accumulation of microtubule-associated protein 2, myelin basic protein, and cleaved caspase-3, which represent axonal and neuronal injury [32].

Cortical Spreading Depolarization, Depression, and Ischemia

Cortical spreading depolarization (CSD) is waves of sustained neuronal depolarization, generally demonstrated as propagating, polyphasic, slow potential changes in an electroencephalogram [2, 4, 36]. CSD is a cortical reaction to various stimuli and is usually associated with the breakdown of ionic gradients across neuronal membranes, where massive neuronal sodium and calcium influx occur along with elevated levels of extracellular potassium and excitatory transmitters [2, 4, 29, 36]. A water shift into a depolarized neural cell owing to the loss of ionic gradients leads to cellular swelling, activation of MMP-9, and breakdown of the BBB [4, 29]. This hyperexcitability is followed by a transient depression of spontaneous electrocortical activity, so-called cortical spreading depression [4, 36]. Cortical spreading depolarization induces a net increase in regional CBF (spreading hyperemia), followed by a protracted hypoperfusion similar to neuronal depression [4, 37]. In cerebral tissue at risk for damage, however, this phenomenon contributes to the ischemia progression that is referred as cortical spreading ischemia [4, 37]. This phenomenon is frequently observed in acute SAH with a bimodal frequency distribution through both the early and the delayed period [37]. There is some speculation that cortical spreading depolarization and ischemia may contribute to development of early brain damage and delayed ischemia in acute SAH [4]. Impairment of ionic distribution, oxyhemoglobin, endothelin-1, reduced NO, and increased glutamate activity may precipitate cortical spreading depolarization in both the early and the late period of SAH [2, 4]. Cortical spreading ischemia may promote microvascular dysfunction, creating cerebral edema and progressive ischemic cortical injury [42]. Local microvascular dysfunction itself also contributes to initiation of spreading ischemia and may act together in both early and delayed brain injury [4].

4.1.2.4 General Medical Complication after SAH

A hypothalamus-mediated adrenergic surge occurs at the onset of SAH as a result of sudden changes in perfusion pressure [29]. This adrenergic surge in the acute phase may be associated with various cardiopulmonary disturbances, including neurogenic pulmonary edema, cardiac wall motion abnormality, arrhythmia, and systemic inflammatory response [29, 35, 38, 39]. Cardiopulmonary complications may synergistically worsen hypoperfusion and hypoxia-related brain injury for those who survived and are associated with a poor clinical outcome [29, 38].

SAH-Induced Cardiac Dysfunction

SAH-induced cardiac dysfunction has been referred to as neurogenic stunned myocardium, neurogenic stress cardiomyopathy, and takotsubo cardiomyopathy [39]. It presents as transient, reversible, diffuse left ventricular dysfunction, transient regional wall motion abnormalities, elevation in cardiac enzymes, and electrocardiogram changes including QTc prolongation and ST-T changes [39]. Electrocardiogram changes can be found in almost all patients with SAH, whereas echocardiographic wall motion abnormalities have been observed in a significant variation of incidence [39]. It occurs due to catecholamine surging at the time of ictus as well as underlying myocardial microvascular dysfunction and genetic polymorphisms. It has been observed more frequently in those with a poor clinical grade at the time of admission [32, 39].

Neurogenic Pulmonary Edema (NPE)

NPE after SAH has also been associated with worse outcomes and death (Fig. 4.4). A massive sympathetic discharge from a sudden increase in intracranial pressure or brain damage may result in a transient increase in pulmonary artery pressure and subsequent hydrostatic pulmonary edema [35, 38]. On the other hand, increased capillary permeability due to a direct sympathetic effect on the capillary endothelium, rather than elevated pulmonary artery pressure, has been suggested as another hypothesis for development of NPE [38]. It is also possible that SAH-related cardiac dysfunction leads to increased left atrial pressure and subsequent pulmonary hypertension, resulting in pulmonary edema [38].

Electrolyte or Metabolic Disturbance

Electrolyte imbalance in sodium and potassium is a frequently encountered clinical issue in the management of patients with acute SAH. Hypernatremia has been found most frequently in subjects suffering from SAH. Its exact mechanism is not fully understood; however, a central origin of diabetes insipidus seems to be the most common cause. Osmotic diuresis by the therapeutic use of mannitol partly plays a role in hypernatremia as well. Hyponatremia develops

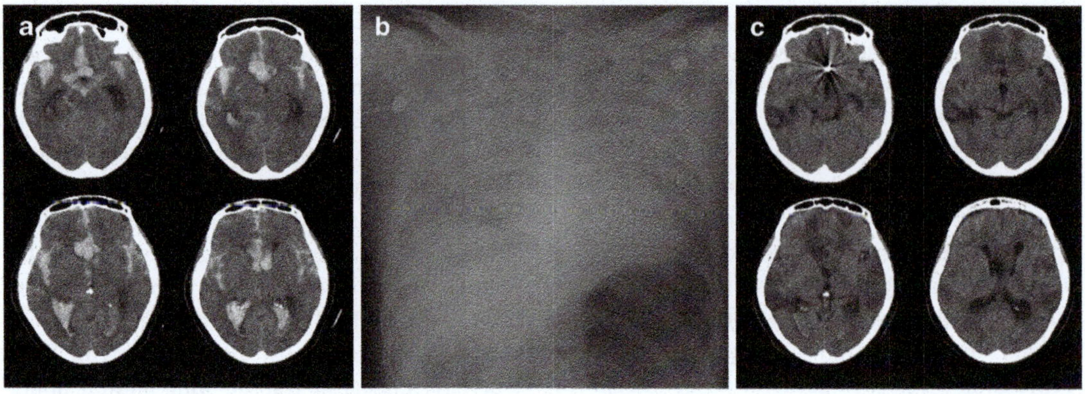

Fig. 4.4 (**a**) A 52-year-old male presents with deep stuporous mental status. The initial brain computed tomography (CT) shows subarachnoid hemorrhage with overt intraventricular hemorrhage. (**b**) The initial chest X-ray demonstrates neurogenic pulmonary edema with diffuse infiltration of haziness on the bilateral lung. (**c**) A brain CT taken on day 14 after ictus shows diffuse multiple low-density lesions representing delayed cerebral ischemia and infarction

in approximately 10–30% of SAH patients. Its underlying mechanisms have been explained by inappropriate secretion of antidiuretic hormone (SIADH) and cerebral salt-wasting syndrome (CSWS) [2]. SIADH is the most common cause of hyponatremia in SAH and water retention with excess secretion of antidiuretic hormone probably due to hypothalamic insult at ictus [2]. CSWS leads to natriuresis, possibly owing to an increase in humoral factors, including brain natriuretic peptide or atrial natriuretic peptide.

Systemic Inflammatory Response Syndrome

Systemic inflammatory response syndrome (SIRS) is a syndrome with noninfectious hyperthermia, leukocytosis along with tachycardia, and tachypnea [29, 35]. SIRS may develop in patients with acute aneurysmal SAH, especially for those with a poor clinical grade, a large burden of clot, larger aneurysm size, and higher blood glucose and blood pressure levels on admission [35, 40]. This may result either from activation of an inflammatory cascade with the upregulated cytokines or release of circulating catecholamine triggered by acute brain injury [32, 35, 40]. Elevated levels of CRP in the early stage after SAH reflect a systemic inflammatory response, triggered by IL-6-mediated hepatic production of acute-phase proteins [32, 35]. Clinical data regarding SAH-related SIRS has demonstrated that the presence of SIRS is associated with the development of vasospasm, hydrocephalus, and other systemic complications with higher mortality and morbidity rates than those without such complications [32, 35, 40]. These findings indicate that SIRS after SAH represents the severity of the initial ictal injury and further progress of tissue damage [32].

4.2 Pathophysiology of Non-aneurysmal Subarachnoid Hemorrhage

Non-aneurysmal SAH is responsible for a minority of spontaneous cases of SAH, representing approximately 6.8–20% of all spontaneous SAH [3, 41, 42]. It has been proposed that the distribution of SAH on CT is related to the likelihood of identifying underlying etiology [41, 43, 44]. CT images of patients who have SAH with an unknown etiology often exhibit an atypical pattern of SAH, including perimesencephalic and convexity SAH, as well as the classic pattern of diffuse SAH [41–43, 45]. It is important to note that 5–17.5% of patients with a classic pattern of subarachnoid clot distribution and negative initial catheter-based angiography might have aneurysms on repeated angiography [41]. In these cases, diagnostic failure to detect aneurysms on initial angiography probably occurs as a result of thrombosis of the aneurysm, local vasospasm, and obliteration of the aneurysm by the rupture. Thus, it is important to exclude underlying pathology as the source of hemorrhage.

Many different sources of bleeding have been suggested in non-aneurysmal SAH, including inflammatory lesions (mycotic aneurysms, vasculitis), vascular anomaly other than aneurysms (spontaneous arterial dissection, vascular malformation, moyamoya disease, venous thrombosis, and cerebral amyloid angiopathy), vascular or neoplastic lesions in the cervical spine, coagulopathies, tumor, and drug use [3, 41, 42, 44–48]. One of the well-known conditions among angiographic negative SAH is the so-called perimesencephalic non-aneurysmal SAH (PNSAH), which accounts for about 26.3–70% of non-aneurysmal SAH [42, 43, 45]. It is widely accepted to distinguish PNSAH, in which SAH is typically concentrated near the pons and midbrain and has a uniformly benign prognosis [41–43, 45], from other types of non-aneurysmal SAH, where it has a more varied degree of distribution and diverse clinical outcomes as well as various underlying etiologies [43].

4.2.1 Perimesencephalic Non-aneurysmal Subarachnoid Hemorrhage

PNSAH can be described as focal SAH accumulated predominantly in the perimesencephalic cisterns, usually at the anterior to the midbrain and pons or, infrequently, in the quadrigeminal cistern, with no more than minimal blood in the Sylvian and interhemispheric fissures and without overt intraventricular hemorrhage [3, 41, 42, 45]. The term PNSAH is widely accepted to describe this entity, though it is also referred to by various terms, such as pretruncal, pre-mesencephalic, or cryptogenic SAH. Approximately 21–77% of patients with SAH with no identifiable cause for the hemorrhage on initial work-up have been reported to have a PNSAH pattern of bleeding on the CT scan [41]. PNSAH has a slight male predominance in contrast to female predominance in aneurysmal SAH; it may be associated with hypertension, diabetes, alcohol abuse, and physical activity such as physical straining at the time of ictus [41]. The origin of the bleeding in PNSAH is still unclear and may be diverse. Suggested etiologies for PNSAH are mainly divided into arterial and venous pathologies; however, the diagnosis of PNSAH should still be a diagnosis of exclusion [42, 45].

4.2.1.1 Rupture of a Small Perforating Artery

It has been suggested that PNSAH is likely to have a non-visualized tiny aneurysm of the perforators around the mesencephalon or basilar artery itself [41, 49]. Although current diagnostic images are able to detect small aneurysms, a very tiny one could be missed on the initial work-up owing to intra-aneurysmal thrombosis, collapse of volume following the rupture, or by its small size itself, which has subsequently sealed [49]. Possible perforators that bleed around the mesencephalon as an explanation for PNSAH include posterior thalamoperforating arteries arising from the P1 segment of the posterior cerebral artery (PCA), the artery of Davidoff and Schechter (a branch of the P2 segment of the PCA), paramedian mesencephalic arteries (branches of the PCA or sometimes the basilar artery), and perforators from lateral surfaces of the upper basilar artery (Fig. 4.5). The diameter of these perforators is measured as 0.24–1.18 mm in an autopsy study [50]. Hence, vascular lesions arising from these small perforators may spontaneously resolve, negating further evaluation and therapeutic intervention. Intramural hematoma of basilar arterial dissection has also been proposed as a possible bleeding mechanism in PNSAH [49].

4.2.1.2 Anatomic Variation in Deep and Perimesencephalic Venous Drainage System

Physical activity involving the Valsalva maneuver at the time of ictus has been suggested as a risk factor for NPSAH, reaching 16–50% across all studies [41, 42]. Physical straining that

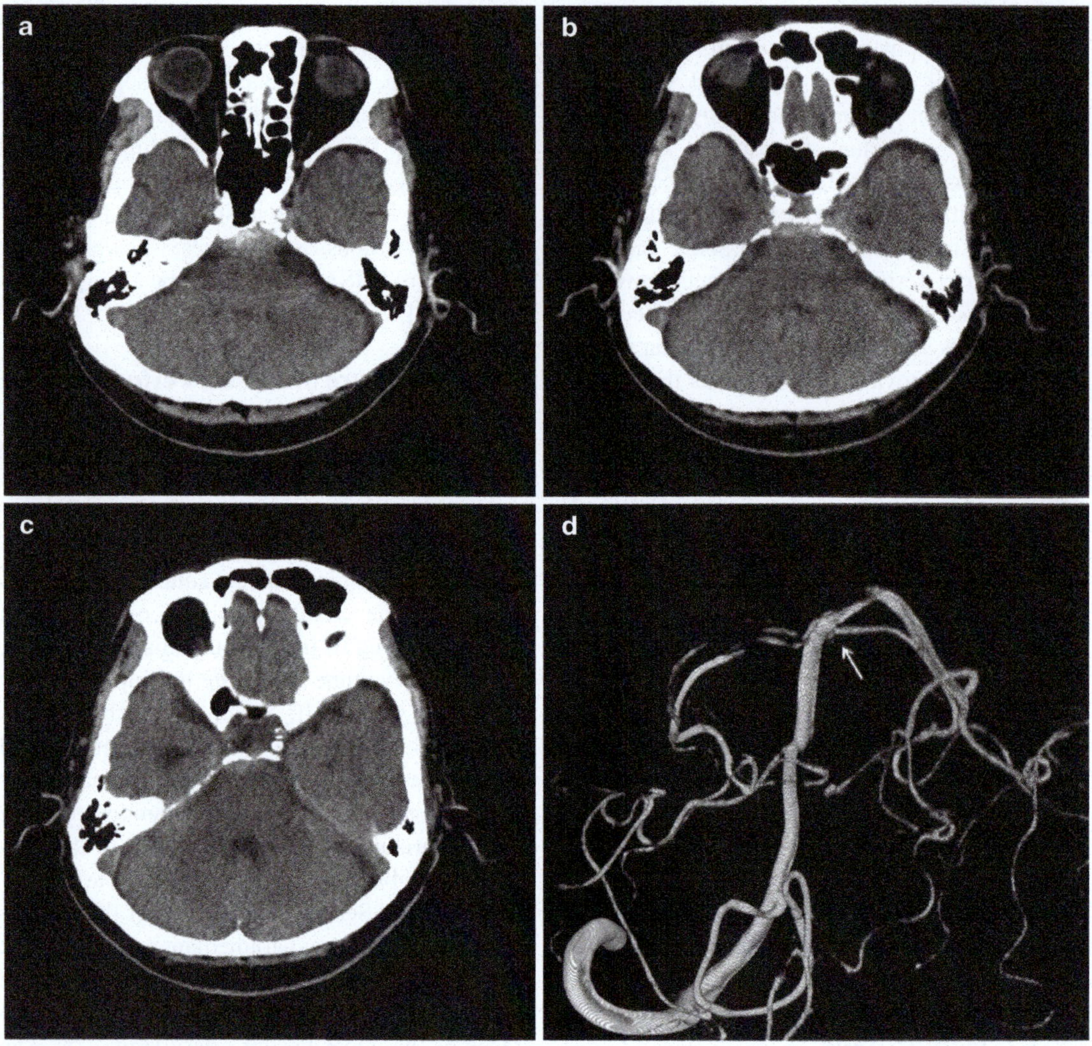

Fig. 4.5 (**a**–**c**) The brain computed tomography (CT) of a 53-year-old male who presented with headache shows focal hemorrhage accumulated predominantly in the prepontine cisterns. (**d**) Three-dimensional rotational angiography reveals a tiny aneurysmal budding near the basilar top (*white arrow*)

increases thoracic pressure and reduces jugular back flow consequently elevates an intracranial venous pressure at the time of ictus [42]. Accordingly, possible venous bleeding from abnormal deep venous drainage has been proposed as one of explanations for PNSAH [41, 42, 45]. Rupture of a vein in the prepontine or interpeduncular cistern is also proposed as a likely cause of bleeding in PNSAH [3].

A variation of the basal vein of Rosenthal (BVR) and its tributaries are being explored as a likely cause of PNSAH [42]. When the BVR drains directly into the dural sinus instead of the vein of Galen, it can be classified as primitive-type BVR [42]. It has been shown that patients with PNSAH have higher rates of primitive-type BVR (40–66%) compared with those having aneurysmal SAH (10–19%) [41, 42]. The direct connection of perimesencephalic veins with the dural sinuses may be more prone to rupture in case of sudden increase of venous pressure [42]. In addition, some of the primitive veins circulate across the tentorial margin, which is more vulnerable to rupture when exposed to torsion or friction [42]. In a normal venous drainage pattern, a small caliber of BVR is more likely to have an association with PNSAH. In addition, anomalies of the venous system, such as stenosis of the vein of Galen and straight sinus, as well as jugular vein occlusion, have been proposed as underlying pathology [41]. However, a limitation in explaining venous theories as the cause of PNSAH is that not all cases of PNSAH have abnormal venous drainage, and PNSAH is less likely to recur even if the anatomic variation is not corrected [42]. Some authors explain that the venous rupture is healed by a fibrous tissue reaction that strengthens the vein walls [42].

4.2.2 Convexal or Cortical Subarachnoid Hemorrhage

Convexal or cortical SAH is a localized clot in the subarachnoid space, adjacent to one or more sulci near the convexity, with no associated blood in the basal cisterns or elsewhere [44, 46, 48]. Due to the high rates of misdiagnosis from a relatively small clot burden and its atypical location of hemorrhage, MRI is considered a better diagnostic tool than CT for localizing acute or subacute convexal SAH, which shows hyperintense and hypointense signals in fluid-attenuated inversion recovery images and T2-weighted images, respectively [46–48].

The clinical course and prognosis of convexal SAH are quite different from those of PNSAH. Convexal SAH can present atypical symptoms, such as transient focal sensorimotor symptoms or epileptic seizure, and has a relatively poor clinical outcome [44, 46, 48]. The underlying cause of convexal SAH includes cerebral venous sinus/cortical vein thrombosis, posterior reversible leukoencephalopathy syndromes, arteriovenous fistula or malformations, hyperperfusion syndrome after revascularization, reversible cerebral vasoconstriction syndrome (RCVS), and cerebral amyloid angiopathy (CAA) [44, 46–48].

4.2.2.1 Reversible Cerebral Vasoconstriction Syndrome (RCVS)

It has been reported that 22% of patients with RCVS have cortical SAH as an early complication, occurring mainly within the first week. One study found that about 60% of the convexal hemorrhage was included in this category [44]. RCVS is characterized by the recurrent thunderclap headache with multiple peripheral narrowing of cerebral arteries. It resolves spontaneously within 1–3 months [48]. This rare disease has been referred to by various names, including isolated angiitis of the central nervous system, isolated benign cerebral vasculitis, central nervous system pseudovasculitis, postpartum angiopathy, migrainous vasospasm, and drug-induced cerebral vasculopathy [48]. SAH due to RCVS frequently presents as a small, localized unilateral or bilateral cortical SAH on MRI and has a female predominance [44, 48]. It is interesting to note that the diffuse vasoconstriction observed in RCVS cannot be explained by vasospasm because the constricted arteries mostly do not have direct contact with the subarachnoid clot. A transient disturbance in the control of vascular tone has been suggested as a pathophysiology of tandem arterial narrowing [48]. As hemorrhage mostly occurs within the first week, it is assumed that abnormal control of cerebrovascular tone involves small distal arteries responsible for hemorrhages in the early phase of the clinical course, which then affects more proximal large arteries later [48]. The use of drugs such as vasoconstrictors may be a risk factor for RCVS [48].

4.2.2.2 Cerebral Amyloid Angiopathy (CAA)

The frequent association of convexal SAH with cortical microbleeds, leukoaraiosis, and superficial siderosis supports the assumption of CAA as a possible etiologic cause for convexal SAH across the studies, especially in patients over 60 years old [44, 46]. In recent studies, 30–40% of CAA-associated convexal SAH had recurrent bleeding on follow-up [44]. A high prevalence of superficial siderosis in pathologically proven CAA also suggests that CAA-associated SAH might be a recurrent event [44, 46].

CAA-related SAH usually presents in patients with focal neurologic symptoms mimicking transient ischemic attack rather than thunderclap headache [44, 46]. Spreading ischemia or focal seizure has been proposed to explain these focal symptoms [46]. It is still unclear whether the bleeding focus of the convexal SAH is the cortical or the leptomeningeal artery. In an autopsy study of CAA-associated hemorrhage, Aß-amyloid deposition was more prominent in the meningeal vessels than in the cortical artery [51]. Based on this report, leptomeningeal vessels might be more responsible for bleeding than cortical arteries in CAA-associated convexal SAH.

4.2.2.3 Cortical Venous Thrombosis

Cortical venous thrombosis (CVT) can present as an isolated SAH. In one study, 6.4% of CVT involving in continuity with dural sinus thrombosis had SAH that was always localized, involving only a few sulci and invariably located adjacent to the thrombosis at the convexities without overt intracerebral hemorrhage [47]. Cortical swelling and edema may be associated with the CVT-related convexal SAH (Fig. 4.6) [47]. Diagnosis of

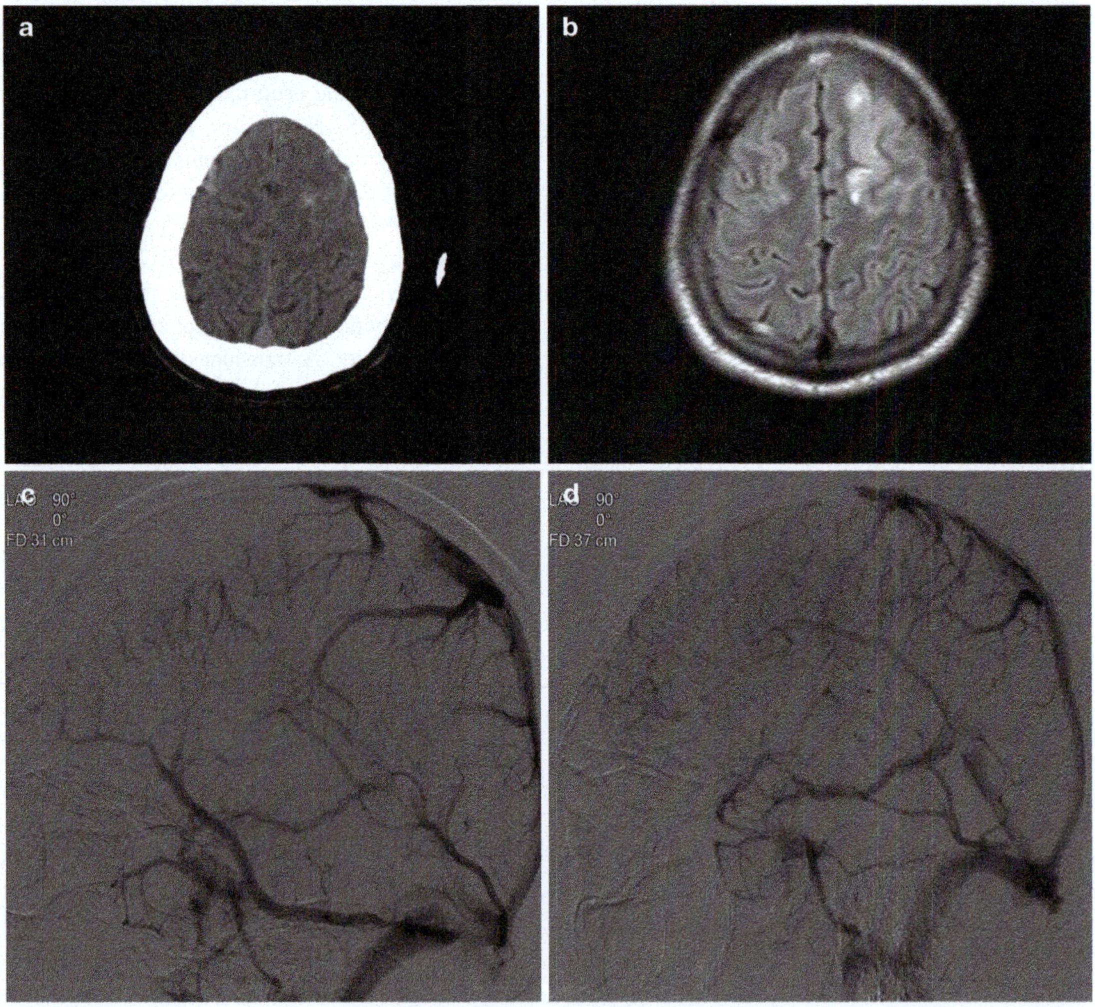

Fig. 4.6 (**a**). The brain computed tomography (CT) of a 23-year-old male who presents with epileptic seizures shows a focal subarachnoid hemorrhage in the bilateral frontal sulci. (**b**) Magnetic resonance image (MRI) shows accompanying frontal lobe edema adjacent to a subarachnoid clot. (**c**) The venous phase of the left internal carotid artery (ICA) angiogram reveals superior sagittal sinus thrombosis with cortical venous thrombosis. (**d**) A right ICA angiogram also shows occlusion of the anterior half of the superior sagittal sinus

an isolated CVT is difficult because of variations in the number and location of the cortical veins. In addition, the presence of cortical SAH further prevents differentiating cortical vein thrombosis from fresh clot [47]. A differential finding between cortical vein thrombosis and cortical SAH in T2-weighted MRI is that cortical vein thrombosis might be seen as a hypointense tubular structure, while SAH appears as a slight hemosiderin deposit. It is suggested that increased venous pressure in the venous thrombosis leads to rupture of the adjacent cortical vein and parenchymal hemorrhage leaks to the subarachnoid space.

4.2.3 Diffuse-Type Subarachnoid Hemorrhage Without Cerebral Aneurysms

A significant number of SAH with no identifiable aneurysm have diffuse, thick subarachnoid clots around the basal and Sylvian cisterns, mimicking the typical pattern of aneurysmal SAH rather than those of focal accumulation of clot in PNSAH [43, 45]. One report showed that about 60% of the patients with angiographically negative SAH fit the diffuse subtype [43]. The origin of the bleeding for these criteria has not been fully established; however, a substantial percentage of these patients has reduced platelet activity with aspirin use even though the underlying pathologies might be similar to the typical PNSAH [45]. As expected, large hemorrhagic volumes are associated with a higher prevalence of hydrocephalus than typical PNSAH; nevertheless, they have lower mortality and a better clinical outcome compared to aneurysmal SAH because of the absence of active arterial bleeding and a lower incidence of rebleeding [43, 45].

4.2.4 Prognosis of Non-aneurysmal Subarachnoid Hemorrhage

In general, PNSAH is considered to have a benign clinical course, a low risk of complications, and a short hospital stay [41, 42, 45]. Incidence of shunt-dependent hydrocephalus and symptomatic vasospasm was reported as 9.6%, which is significantly less than aneurysmal SAH [43]. It is expected that 97% of patients with PNSAH will be able to live independently at the time of discharge [41, 43].

Non-perimesencephalic diffuse SAH has some risk of having an underlying cause for the hemorrhage, such as coagulopathy or platelet dysfunction, mostly secondary to anticoagulant or antiplatelet agent [41, 45]. One study reported 7.4% of the patients with non-aneurysmal SAH had an antithrombotic medication [41]. The patients with this entity may be more likely to have a larger clot burden and a poorer outcome [41, 45]. Patients with diffuse aneurysmal bleeding patterns have a significantly higher rate of complications than PNSAH, even though their mortality and morbidity rates vary substantially across studies. These inconsistent clinical results of non-aneurysmal diffuse SAH are drawn from previously published studies performed in different decades and countries. The differences may stem from overestimation of the true complication rates because some of them might include angiographic occult aneurysmal SAH before the introduction of high-quality digital subtraction angiography and three-dimensional rotational angiography.

It has been reported that more hemorrhage on CT than is typical for PNSAH is related to an increased risk of hydrocephalus [45]. In comparison with PNSAH, diffuse-type non-aneurysmal SAH has an increased incidence of hydrocephalus (50.8% vs. 9.6%) and symptomatic vasospasm (28.6% vs. 9.6%) [43]. Only 76% of diffuse-type non-aneurysmal SAH has been reported to achieve complete recovery and independent living in the same reports [43].

The prognosis of patients who have isolated convexal hemorrhage has also been reported to be poor, at least for the elderly, even in the absence of recurrent hemorrhage [44, 46, 48]. In recent clinical series, previous bleeding and extensive white matter hyperintensities were significantly associated with increased disability. Furthermore, high rates of subsequent ischemic infarctions and intracerebral hemorrhage have been reported to contribute to unfavorable outcomes in these patients [48].

References

1. Andreasen TH, Bartek J Jr, Andresen M, et al. Modifiable risk factors for aneurysmal subarachnoid hemorrhage. Stroke. 2013;44:3607–12.
2. Sehba FA, Hou J, Pluta RM, et al. The importance of early brain injury after subarachnoid hemorrhage. Prog Neurobiol. 2012;97:14–37.
3. van Gijn J, Kerr RS, Rinkel GJ. Subarachnoid hemorrhage. Lancet. 2007;369:306–18.
4. van Lieshout JH, Dibué-Adjei M, Cornelius JF et al (2017) An introduction to the pathophysiology of aneurysmal subarachnoid hemorrhage. Neurosurg Rev: https://doi.org/10.1007/s10143-017-0827-y. [Epub ahead of print].
5. Boogaarts HD, van Lieshout JH, van Amerongen MJ, et al. Aneurysm diameter as a risk factor for pretreatment rebleeding: a meta-analysis. J Neurosurg. 2015;122:921–8.
6. Can A, Du R. Association of hemodynamic factors with intracranial aneurysm formation and rupture: systematic review and meta-analysis. Neurosurgery. 2016;78:510–20.
7. Kassam AB, Horowitz M, Chang YF, et al. Altered arterial homeostasis and cerebral aneurysms: a molecular epidemiology study. Neurosurgery. 2004;54:1450–60.
8. Meng H, Wang Z, Hoi Y, et al. Complex hemodynamics at the apex of an arterial bifurcation induces vascular remodeling resembling cerebral aneurysm initiation. Stroke. 2007;38:1924–31.
9. Skirgaudas M, Awad IA, Kim J, et al. Expression of angiogenesis factors and selected vascular wall matrix proteins in intracranial saccular aneurysms. Neurosurgery. 1996;39:537–47.
10. Xiang J, Tutino VM, Snyder KV, et al. CFD: computational fluid dynamics or confounding factor dissemination? The role of hemodynamics in intracranial aneurysm rupture risk assessment. Am J Neuroradiol. 2014;35:1849–57.
11. Wiebers DO, Whisnant JP, Huston J III, et al. Unruptured intracranial aneurysms: natural history, clinical outcome, and risks of surgical and endovascular treatment. Lancet. 2003;362:103–10.
12. Nahed BV, Bydon M, Ozturk AK, et al. Genetics of intracranial aneurysms. Neurosurgery. 2007;60:213–25.
13. Peters DG, Kassam A, St. Jean PL, et al. Functional polymorphism in the matrix metalloproteinase-9 promoter as a potential risk factor for intracranial aneurysm. Stroke. 1999;30:2612–6.
14. Hussain I, Duffis EJ, Gandhi CD, et al. Genome-wide association studies of intracranial aneurysms: an update. Stroke. 2013;44:2670–5.
15. Larsen CC, Astrup J. Rebleeding after aneurysmal subarachnoid hemorrhage: a literature review. World Neurosurg. 2012;79:307–12.
16. Bridinski W, Zhu YQ, Lanzino G, et al. Risk factors for growth of intracranial aneurysms: a systematic review and meta-analysis. AJNR Am J Neuroradiol. 2016;37:615–20.
17. Villablanca JP, Duckwiler GR, Jahan R, et al. Natural history of asymptomatic unruptured cerebral aneurysms evaluated at CT angiography: growth and rupture incidence and correlation with epidemiologic risk factors. Radiology. 2013;269:258–65.
18. Beckes D, Rinkel GJ, Laban KG, et al. Patient- and aneurysm-specific risk factors for intracranial aneurysm growth. A systematic review and meta-analysis. Stroke. 2016;47:951–7.
19. Juvela S, Poussa K, Porras M. Factors affecting formation and growth of intracranial aneurysms: a long-term follow-up study. Stroke. 2001;32:485–91.
20. Morita A, Kirino T, Hashi K, et al. The natural course of unruptured cerebral aneurysms in a Japanese cohort. New Engl J Med. 2012;366:2474–82.
21. Wermer MJ, van der Schaaf IC, Algra A, et al. Risk of rupture of unruptured intracranial aneurysms in relation to patient and aneurysm characteristics: an updated meta-analysis. Stroke. 2007;38:1404–10.
22. Guo LM, Zhou HY, Xu JW, et al. Risk factors related to aneurysmal rebleeding. World Neurosurg. 2011;76:292–8.
23. Tanno Y, Homma M, Oinuma M, et al. Rebleeding from ruptured intracranial aneurysms in north Eastern Province of Japan. A cooperative study. J Neurol Sci. 2007;258:11–6.
24. Aoyagi N, Hayakawa I. Study on early re-rupture of intracranial aneurysms. Acta Neurochir. 1996;138:12–8.
25. van Asch CJ, van der Schaaf IC, Rinkel GJ. Acute hydrocephalus and cerebral perfusion after aneurysmal subarachnoid hemorrhage. AJNR Am J Neuroradiol. 2010;31:67–70.
26. Chen S, Luo J, Reis C, et al. Hydrocephalus after subarachnoid hemorrhage: pathophysiology, diagnosis, and treatment. Biomed Res Int. 2017;2017:8584753.
27. Wilson CD, Safavi-Abbasi S, Sun H, et al. Meta-analysis and systematic review of risk factors for shunt dependency after aneurysmal subarachnoid hemorrhage. J Neurosurg. 2017;126:586–95.
28. Yolas C, Ozdemir NG, Kanat A, et al. Uncovering a new cause of obstructive hydrocephalus following subarachnoid hemorrhage: choroidal artery vasospasm-related ependymal cell degeneration and aqueductal stenosis-first experimental study. World Neurosurg. 2016;90:484–91.
29. Foreman B. The pathophysiology of delayed cerebral ischemia. J Clin Neurophysiol. 2016;33:174–82.
30. Kanat A, Turkmenoglu O, Aydin MD, et al. Toward changing of the pathophysiologic basis of acute hydrocephalus after subarachnoid hemorrhage: a preliminary experimental study. World Neurosurg. 2013;34:390–5.
31. Vergouwen MD, Vermeulen M, van Gijn J, et al. Definition of delayed cerebral ischemia after aneurysmal subarachnoid hemorrhage as an outcome event in clinical trials and observational studies:

proposal of a multidisciplinary research group. Stroke. 2010;41:2391–5.
32. Zheng VZ, Wong GK. Neuroinflammation responses after subarachnoid hemorrhage: a review. J Clin Neurosci. 2017;42:7–11.
33. Ecker A, Riemenschneider PA. Arteriographic demonstration of spasm of the intracranial arteries, with special reference to saccular arterial aneurysms. J Neurosurg. 1951;8:660–7.
34. Fisher CM, Kistler JP, Davis JM. Relation of cerebral vasospasm to subarachnoid hemorrhage visualized by computerized tomographic scanning. Neurosurgery. 1980;6:1–9.
35. Dhar R, Diringer MN. The burden of the systemic inflammatory response predicts vasospasm and outcome after subarachnoid hemorrhage. Neurocrit Care. 2008;8:404–12.
36. Dreier JP, Woitzik J, Fabricius M, et al. Delayed ischaemic neurological deficits after subarachnoid haemorrhage are associated with clusters of spreading depolarizations. Brain. 2006;129:3224–37.
37. Dreier JP, Major S, Manning A, et al. Cortical spreading ischaemia is a novel process involved in ischaemic damage in patients with aneurysmal subarachnoid haemorrhage. Brain. 2009;132:1866–81.
38. Friedman JA, Pichelmann MA, Piepgras DG, et al. Pulmonary complications of aneurysmal subarachnoid hemorrhage. Neurosurgery. 2003;52:1025–31.
39. Kerro A, Woods T, Chang JJ. Neurogenic stunned myocardium in subarachnoid hemorrhage. J Crit Care. 2017;38:27–34.
40. Yoshimoto Y, Tanaka Y, Hoya K. Acute systemic inflammatory response syndrome in subarachnoid hemorrhage. Stroke. 2001;32:1989–93.
41. Kapadia A, Schweizer TA, Spears J, et al. Nonaneurysmal perimesencephalic subarachnoid hemorrhage: diagnosis, pathophysiology, clinical characteristics, and long-term outcome. World Neurosurg. 2014;82:1131–43.
42. Rouchaud A, Lehman VT, Murad MH, et al. Nonaneurysmal perimesencephalic hemorrhage is associated with deep cerebral venous drainage anomalies: a systematic literature review and meta-analysis. AJNR Am J Neuroradiol. 2016;37:1657–63.
43. Hui F, Tumialán L, Tanaka T, et al. Clinical differences between angiographically negative, diffuse subarachnoid hemorrhage and perimesencephalic subarachnoid hemorrhage. Neurocrit Care. 2009;11:64–70.
44. Kumar S, Goddeau RP Jr, Selim MH, et al. Atraumatic convexal subarachnoid hemorrhage: clinical presentation, imaging patterns, and etiologies. Neurology. 2010;74:893–9.
45. Naidech AM, Rosenberg NF, Maas MB, et al. Predictors of hemorrhage volume and disability after perimesencephalic subarachnoid hemorrhage. Neurology. 2012;78:811–5.
46. Beitzke M, Gattringer T, Enzinger C, et al. Clinical presentation, etiology, and long-term prognosis in patients with nontraumatic convexal subarachnoid hemorrhage. Stroke. 2011;42:3055–60.
47. Boukobza M, Crassard I, Bousser MG, et al. Radiological findings in cerebral venous thrombosis presenting as subarachnoid hemorrhage: a series of 22 cases. Neuroradiology. 2016;58:11–6.
48. Ducros A, Boukobza M, Porcher R, et al. The clinical and radiological spectrum of reversible cerebral vasoconstriction syndrome. A prospective series of 67 patients. Brain. 2007;130:3091–101.
49. Matsumaru Y, Yanaka K, Muroi A, et al. Significance of a small bulge on the basilar artery in patients with perimesencephalic nonaneurysmal subarachnoid hemorrhage: report of two cases. J Neurosurg. 2003;98:426–9.
50. Park SQ, Bae HG, Yoon SM, et al. Morphological characteristics of the Thalamoperforating arteries. J Korean Neurosurg Soc. 2010;47:36–41.
51. Takeda S, Yamazaki K, Miyakawa T, et al. Cerebral amyloid angiopathy initially occurs in the meningeal vessels. Neuropathology. 2017;37:502–8.
52. Etminan N, Dreier R, Buchholz BA, et al. Age of collagen in intracranial saccular aneurysms. Stroke. 2014;45:1757–63.

Pathophysiology of Arteriovenous Anomaly-Related Hemorrhage

5

Jae H. Choi and John Pile-Spellman

Brain arteriovenous malformations (AVMs) and dural arteriovenous fistulas (DAVFs, sometimes referred to as dural AVM) belong to the group of intracranial vascular malformations (IVMs). Although uncommon, they are important causes of intracranial hemorrhage [1–3]. Brain AVMs are the most frequent IVMs, whereas DAVFs are the least frequent.

The detection rates from population-based studies for brain AVMs range between 1.1/100,000 person-years (Olmsted County, Minnesota, USA) [2] and 1.34/100,000 person-years (NY Islands, NY, USA) [4]. Brain AVMs may present with hemorrhage, most commonly in the third and fourth decade of life with equal distribution between both sexes (incidence rate of 0.51/100,000 person-years in the NY Islands and 0.7/100,000 person-years in Olmsted County). A pooled patient-level meta-analysis over more than 6000 patient-years of follow-up revealed an average annual hemorrhage rate of 2.3% (95% confidence interval (CI) 2.0–2.7%) in patients with brain AVMs [5]. The only randomized controlled trial comparing the outcome in patients with unruptured brain AVMs (all deemed treatable with invasive means) following medical therapy versus eradication therapy found a bleeding rate of 5.6% in the medical group over 33 months of follow-up (A Randomized trial of Unruptured Brain Arteriovenous Malformations, ARUBA) [6].

DAVFs make up 6–15% of IVMs with age- and gender-adjusted detection rates of 0.15 to 0.43/100,000/year (Olmsted County) [2] and a crude detection rate of 0.16/100,000/year (95% CI, 0.08–0.27) in a Scottish population [1]. Hospital-based cohort studies found annual hemorrhage rates of 4.5–35% with no clear preference for either gender owing the large variability to significant selection bias [7–10]. DAVFs typically present in the fifth and sixth decade of life.

AVMs and DAVFs are characterized by direct connections between the artery and vein, lacking capillaries and often times smaller arterioles and venules [3, 11]. The angioarchitecture may be complex in a brain AVM, consisting of (1) multiple feeding arteries usually from branches of intracerebral vessels; (2) a tangled conglomerate of abnormal vessels, the nidus, located in the brain parenchyma or cortex; and (3) draining veins. DAVFs may consist of multiple AV connections, so-called shunts or fistulas [12, 13].

J. H. Choi (✉)
Center for Unruptured Brain Aneurysms, Neurological Surgery, P.C, Lake Success, NY, USA

Department of Neurology, State University of New York, Downstate Medical Center, Brooklyn, NY, USA

Hybernia Medical, LLC, Uniondale, NY, USA

J. Pile-Spellman
Center for Unruptured Brain Aneurysms, Neurological Surgery, P.C, Lake Success, NY, USA

Hybernia Medical, LLC, Uniondale, NY, USA

S.-H. Lee (ed.), *Stroke Revisited: Hemorrhagic Stroke*, Stroke Revisited,
https://doi.org/10.1007/978-981-10-1427-7_5

However, DAVFs typically located along the dura do not form a nidus, receive their blood supply usually from meningeal artery branches, and drain directly or via cortical and leptomeningeal veins into the venous sinuses. Aneurysms may be found along the feeding arteries and within the nidus [14, 15].

AVMs are considered congenital anomalies and may evolve over time. Some genetic disorders, such as hereditary hemorrhagic telangiectasia, are associated with the occurrence of brain AVMs. Most DAVFs are probably idiopathic. However, their occurrence has been associated with preceding trauma, venous thrombosis, and venous stenosis. The clinical outcome following rupture of an AVM or DAVF is usually more benign compared to the outcome following aneurysmal subarachnoid hemorrhage or primary intracerebral hemorrhage [16–18]. However, any IVM-related bleeding event carries a certain risk of mortality and morbidity which has been found to depend on various clinical and anatomical factors.

The present chapter attempts to review clinical and anatomical factors, as well as physiological and molecular mechanisms, that are related to hemorrhage from brain AVMs and DAVFs. Conceptual diagrams of pathophysiology of AVM-related hemorrhages and DAVF-related hemorrhages are described in Fig. 5.1.

5.1 Pathophysiology of Arteriovenous Malformation-Related Hemorrhage

Brain AVMs consist of three distinct anatomical parts [3, 11, 19]. First, there are arterial feeders that may arise from any of the intracranial vessels. AVM-feeding arteries may follow on to nurture the brain tissue after contributing to the AVM's blood supply as en passage vessels. Second, a complex tangled bundle of abnormal vessels makes up the nidus that may be located in any part of the brain parenchyma. A supratentorial location of the lesion is most common. However, these abnormal vessels, lacking capillaries, are not part of neurovascular units and thus do not actively contribute to tissue metabolism. The perinidal hemodynamic and metabolic physiology may be complex as there is evidence for functional reorganization, metabolic redistribution, and displacement of adjacent tissue which may result in non-hemorrhagic focal neurological deficits [20–23]. The absence of critical brain tissue within the lesion may help explain the relatively benign clinical outcome following AVM bleed compared to the consequences often seen after intracerebral hemorrhage [6, 16, 17, 24, 25]. The nidus may connect to the ventricular system and lead to ventricular hemorrhage in case of a rupture. Finally, blood from the nidus may drain into superficial or deep cerebral veins or both. Aneurysms may be associated with the AVM and found along feeding arteries (flow-related aneurysms) and within the nidus (intranidal aneurysms) [14, 15]. The hemodynamic pattern of an AVM is characterized by low-resistance and either high-flow or low-flow shunt [26].

The source of AVM-related hemorrhages may be located in any of the three anatomical parts [16, 27, 28]. However, hemorrhage usually originates from parts of the nidus or the draining vein (Figs. 5.2, 5.3, and 5.4). The arterial source is often a flow-related aneurysm (subarachnoid hemorrhage). Brain AVMs are classified using the Spetzler-Martin scale (SMS) with scores ranging from 1 to 5 (Table 5.1; see ref. [19]. The SMS classifies AVMs according to size, eloquent versus non-eloquent location, and venous drainage type. A high SMS score is associated with increased risk for permanent neurological deficit after surgery.

Hemorrhagic presentation is the most important independent risk factor for future AVM-related bleeds: hazard ratio (HR) of 5.38 (95% CI 2.64–10.96), the Columbia AVM database (C-AVM) [29]; HR 3.86 (95% CI 2.42–6.14), Multicenter AVM Research Study (MARS) with pooled 4-cohort patient-level meta-analysis [5]; and HR 3.2 (95% CI 2.1–4.3), literature review and meta-analysis (Lit-Meta) [30]. This is not difficult to comprehend, as a hemorrhagic event may be an indication for a structural or hemodynamic instability of the lesion. Thus, early eradication therapy

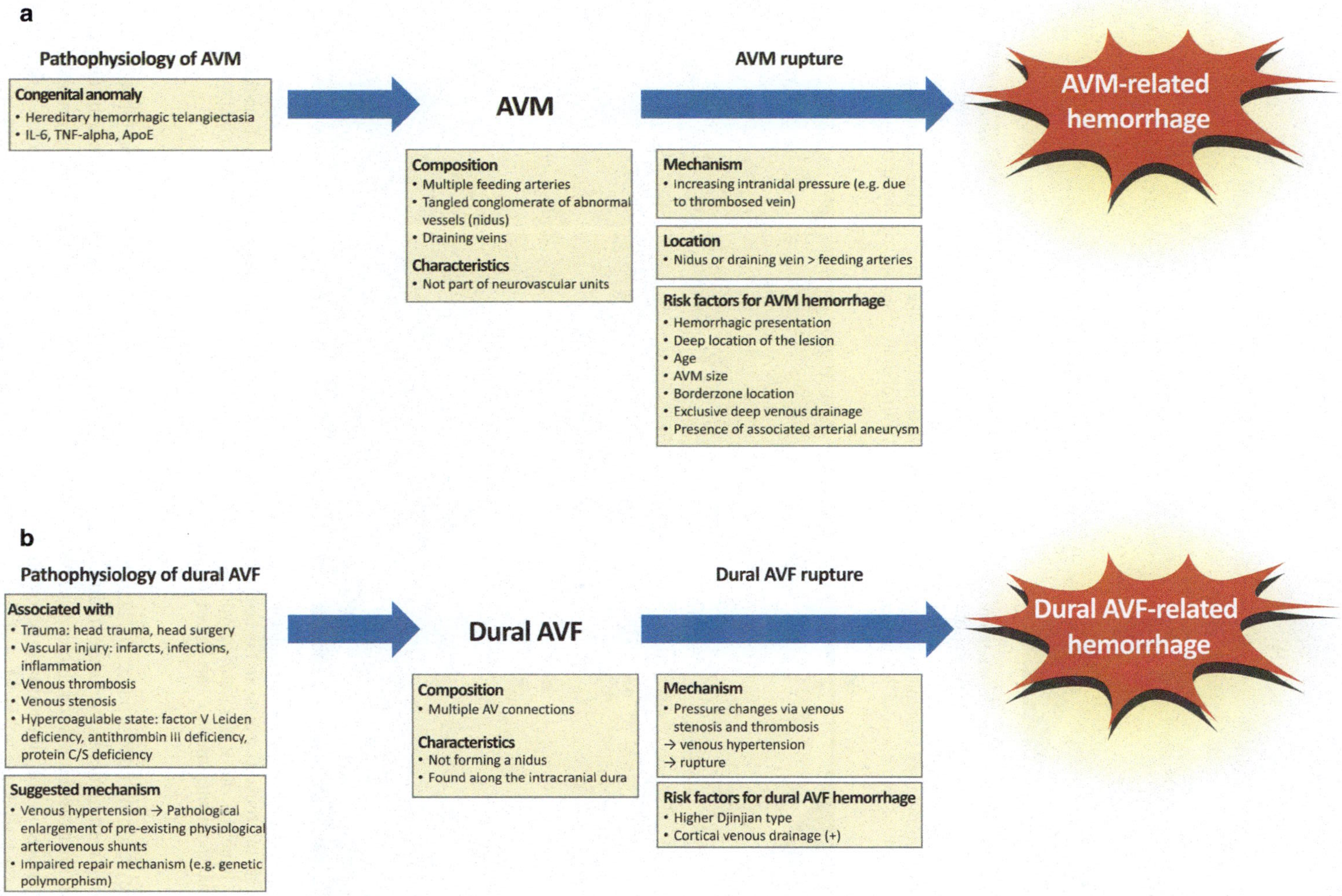

Fig. 5.1 (**a**) Pathophysiology of arteriovenous malformation (AVM)-related hemorrhage. (**b**) Pathophysiology of dural arteriovenous fistula (AVF)-related hemorrhage

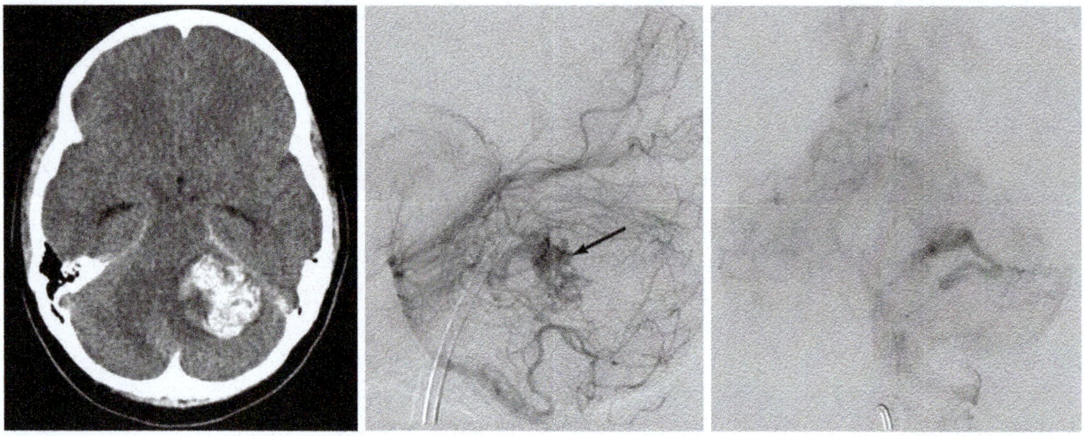

Fig. 5.2 CASE 1. Infratentorial brain AVM with presumed nidal bleed (left) in a 16-year-old girl. The patient awoke early morning with a sharp pain in the back of her head which progressed over the next couple of hours with development of numbness of her lower lip and tongue, later followed by development of visual disturbance and finally, becoming obtunded. Left vertebral artery injection (middle) showing AVM (black arrow) fed by the posterior inferior cerebellar artery and the superior cerebellar artery with drainage into the superior petrosal veins (right)

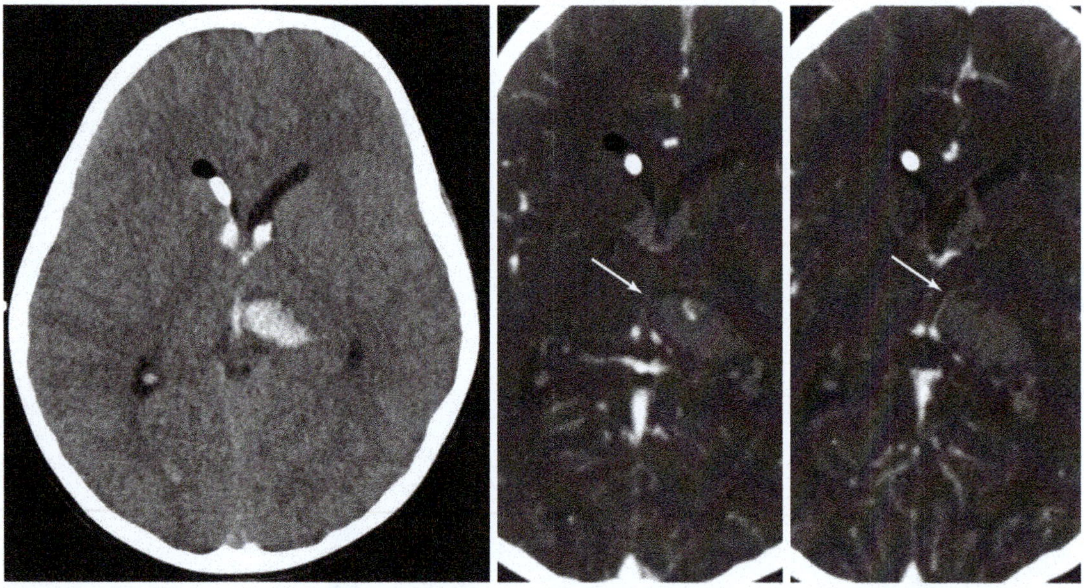

Fig. 5.3 CASE 2. Ruptured left thalamic brain AVM in a 6½ years old found comatose in his bed in the morning (left). Intubated, he was localizing with his left arm. External ventricular drainage was placed for hydrocephalus. CT angiogram shows a thin area of curve linear enhancement in the anterior aspect of the thalamus representing a small AVM (white arrow; middle/right)

is the recommended course of action in AVM patients with hemorrhagic presentation [31].

Another often cited risk factor for AVM-related hemorrhage is deep location of the lesion: HR 3.25 (95% CI 1.30–8.16), C-AVM, and HR 2.4 (95% CI 1.4–3.4), Lit-Meta. This may be related to the fact that deep lesions usually drain into the deep cerebral veins. Hereby, exclusively deep drainage patterns have been found to be independent risk factors for future hemorrhage: HR 2.39 (95% CI 1.01–5.67),

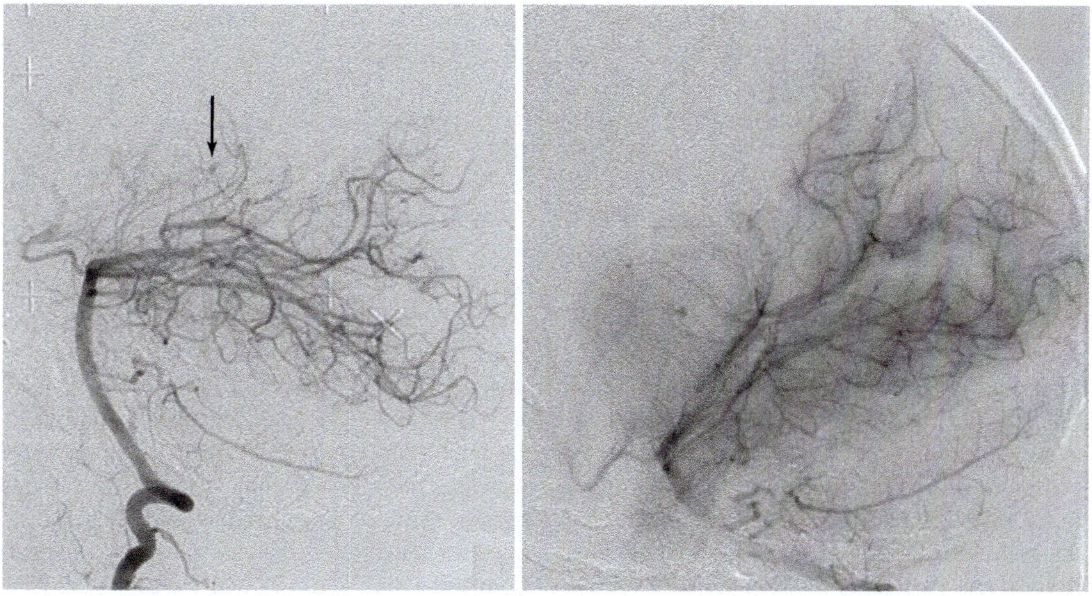

Fig. 5.4 CASE 2. Ruptured left thalamic brain AVM. Left vertebral artery injection shows tiny arteriovenous malformation (black arrow) in the thalamus (left). AVM after partial obliteration (right). Patient underwent Gamma Knife radiosurgery with total obliteration of the lesion

Table 5.1 The Spetzler-Martin brain arteriovenous malformation (AVM) scale

Characteristic of brain AVM		Points
Size	Small (diameter < 3 cm)	1
	Medium (diameter 3–6 cm)	2
	Large (diameter > 6 cm)	3
Location	Non-eloquent	0
	Eloquent[a]	1
Venous drainage	Superficial only	0
	Any deep	1

High scores (range 1–5) are associated with an elevated risk of permanent neurological deficit after resection surgery. Reproduced by permission of *Journal of Neurosurgery* [19]

[a]Language, visual cortex, sensorimotor, basal ganglia, brainstem, cerebellar peduncles or nuclei.

C-AVM, and HR 2.4 (95% CI 1.1–3.8), Lit-Meta. In fact, the presence of both deep location and deep drainage was associated with the highest hemorrhage rates (annual rate of 34.3%) versus deep location (14.8%), deep drainage (11.4%), and absence of these factors (4.5%) (C-AVM). Increasing intranidal pressure is assumed to be one key mechanism for rupture [27, 28, 32]. In principle, this intralesional pressure elevation may be caused by changes in any part of the AVM. For instance, a thrombosed vein causes venous stenosis which in turn leads to venous hypertension aggravated by continuous high arterial inflow [33]. The tipping point then constitutes a hemorrhagic event.

Age has been found to be associated with AVM hemorrhage: HR 1.05 per year (95% CI 1.03–1.08), C-AVM, and HR 1.34 per decade (95% CI 1.17–1.53), MARS. This may be related to a common aging process with decreasing capacity for and failure of vascular repair and hemodynamic compensation.

The risk for future AVM hemorrhage following an initial presentation and diagnostic event is distinguished from the risk of the initial AVM bleed. The average annual hemorrhage rate during follow-up was 2.8% (95% CI 1.7–3.9) in C-AVM and 2.3% (95% CI 2.0–2.7) in MARS. The future bleeding rate for patients presenting with hemorrhage was higher (4.8% (95% CI 3.9–5.9) than the rate for those without initial bleed (1.3% (95% CI 1.0–1.7) in MARS. Similarly,

ARUBA showed a low hemorrhage risk in patients with unruptured brain AVMs with 5.6% over a 33-month follow-up period [6]. The risk factors for initial AVM bleed were found to include AVM size (OR 0.97 (95% CI 0.96–0.98), deep brain location (OR 2.14 (95% CI 1.09–4.22), borderzone location (OR 0.40 (95% CI 0.26–0.60), exclusive deep venous drainage (OR 1.84 (95% CI 1.11–3.07), and presence of associated arterial aneurysms (OR 2.70 (95% CI 1.72–4.24) in C-AVM.

Brain AVMs are rare congenital conditions [34, 35]. This makes epidemiological studies and investigations of the natural history of the disease extremely difficult. In addition, the risk for hemorrhagic events commonly triages the patient into the pathway of eradication therapy. Thus, most studies are hampered at least by referral and selection bias. ARUBA is the only randomized controlled trial to investigate the nature of the disease before rupture and to compare this with the clinical course following early invasive treatment. The results show an early and sustained improved outcome in patients who do not undergo invasive treatment compared to those who do.

Molecular mechanisms involved in the pathogenesis of brain AVMs include angiogenetic and inflammatory pathways [36]. The etiology of brain AVMs remains unknown. However, knowledge gained from studies of genetic diseases that manifest in the occurrence of AVMs, such as hereditary hemorrhagic telangiectasia (HHT), an autosomal dominant disorder, gives insight into potential mechanisms of morphological change and growth of the AVM that may lead to clinical events, such as hemorrhage [37]. HHT is also known as Rendu-Osler-Weber syndrome. Known gene mutations code for endoglin (ENG, HHT1) and activin receptor-like kinase 1 (ALK1, HHT2) [38, 39]. ENG and ALK1 are part of the TGF-beta receptor complex (transforming growth factor beta) and are located on surfaces of cells, such as white cells and endothelial cells. TGF-beta is a cytokine that induces cell proliferation, differentiation, and cell activation. Polymorphism in genes involved in inflammation and atherosclerosis has been identified as candidates involved in the evolution of AVMs. Affected genes include IL-6, TNF-alpha, and ApoE [40–42].

5.2 Pathophysiology of Dural Arteriovenous Fistula-Related Hemorrhage

DAVFs consist of a single or multiple fistula or shunts, direct connections between the artery and vein [3, 43, 44]. As in AVMs, capillaries are absent. Unlike AVMs, no nidus is found. DAVFs are found along the intracranial dura usually with feeders from dural branches of the external carotid artery or vertebral artery. The internal carotid artery may be involved in carotid-cavernous fistula (CCF) either directly or via its dural branches (indirect CCF). Venous drainage occurs either directly into a venous sinus or via cortical or leptomeningeal veins. DAVF-related hemorrhage may result in parenchymal, subarachnoid, or ventricular bleeds (Figs. 5.5 and 5.6). The risk of hemorrhage varies widely and depends on specific angiographical features. According to angiographical findings, DAVFs are classified using two widely used systems.

The Cognard type classification is a revised adaptation of the Djinjian system (Tables 5.2 and 5.3) [45, 46]. The Djinjian system classifies DAVFs into four types. Type I DAVFs drain directly into a dural sinus. Type II DAVFs drain into the dural sinus with retrograde drainage flow. Type III DAVFs drain into leptomeningeal veins. Type IV DAVFs are like type III with venous ectasia. Cognard modified the Djinjian system by adding the presence of cortical venous drainage or CVD (Cognard Type IIb, IIa + b, III, IV, V).

The Borden- Shucart system is a further simplified classification system for DAVFs (Table 5.4) [47]. Type I DAVFs drain into the dural sinus and have no CVD. Type II DAVFs are like type I with CVD. Type III DAVFs drain into leptomeningeal veins and have CVD.

It has been found that higher-grade DAVFs have an increased risk for hemorrhagic presentation and non-hemorrhagic neurological deficits. In a multicenter pooled analysis of 295 patients with DAVFs (M-Center), patients with Djinjian

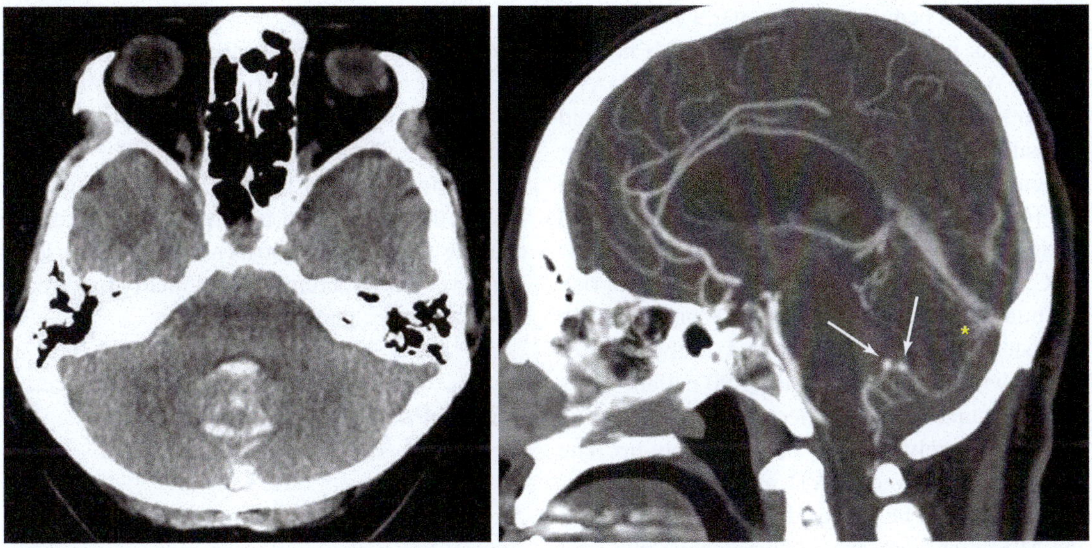

Fig. 5.5 CASE 3. Dural AVM with presumed feeding artery aneurysm bleed in a 72-year-old woman presenting with severe headache, meningism, and somnolence. Initial CT shows subarachnoid and intraventricular blood (left). CT angiogram shows small posterior inferior cerebellar artery aneurysms (white arrows) associated with surrounding hemorrhage and the dural AVM (yellow asterisk) (right)

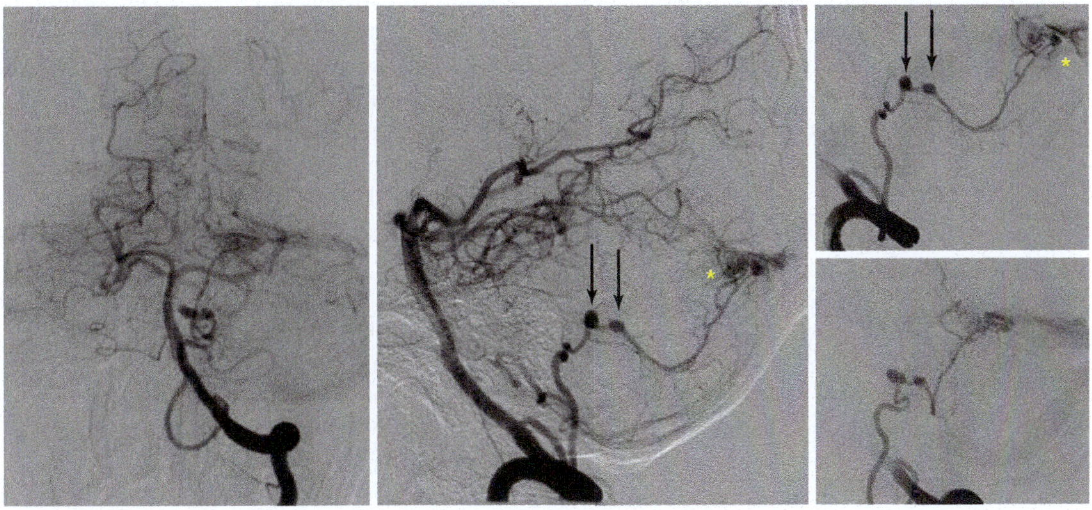

Fig. 5.6 CASE 3. Dural AVM with presumed feeding artery aneurysm bleed. Left vertebral artery injection shows AVM (yellow asterisk) fed by the posterior inferior cerebellar artery and the superior cerebellar artery with drainage into the torcula (left/middle). Two small aneurysms (black arrows) are seen at the inflection point, associated with the previously seen subarachnoid hemorrhage (middle/right)

type II (n = 66), III (n = 74), and IV (n = 29) DAVFs presented with hemorrhage in 6%, 22%, and 28%, respectively [18]. The annual bleeding rates during follow-up (177 lesion-years) were 3.4%, 4.0%, and 9.1% for types II, III, and IV, respectively. None of the patients with Djinjian type I (n = 126) DAVF bled. Furthermore, the study found that hemorrhagic presentation (HR 17.67 (95% CI 2.99–117)) and leptomeningeal drainage (HR 10.39 (95% CI 1.11–1384) were predictors of future hemorrhage. In fact, patients with asymptomatic Djinjian type II-IV DAVFs had an annual hemorrhage rate of 2.9% vs. 46.2% in patients who initially presented with hemorrhage. A single-center study (n = 85 DAVF patients with cortical venous drainage) found annual hemorrhage rates of 7.4% and 1.5% for patients with hemorrhagic presentation and without [48]. Only one patient with hemorrhage died during the study period (58.5 patient-years).

CVD has been considered to increase the risk of future hemorrhage. In 20 DAVF patients with persistent CVD 7 suffered a bleed (of those 3 presented with hemorrhage) during 90 patient-years of follow-up [49]. Ten patients (50%) either died or were severely disabled during follow-up. The relationship between CVD and risk of hemorrhage may also be reflected in the findings from the M-Center study where hemorrhage risk rose with increasing Djinjian type DAVFs.

Apart from drainage site and direction, the location of the lesion has been associated with hemorrhage risk. In the M-Center study, 78% and 75% of Djinjian type III and IV DAVFs were located in the tentorium or cerebral convexity whereas only 5% and 3% of type I and II were. In contrast, type I and II DAVFs were located mostly in the transverse/sigmoid sinus and cavernous sinus (76% and 80%). However, the presence of CVD may influence the risk of hemorrhage independently from the location as only 30% of the 10 patients who died or were severely disabled had DAVFs with tentorial location [9].

The final pathway leading to hemorrhage may be like that considered for brain AVMs. Pressure changes via venous stenosis and thrombosis leading to venous hypertension and finally rupture are a potential mechanism [49].

Table 5.2 The Djinjian classification for dural arteriovenous fistula (DAVF) [46]

Type	Drainage site	Drainage flow	Venous ectasia
I	Dural sinus	Antegrade	
II	Dural sinus	Retrograde	
III	Leptomeningeal vein		No
IV	Leptomeningeal vein		Yes

5.3 Pathogenesis of Arteriovenous Fistula

Although most DAVFs are considered idiopathic, associations with trauma, thrombosis, or atherosclerosis are widely accepted [3, 44, 50]. In conjunction with thrombosis, the presence of hypercoagulable states has been reported, such as factor V Leiden, antithrombin III deficiency, and protein C/S deficiencies [50–52]. Preceding traumatic events may include head trauma and head surgery but also vascular injury mechanisms from infarcts, infections, and inflammation [36, 53–55].

Thrombosis of a cerebral sinus vein or leptomeningeal veins may lead to pressure elevation proximal to the obstruction (venous hypertension) and result in pathological enlargement of

Table 5.4 The Borden-Shucart classification for dural arteriovenous fistula (DAVF) [47]

Type	Drainage site	CVD
I	Dural sinus	No
II	Dural sinus	Yes
III	Leptomeningeal vein	Yes

CVD cortical venous drainage.

Table 5.3 The Cognard classification for dural arteriovenous fistula (DAVF) [45]

Type	Drainage site	Drainage flow	CVD	Venous ectasia
I	Dural sinus	Antegrade	No	
IIa	Dural sinus	Retrograde	Yes	
IIb	Dural sinus	Antegrade	Yes	
IIa + b	Dural sinus	Retrograde	Yes	
III	Leptomeningeal vein		Yes	No
IV	Leptomeningeal vein		Yes	Yes
V	Leptomeningeal vein	Spinal perimed. vein*	Yes	

CVD cortical venous drainage.
*spinal perimedullary vein.

pre-existing physiological arteriovenous shunts. Furthermore, local pressure and flow changes may promote neoangiogenetic mechanisms leading to development of arteriovenous shunts [56]. Finally, if biological repair mechanisms are affected, e.g., due to genetic polymorphism, vascular injury may follow a pathologic response-to-injury pathway, leading to impaired or incomplete repair with increased odds for the formation of intracranial vascular malformations [36].

References

1. Al-Shahi R, Bhattacharya JJ, Currie DG, et al. Population-based detection of intracranial vascular malformations in adults; the Scottish intracranial vascular malformation study (SIVMS). Stroke. 2003;34:1163–9.
2. Brown RD, Wiebers DO, Torner JC, et al. Frequency of intracranial hemorrhage as a presenting symptom and subtype analysis: a population-based study of intracranial vascular malformations in Olmsted County, Minnesota. J Neurosurg. 1996;85:29–32.
3. Stapf C, Mohr JP, Hartmann A, et al. Arteriovenous malformations and other vascular anomalies. In: Mohr JP, editor. Stroke: pathophysiology, diagnosis, and management, 5th edn. Philadelphia: Elsevier; 2011. p. 616–42.
4. Stapf C, Mast H, Sciacca RR, et al. The New York Islands AVM study design, study progress, and initial results. Stroke. 2003;34:29–33.
5. Kim H, Al-Shahi Salman R, McCulloch CE, et al. Untreated brain arteriovenous malformation patient-level meta-analysis of hemorrhage predictors. Neurology. 2014;83:590–7.
6. Mohr JP, Parides MK, Stapf C, et al. Medical management with or without interventional therapy for unruptured brain arteriovenous malformations (ARUBA): a multicentre, non-blinded, randomised trial. Lancet. 2014;9917:614–21.
7. Davies MA, Ter Brugge K, Willinsky R, et al. The natural history and management of intracranial dural arteriovenous fistulae. Part 2: aggressive lesions. Interv Neuroradiol. 1997;3:303–11.
8. Shin NY, Kwon YS, Ha SY, et al. Venous angioarchitectural features of intracranial dural arteriovenous shunt and its relation to the clinical course. Neuroradiology. 2013;55:1119–27.
9. van Dijk JM, terBrugge KG, Willinsky RA, et al. Clinical course of cranial dural arteriovenous fistulas with long-term persistent cortical venous reflux. Stroke. 2002;33:1233–6.
10. Newton TH, Cronqvist S. Involvement of dural arteries in intracranial arteriovenous malformations. Radiology. 1969;93:1071–8.
11. Choi JH, Mohr JP. Brain arteriovenous malformations in adults. Lancet Neurol. 2005;4:299–308.
12. Borden JA, Wu JK, Shucart WA. A proposed classification for spinal and cranial dural arteriovenous malformations and implications for treatment. J Neurosurg. 1995;82:166–79.
13. Brown RD, Flemming KD, Meyer FB, et al. Natural history, evaluation, and management of intracranial vascular malformations. Mayo Clin Proc. 2005;80:269–81.
14. Stapf C, Mohr JP, Pile-Spellman J, et al. Concurrent arterial aneurysms in brain arteriovenous malformations with haemorrhagic presentation. J Neurol Neurosurg Psychiatry. 2002;73:294–8.
15. Gross BA, Ropper AE, Du R. Cerebral dural arteriovenous fistulas and aneurysms. Neurosurg Focus. 2012;32:E2.
16. Choi JH, Mast H, Sciacca RR, et al. Clinical outcome after first and recurrent hemorrhage in patients with untreated brain arteriovenous malformation. Stroke. 2006;37:1243–7.
17. van Beijnum J, Lovelock CE, Cordonnier C, et al. Outcome after spontaneous and arteriovenous malformation-related intracerebral haemorrhage: population-based studies. Brain. 2009;132:537–43.
18. Gross BA, Albuquerque FC, McDougall CG, et al. A multi-institutional analysis of the untreated course of cerebral dural arteriovenous fistulas. J Neurosurg. 2017:15:1–6.
19. Spetzler RF, Martin NA. A proposed grading system for arteriovenous malformations. J Neurosurg. 1986;65:476–83.
20. Marshall RS, Hacein-Bey L, Young WL, et al. Functional reorganization induced by endovascular embolization of a cerebral AVM. Hum Brain Mapp. 1996;4:168–73.
21. Meyer B, Schaller C, Frenkel C, et al. Distributions of local oxygen saturation and its response to changes of mean arterial blood pressure in the cerebral cortex adjacent to arteriovenous malformations. Stroke. 1999;30:2623–30.
22. Young WL, Pile-Spellman J, Prohovnik I, et al. Evidence for adaptive autoregulatory displacement in hypotensive cortical territories adjacent to arteriovenous malformations. Neurosurgery. 1994;34:601–10.
23. Choi JH, Mast H, Hartmann A, et al. Clinical and morphological determinants of focal neurological deficits in patients with unruptured brain arteriovenous malformation. J Neurol Sci. 2009;287:126–30.
24. Burchiel KJ, Clarke H, Ojemann GA, et al. Use of stimulation mapping and corticography in the excision of arteriovenous malformations in sensorimotor and language-related neocortex. Neurosurgery. 1989;24:322–7.
25. Alkadhi H, Kollias SS, Crelier GR, et al. Plasticity of the human motor cortex in patients with arteriovenous malformations: a functional MRI study. AJNR. 2000;21:1423–33.

26. Mast H, Mohr JP, Thompson JLP, et al. Transcranial doppler ultrasonography in cerebral arteriovenous malformations. Stroke. 1995;26:1024–7.
27. Marks MP, Lane B, Steinberg GK, et al. Hemorrhage in intracerebral arteriovenous malformations: angiographic determinants. Radiology. 1990;176:807–13.
28. Hoang Duong D, Young WL, Vang MC, et al. Feeding artery pressure and venous drainage pattern are primary determinants of hemorrhage from cerebral arteriovenous malformations. Stroke. 1998;29:1167–76.
29. Stapf C, Mast H, Sciacca RR, et al. Predictors of hemorrhage in patients with untreated brain arteriovenous malformation. Neurology. 2006;66:1350–5.
30. Gross BA, Du R. Natural history of cerebral arteriovenous malformations: a meta-analysis. J Neurosurg. 2013;118:437–43.
31. Derdeyn CP, Zipfel GJ, Albuquerque FC, et al. Management of brain arteriovenous malformations. Stroke. 2017;48:e200–24.
32. Miyasaka Y, Yada K, Ohwada T, et al. An analysis of the venous drainage system as a factor in hemorrhage from arteriovenous malformations. J Neurosurg. 1992;76:239–43.
33. Vinuela F, Nombela L, Roach MR, et al. Stenotic and occlusive disease of the venous drainage system of deep brain AVMs. J Neurosurg. 1985;63:180–4.
34. Suh DC, Alvarez H, Bhattacharya JJ, et al. Intracranial hemorrhage within the first two years of life. Acta Neurochir. 2001;143:997–1004.
35. Abdulrauf SI, Malik GM, Awad IA. Spontaneous angiographic obliteration of cerebral arteriovenous malformations. Neurosurgery. 1999;44:280–7.
36. Kim H, Pawlikowska L, Young WL (2011) Genetics and vascular biology of brain vascular malformations. In: Mohr JP (ed) Stroke: Pathophysiology, diagnosis, and management, 5th edn. Elsevier, Philadelphia, 169–186.
37. Abdalla SA, Letarte M. Hereditary haemorrhagic telangiectasia: current views on genetics and mechanisms of disease. J Med Genet. 2006;43:97–110.
38. McAllister KA, Grogg KM, Johnson DW, et al. Endoglin, a TGF-beta binding protein of endothelial cells, is the gene for hereditary haemorrhagic telangiectasia type 1. Nat Genet. 1994;8:345–51.
39. Johnson DW, Berg JN, Baldwin MA, et al. Mutations in the activin receptor-like kinase 1 gene in hereditary haemorrhagic telangiectasia type 2. Nat Genet. 1996;13:189–95.
40. Pawlikowska L, Tran MN, Achrol AS, et al. Polymorphisms in genes involved in inflammatory and angiogenic pathways and the risk of hemorrhagic presentation of brain arteriovenous malformations. Stroke. 2004;35:2294–300.
41. Achrol AS, Pawlikowska L, McCulloch CE et al (2006) Tumor necrosis factor-alpha-238G>A promoter polymorphism is associated with increased risk of new hemorrhage in the natural course of patients with brain arteriovenous malformations. Stroke 37:231–234.
42. Achrol AS, Kim H, Pawlikowska L et al (2007) Association of tumor necrosis factor-alpha-238G>A and Apolipoprotein E2 polymorphisms with intracranial hemorrhage after brain arteriovenous malformation treatment. Neurosurgery 61:731–739.
43. Zipfel GJ, Shah MN, Refal D, et al. Cranial dural arteriovenous fistulas: modification of angiographic classification scales based on new natural history data. Neurosurg Focus. 2009;26:E14.
44. Gandhi D, Chen J, Pearl M, et al. Intracranial dural arteriovenous fistulas: classification, imaging findings, and treatment. AJNR. 2012;33:1007–13.
45. Cognard C, Gobin YP, Pierrot L, et al. Cerebral dural arteriovenous fistulas: clinical and angiographic correlation with a revised classification of venous drainage. Radiology. 1995;194:671–80.
46. Djinjian R, Merland JJ. Meningeal arteriovenous fistulae. In: Djinjian R, editor. Super-selective arteriography of the external carotid artery. New York: Springer; 1978. p. 405–536.
47. Borden JA, Wu JK, Shucart WA. A proposed classification for spinal and cranial dural arteriovenous fistulous malformations and implications for treatment. J Neurosurg. 1995;82:166–79.
48. Soderman M, Pavic L, Edner G, et al. Natural history of dural arteriovenous shunts. Stroke. 2008;39:1735–9.
49. Cognard C, Casasco A, Toevi M, et al. Dural arteriovenous fistulas as a cause of intracranial hypertension due to impairment of cranial venous outflow. J Neurol Neurosurg Psychiatry. 1998;65:308–31.
50. Izumi T, Miyachi S, Hattori K, et al. Thrombophilic abnormalities among patients with cranial dural arteriovenous fistulas. Neurosurgery. 2007;61:262–8.
51. Saito A, Takahashi N, Furuno Y, et al. Multiple isolated sinus dural arteriovenous fistulas associated with antithrombin iii deficiency-case report. Neurol Med Chir. 2008;48:455–9.
52. Safavi-Abbasi S, Di Rocco F, Nakaji P, et al. Thrombophilia due to factor V and factor II mutations and formation of a dural arteriovenous fistula: case report and review of a rare entity. Skull Base. 2008;18:135–43.
53. Chung SJ, Kim JS, Kim JC, et al. Intracranial dural arteriovenous fistulas: analysis of 60 patients. Cerebrovasc Dis. 2002;13:79–88.
54. Cooper CJ, Said S, Nunez A, et al. Dural arteriovenous fistula discovered in patient presenting with recent head trauma. Am J Case Rep. 2013;14:444–8.
55. Nabors MW, Azzam CJ, Albanna FJ, et al. Delayed postoperative dural arteriovenous malformations: report of two cases. J Neurosurg. 1987;66:768–72.
56. Kojima T, Miyachi S, Sahara Y, et al. The relationship between venous hypertension and expression of vascular endothelial growth factor: hemodynamic and immunohistochemical examinations in a rat venous hypertension model. Surg Neurol. 2007;68:277–84.

Pathophysiology of Moyamoya Disease

6

Seung-Ki Kim, Ji Yeoun Lee, and Kyu-Chang Wang

6.1 Introduction

Moyamoya disease (MMD) is an occlusive cerebrovascular disease that is characterized by idiopathic and progressive stenosis of the distal portion of major intracranial arteries with abnormal basal collaterals ("moyamoya" vessels) [1]. The internal carotid artery (ICA) and its major branches (anterior carotid artery [ACA] and middle cerebral artery [MCA]) are mainly involved, but basilar artery (BA) and posterior cerebral artery (PCA) stenosis is also detected in some patients, especially during follow-up [2]. When the vascular changes are associated with well-recognized conditions, it is called moyamoya syndrome (MMS). As the disease is defined by the radiological morphology of vessels, MMD may not be a homogeneous entity but may instead comprise a heterogeneous group of conditions.

S.-K. Kim (✉) · K.-C. Wang
Department of Neurosurgery, Seoul National University Hospital, Seoul National University College of Medicine, Seoul, South Korea
e-mail: nsthomas@snu.ac.kr

J. Y. Lee
Department of Anatomy, Seoul National University College of Medicine, Seoul, South Korea

Department of Neurosurgery, Seoul National University Hospital, Seoul, South Korea

A diagnosis is made based on symptoms and radiologic evaluation. The vessel morphology and presence of infarction are evaluated using brain magnetic resonance imaging (MRI) and magnetic resonance angiography (MRA) [3, 4]. Transfemoral cerebral angiography is the gold standard modality to confirm the diagnosis. The regional blood flow status of the brain is usually checked with perfusion MRI or single photon emission computed tomography (SPECT).

The prevalence of MMD shows a bimodal age pattern: once in mid-childhood and again during the late 40s [3]. The presentation and treatment policy of pediatric and adult MMD are different. Hemorrhagic presentation is very rare in children, but it is not uncommon in adult patients [5].

The common sites of intracranial hemorrhage are the basal ganglia, thalamus, and near the lateral ventricle wall, so possible role of moyamoya vessels has been suspected. Some reports have shown that in cases with no moyamoya vessel dilatation, other arteries such as anterior choroidal artery or posterior communicating artery supplying the hemorrhage area showed dilatation [6]. According to morphometric evaluation using autopsy specimens, the dilated arteries in MMD seem to have fibrosis and attenuation of the media, with irregular segmentation of the elastic lamina. Under the condition of hemodynamic

S.-H. Lee (ed.), *Stroke Revisited: Hemorrhagic Stroke*, Stroke Revisited,
https://doi.org/10.1007/978-981-10-1427-7_6

stress or aging, the attenuated walls in these dilated arteries may be predisposing factor for microaneurysm formation. The rupture of the microaneurysm is hypothesized to cause bleeding in MMD patients [7].

For pediatric patients, indirect revascularization is the primary treatment of choice, but in adults, it is controversial whether indirect revascularization is equivalent to direct bypass procedures [5, 8–14].

Much work has been done to elucidate the pathophysiology of MMD over the years. Due to the inaccessibility of the involved vessel during surgery, blood, cerebrospinal fluid (CSF), and urine have been used for molecular and genomic analyses. The attempts to establish an animal model of the disease have yet to be successful, but recent technical advances in genomic analysis have shed light on the field. This chapter covers the current knowledge of the pathophysiology of MMD in various aspects: proteins (growth factors and cytokines), cells, autoimmunity, biomechanics, and genes.

6.2 Pathology

Autopsy specimens of the stenotic arteries revealed that the fibrocellular thickening of the intima, an irregular undulation ("waving") of the internal elastic lamina, and attenuation of media are the main histopathological findings of MMD. Smooth muscle cell hyperplasia is typically found in the thickened intima. These smooth muscle cells are considered to be the synthetic type and to migrate from the media [15–17]. In contrast to atherosclerosis, inflammatory cell infiltration and the presence of lipid-laden foamy macrophages are not found in the stenotic vessels of MMD.

The moyamoya vessels, the basal collaterals that are dilated perforating arteries, show fibrin deposits in the wall, fragmented elastic lamina, attenuated media, and the formation of microaneurysm [16, 18].

6.3 Cytokines

As the hallmark of the vessel pathology is the proliferation of smooth muscle cells in the intima of the arteries, the involvement of growth factors has been suspected. In addition, both the formation of basal collaterals during disease progression and the extensive neovascularization that is seen after indirect bypass surgery, which involves the mere relocation of a vascularized tissue on the surface of the brain cortex, imply the potential role of an aberrant "abundance" of angiogenic factors in MMD patients [19]. Hence, one of the earliest studies to investigate the pathophysiology of MMD examined the expression levels of various cytokines that were quantified in the CSF, serum, or tissue of MMD patients.

Increased levels of growth factors such as basic fibroblast growth factor (bFGF), hepatocyte growth factor (HGF), hypoxia-inducing factor-1α (HIF-1α), granulocyte colony-stimulating factor (GCSF), transforming growth factor-β (TGF-β), and vascular endothelial growth factor (VEGF) have been observed in the CSF and serum of MMD patients [20–24].

The cytokines associated with angiogenesis and vascular repair have also been evaluated. Matrix metalloproteinases-9 (MMP-9) was increased, and the tissue inhibitor of metalloproteinase (TIMP1) was decreased in the serum of MMD patients, suggesting a disruption in the balance between the two. The imbalance may cause aberrant vascular smooth muscle cell dynamics, which can lead to MMD [20, 21].

Increased levels of the cellular retinoic acid-binding protein-1 (CRABP-1) were detected in the CSF of MMD patients [23]. CRABP-1 is one of the proteins that mediates the biological activity of retinoic acid (RA) and may provide a link between RA signaling and MMD pathogenesis. As retinoids are known to negatively regulate growth factor-stimulated vascular smooth muscle cell proliferation and differentiation, it can be hypothesized that increases in CRABP-1 may inhibit the RA signaling action, resulting in an increase in vascular smooth muscle cell proliferation [23].

It should be noted that although an abundant amount of data implies an important role for the various cytokines in MMD, there is possibility that the differences in the expression levels of cytokines may actually be a compensatory response to the pathology rather than the cause.

6.4 Circulating Progenitor Cells

Investigating the vessel wall cells (endothelial-lineage or smooth muscle type) of MMD patients may be a direct approach to evaluate the pathogenesis of the disease. However, it is nearly impossible to obtain the cells directly from patients. Fortunately, vascular progenitor cells can be derived from the peripheral blood of patients, thus providing an experimental cell model (Fig. 6.1) [25].

Endothelial progenitor cells (EPCs) have been evaluated extensively in many vascular diseases before MMD because these cells are known to originate from the bone marrow and help maintain the vasculature and blood flow in infarcted areas [26–30]. EPCs are commonly characterized by the expression of the surface proteins CD34, CD133, and vascular endothelial growth factor receptor-2 (VEGFR-2). Some studies also consider CD45 and CD114 to be additional markers for defining EPC [31, 32]. Two studies have reported on the EPC count in the peripheral blood of MMD patients. One study, which included mainly adult patients, showed that MMD patients had more EPCs than the normal controls did [29], whereas another study with pediatric patients demonstrated a decreased number of EPCs in patients [33]. The contradictory results may be due to differences in the patients' age groups or in the markers used to isolate EPCs [34]. Additionally, the number of colony-forming units (CFU) of EPCs was shown to be decreased and that of outgrowth cells was increased in MMD patients; these changes were more profound in those patients with advanced diseases. Further, the tube formation ability was significantly decreased in the late EPCs from MMD patients, suggesting the dysfunction of the EPCs of MMD patients [29, 33]. More direct evidence on the contribution of EPCs in MMD was provided when cells expressing CD34 and VEGFR2 were found in the thickened intima of distal ICA samples collected from MMD patients [35].

The role of EPCs in MMD was further analyzed in a recent study that compared the gene expression profiles of EPCs from MMD patients and normal controls. A downregulation of retinaldehyde dehydrogenase 2 (Raldh2), which is one of the enzymes in the physiological process

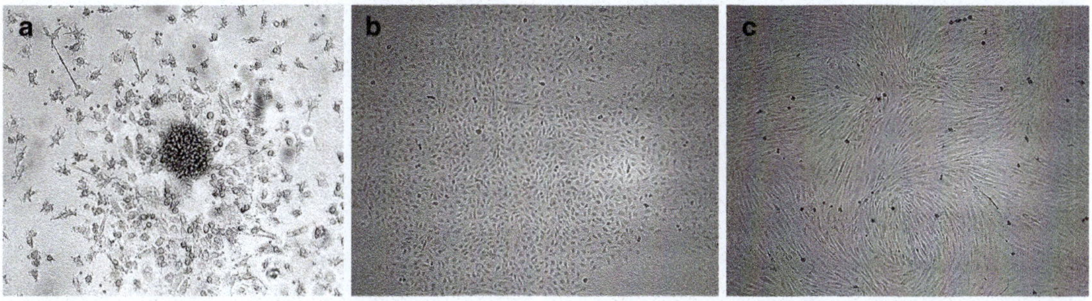

Fig. 6.1 Vascular progenitor cells. (**a**) Early endothelial progenitor cells (EPCs), also called colony-forming units or cell clusters (×200). This cell cluster is composed of a central core of round cells that are surrounded by spindle-shaped cells. (**b**) Late EPCs, also known as endothelial outgrowth cells (×40). The cells are arranged in cobblestone-like formations. (**c**) Smooth muscle progenitor cells (SPCs) (×40). These cells appear elongated and have a typical hill-and-valley appearance. Adapted from Journal of Korean Neurosurgical Society [25]

to convert RA from retinol, was noted. Based on the previous link between RA signaling and MMD, the effect of Raldh2 on the function of EPCs was analyzed. It was shown that decreased levels of Raldh2 in normal EPCs resulted in poor tube formation, similar to EPCs from MMD. Furthermore, the disrupted tube formation capacity was restored by supplementation with exogenous RA in both MMD EPCs and the normal EPCs with downregulated Raldh2 [36].

The possible role of smooth muscle progenitor cells (SPCs) in MMD has recently been evaluated to determine the origin of smooth muscle cell hyperplasia in the thickened intima. SPCs differ from EPCs in the appearance of the outgrowth cells, namely, "hill-and-valley" for the former and "cobblestone" for the latter (Fig. 6.1) [37]. Additionally, SPCs stain positive for smooth muscle-specific markers, such as smooth muscle actin-α, smooth muscle myosin heavy chain (MHC), and calponin [38]. The SPCs from MMD expressed lower levels of platelet-derived growth factor receptor (PDGF)-α, MHC, and calponin than did normal controls. Furthermore, in the tube formation assay, MMD SPCs made more irregular and thick tubes, reminiscent of the pathologic arteries in MMD patients (Fig. 6.2) [39]. These findings suggest that SPCs of MMD patients may have a defect in the cell maturation process that results in dysfunctional vasculogenesis.

A recent study investigated the interaction between the precursors of the two major cellular components' vessel walls. The results showed that EPCs are mostly responsible for the dysfunction of both EPCs and SPCs in MMD and that the enhanced migration of the SPCs to the EPCs is mediated by the release of chemokine (C-C motif) ligand 5 (CCL5) by the EPCs [40].

6.5 Immunologic Factors

The role of immune function in the pathogenesis in MMD has been hypothesized based on its association with immune diseases [41]. Many studies have reported on cases of MMS associated with Graves' disease, an autoimmune disease that causes hyperthyroidism [42]. A recent meta-analysis on the literature has clearly demonstrated a close relationship between thyroid function and MMS [43]. Most of the cases were females, and most of the patients were suffering from active hyperthyroidism when they were diagnosed with MMS. Moreover, recurrence or aggravation of the MMS symptoms was more common in patients with poorly controlled thy-

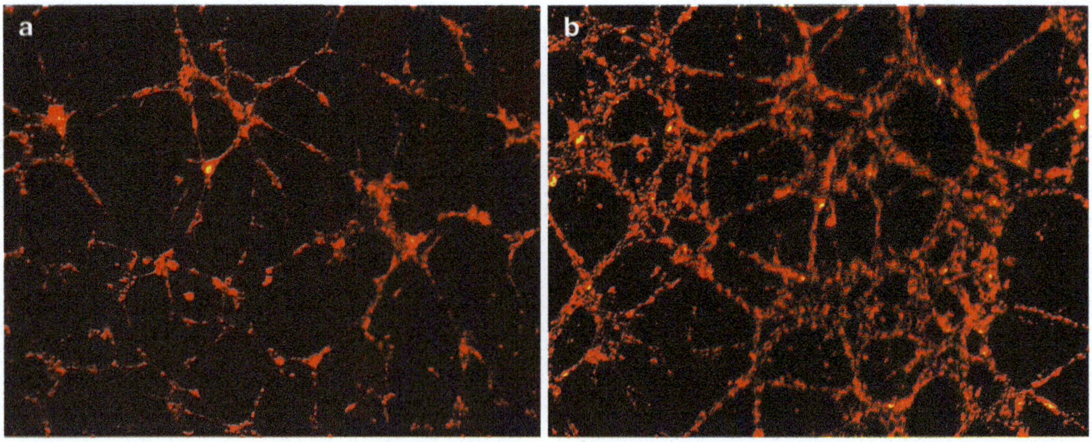

Fig. 6.2 The networks formed by smooth muscle progenitor cells (SPCs). Photomicrographs showing immunofluorescence staining and tubule formation of SPCs on Matrigel. The cells are labeled with red fluorescent dye (PKH26). Compared with the SPCs obtained from a healthy volunteer (**a**), the SPCs obtained from a moyamoya disease patient (**b**) have rather irregularly arranged tubules of varying sizes. In some areas, thickened tubules are noted. Adapted from Journal of Korean Neurosurgical Society [25]

roid function [43]. The fact that abnormal cerebrovascular autoregulation associated with sympathetic nerve excitation has been known to occur in patients with hyperthyroidism suggests a potential mechanism underlying the role of autoimmunity in MMD pathogenesis [44]. However, the possibility that hemodynamic stress caused by the thyrotoxicosis instead of autoimmune dysfunction still stands as the cause of vascular changes in these patients.

Antiphospholipid syndrome (APS) consists of various conditions that are caused by the presence of antiphospholipid (APL) autoantibodies, and systemic lupus erythematosus (SLE) is a representative disease in APS. MMS patients with SLE or increased APL autoantibodies have been reported [45]. Also some SLE patients with "lupus headaches" have been investigated for the possibility of underlying cerebral ischemia and MMS-like changes [46].

Studies to search for more direct evidence of the involvement of immunity in MMD have been performed over the last several years. An increase in the number of thyroid-related autoantibodies (but with normal thyroid function) in MMD patients has been demonstrated in both Asians and Caucasians. The recent reports are different from previous ones, in which the patients showed both hyperthyroidism and increased autoantibodies, thus providing supportive evidence that autoimmunity, instead of thyroid dysfunction, may be the main contributor in MMS [42].

6.6 Biomechanical Factors

The regional predilection of MMD to only involve the distal portion of major intracranial arteries (ICA and BA) is a distinguishing characteristic of the disease [44]. However, most studies on the pathophysiology of MMD have only been able to investigate systemic factors, which does not address the question of why certain arteries are involved. Biomechanical factors, including hemodynamic changes and the properties of the intracranial vasculature, have been hypothesized as one of the etiologies [4]. Many techniques, such as perfusion MRI, SPECT, and transcranial Doppler, have been used to predict the regional blood perfusion and hemodynamic changes in MMD, but the data were only useful for detecting the "resulting" changes in regional cerebral perfusion [47–49].

Computerized mathematical models have been used to analyze the hemodynamics of cerebral arteries [50]. Only one study is available in the literature, and it utilized computational modeling to elucidate the underlying mechanism of the regional specificity of MMD [51]. Based on data obtained for cardiovascular diseases, the authors hypothesized that a chronic, constant state of relatively low shear stress causing turbulent flow to the vessel wall may result in the stimulation and proliferation of smooth muscle cells of the intima of the vessel. After establishing models of ICA and BA with the respective distal branches of ACA/MCA and PCA, the shear stress at various points, including the predisposing areas of stenosis at the bifurcation of distal branches, was determined. The stimulation results revealed that the predisposed areas showed lower values of shear stress than do regions of ICA or BA that are more distant from the bifurcation. Although the computational models have a critical limitation in recapitulating the real in vivo phenomenon, this study is noteworthy because it shows the potential biomechanics to explain the regional predilection of MMD. A retrospective clinical investigation on the delayed involvement of PCA suggested that a smaller angle between PCA and BA is significantly associated with the progressive stenosis of PCA [52]. This is in line with the computational modeling, as a smaller angle between the vessels may result in less shear stress.

6.7 Genetics

A strong predisposition for ethnicity and the existence of familial cases (10–15%) suggest a genetic susceptibility of the disease [34, 44]. Different modes of inheritance have been proposed, including an autosomal dominant pattern with incomplete penetrance in several parent-child cases and an autosomal recessive pattern in sibling pedigrees [53]. Various technical methods have been applied and have provided clues (candidate loci or gene) for the genetic etiology since the late 1990s. The interpretation of the genetic findings was difficult because the results were infrequently replicated in following studies. Additionally, genetic analysis on Caucasians has yet to be successful in identifying associated genes. Recent high-throughput genomic analysis has yielded a gene (*Ring finger 213* [RNF213]) with a strong robust association, but the mechanism of the mutation in the pathogenesis of MMD remains unknown.

Linkage studies using genome-wide markers or previously reported loci have revealed several candidate loci: 3p24-26, 6q25, 8q21-22, 12p12-13, and 17q25 [54–57]. Only the 17q25 locus was replicated, and further genome-wide linkage analysis narrowed the candidate locus to 17q25.3. Many case-controlled association studies were performed and screened genes based on various hypotheses about the pathogenesis of the disease. As the possible contribution of autoimmune dysfunction in MMD has been suggested, the association of human leukocyte antigen (HLA)-related genes was investigated first. A significant association with HLA B51 and HLA B51-DR4 was shown in Japanese patients and HLA B35 in Korean patients [58–60]. In European patients, the HLA DRB1*03, DRB1*13, DRA*02, DRB*08, and DQB1*03 antigens were more frequent in patients than they were in controls [61].

The next set of genes of interest was based on the increase in the amount of growth factors and cytokines in the blood, CSF, urine, or tissues of patients. Some studies found associations with single-nucleotide polymorphisms (SNPs) in PDGFR-β promoter or TGF-β [62]. Additionally, associations with SNPs in genes related to MMPs and their tissue inhibitors have been demonstrated (TIMP2, MMP2, MMP3 genes or their promoters) [22, 63].

In 2011, two groups reported the RNF213 gene located in chromosome 17q25.3 as the strongest susceptibility gene for MMD in East Asian (Japanese and Korean) patients using two different approaches (genome-wide association study [GWAS] or whole-exome sequencing [WES]) [64, 65]. A GWAS detected a variant of the RNF213 (p.R4810K) in 95% of familial MMD patients, with 80% in sporadic cases, and demonstrated that the variant strongly increased the risk to develop MMD, with an odds ratio (OR) greater than 190 [65]. Another study utilizing genome-wide linkage analysis and WES in eight multigenerational families revealed that all of the probands had this variant. The variant was also detected in 1.4–2.4% of normal Asian controls, thus providing a possible explanation for the extreme ethnic gradient in disease prevalence [64]. The potentially strong contribution of the variant was further supported by the fact that patients with homozygous mutations of the p. R4810K variant have an earlier age of onset and more severe phenotypes than do those with heterozygous mutations [66]. Recent studies have also revealed novel variants in RNF213 in a small number of Caucasian and Chinese cases [67].

RNF213 encodes for a cytosolic protein with a really interesting new gene (RING) finger domain and a pair of two ATPase associated with a variety of cellular activities (AAA) positive ATPase modules and is speculated to have ubiquitin ligase activity [68]. The functional consequence of the mutation in RNF213 is under intensive evaluation. In an in vitro functional study, the mutation had no effect on the transcription level or ubiquitin ligase activity of the protein [64]. However, in a more recent study, the vascular endothelial cells derived from induced pluripotent stem cells were compared between normal controls and both MMD patients and RNF213 mutant carriers [69]. The latter group showed decreased angiogenic activity compared with the former. Additional experiments have shown the association of RNF213 with securin, the interferon (IFN)-beta signaling pathway, and PI3 kinase-AKT pathway in endothelial cells [69]. A series of in vivo experiments using genetically engineered animals have been performed. Knockdown of RNF213 in zebrafish resulted in abnormal vascular development, showing irregular wall formation and abnormal sprouting vessels [64]. However, RNF213-deficient mice did not show any anatomical or histopathological evidence of MMD in the brain vasculature under physiological conditions [70]. Another experiment with mice harboring the p.R4810K mutation was not successful in developing MMD under normal conditions [71]. Recently, the environmental setting was added as a crucial component in the experiment by exposing the RNF213-deficient mice to a chronic, ischemic insult. Post-ischemic angiogenesis was found to be enhanced in RNF213-deficient mice in response to chronic hind limb ischemia [72]. Nevertheless, because the role of RNF213 as the causative mutation has not been demonstrated, despite its robustness, the possibility that another causative gene is still to be found should be considered by evaluating the entire genome using whole-genome sequencing.

Investigation of the genes known to be related to other vascular diseases (e.g., coronary artery disease, stroke) or associated diseases in MMS (achalasia) has shown other potential genes. Smooth muscle alpha-actin (ACTA2) is a major component of the contractile apparatus of smooth muscle cells, and mutations of the ACTA2 gene have been known to cause familial thoracic aortic aneurysm and dissections. It was also found to be associated with pseudo-moyamoya angiopathy [73]. Mutations of the guanylate cyclase soluble subunit alpha-3 (GUCY1A3) gene have been found in MMD patients with achalasia. Loss of function mutations of this gene lead to alterations of the nitric oxide pathway in smooth muscle cells, thus supporting the possible pathogenetic mechanism of MMD [74].

Conclusions

MMD is probably caused by a combination of complex etiologies, genetics, and environmental factors. Genetic susceptibility, including RNF213 and many other factors such as the RA pathway, autoimmune process, environmental factors, and hemodynamic stress, may be related to increased levels of growth factors and cytokines. Through mechanisms that are still to be elucidated, the systemic factors and conditions may lead to the proliferation and migration of SMC into the vessel wall, thereby causing thickening of the intima. The low shear stress in the bifurcation regions may lead to the involvement of only the distal ICA and BA in MMD. Establishing an animal model will shed light on integration of the various, independent factors.

References

1. Suzuki J, Takaku A. Cerebrovascular "moyamoya" disease. Disease showing abnormal net-like vessels in base of brain. Arch Neurol. 1969;20:288–99.
2. Lee JY, Choi YH, Cheon JE, et al. Delayed posterior circulation insufficiency in pediatric moyamoya disease. J Neurol. 2014;261:2305–13.
3. Fukui M. Guidelines for the diagnosis and treatment of spontaneous occlusion of the circle of Willis ('moyamoya' disease). Research Committee on Spontaneous Occlusion of the Circle of Willis (Moyamoya Disease) of the Ministry of Health and Welfare, Japan. Clin Neurol Neurosurg. 1997; 99(Suppl 2):S238–240.
4. Lee M, Zaharchuk G, Guzman R, et al. Quantitative hemodynamic studies in moyamoya disease: a review. Neurosurg Focus. 2009;26:E5.
5. Kim SK, Wang KC, Kim IO, et al. Combined encephaloduroarteriosynangiosis and bifrontal encephalogaleo (periosteal) synangiosis in pediatric moyamoya disease. Neurosurgery. 2008;62:1456–64.
6. Morioka M, Hamada JI, Kawano T, et al. Angiographic dilatation and branch extension of the anterior choroidal and posterior communicating arteries are predictors of hemorrhage in adult Moyamoya patients. Stroke. 2002;34:90–5.
7. Yamashita M, Oka K, Tanaka K. Histopathology of the brain vascular network in moyamoya disease. Stroke. 1983;14:50–8.
8. Imaizumi T, Hayashi K, Saito K, et al. Long-term outcomes of pediatric moyamoya disease monitored to adulthood. Pediatr Neurol. 1998;18:321–5.
9. Hirotsune N, Meguro T, Kawada S, et al. Long-term follow-up study of patients with unilateral moyamoya disease. Clin Neurol Neurosurg. 1997;99(Suppl 2):S178–81.
10. Golby AJ, Marks MP, Thompson RC, et al. Direct and combined revascularization in pediatric moyamoya disease. Neurosurgery. 1999;45:50–8.
11. Ozgur BM, Aryan HE, Levy ML. Indirect revascularisation for paediatric moyamoya disease: the EDAMS technique. J Clin Neurosci. 2006;13:105–8.
12. Rashad S, Fujimura M, Niizuma K, et al. Long-term follow-up of pediatric moyamoya disease treated by combined direct-indirect revascularization surgery: single institute experience with surgical and perioperative management. Neurosurg Rev. 2016;39:615–23.
13. Sainte-Rose C, Oliveira R, Puget S, et al. Multiple bur hole surgery for the treatment of moyamoya disease in children. J Neurosurg. 2006;105:437–43.

14. Ueki K, Meyer FB, Mellinger JF. Moyamoya disease: the disorder and surgical treatment. Mayo Clin Proc. 1994;69:749–57.
15. Lin R, Xie Z, Zhang J, et al. Clinical and immunopathological features of Moyamoya disease. PLoS One. 2012;7:e36386.
16. Kuroda S, Houkin K. Moyamoya disease: current concepts and future perspectives. Lancet Neurol. 2008;7:1056–66.
17. Takagi Y, Kikuta K, Nozaki K, et al. Histological features of middle cerebral arteries from patients treated for Moyamoya disease. Neurol Med Chir (Tokyo). 2007;47:1–4.
18. Czabanka M, Pena-Tapia P, Schubert GA, et al. Characterization of cortical microvascularization in adult moyamoya disease. Stroke. 2008;39:1703–9.
19. Kim SJ, Son TO, Kim KH, et al. Neovascularization precedes occlusion in moyamoya disease: angiographic findings in 172 pediatric patients. Eur Neurol. 2014;72:299–305.
20. Fujimura M, Watanabe M, Narisawa A, et al. Increased expression of serum matrix Metalloproteinase-9 in patients with moyamoya disease. Surg Neurol. 2009;72:476–80.
21. Kang HS, Kim JH, Phi JH, et al. Plasma matrix metalloproteinases, cytokines and angiogenic factors in moyamoya disease. J Neurol Neurosurg Ps. 2010;81:673–8.
22. Kang HS, Kim SK, Cho BK, et al. Single nucleotide polymorphisms of tissue inhibitor of metalloproteinase genes in familial moyamoya disease. Neurosurgery. 2006;58:1074–80.
23. Kim SK, Yoo JI, Cho BK, et al. Elevation of CRABP-I in the cerebrospinal fluid of patients with Moyamoya disease. Stroke. 2003;34:2835–41.
24. Park YS, Jeon YJ, Kim HS, et al. The role of VEGF and KDR polymorphisms in moyamoya disease and collateral revascularization. PLoS One. 2012;7:e47158.
25. Kang HS, Wang KC, Kim SK. Circulating vascular progenitor cells in Moyamoya disease. J Korean Neurosurg Soc. 2015;57:428–31.
26. Fadini GP, Agostini C, Avogaro A. Endothelial progenitor cells in cerebrovascular disease. Stroke. 2005;36:1112–3.
27. Fadini GP, Coracina A, Baesso I, et al. Peripheral blood CD34+KDR+ endothelial progenitor cells are determinants of subclinical atherosclerosis in a middle-aged general population. Stroke. 2006;37: 2277–82.
28. Ghani U, Shuaib A, Salam A, et al. Endothelial progenitor cells during cerebrovascular disease. Stroke. 2005;36:151–3.
29. Jung KH, Roh JK. Circulating endothelial progenitor cells in cerebrovascular disease. J Clin Neurol. 2008;4:139–47.
30. Vasa M, Fichtlscherer S, Aicher A, et al. Number and migratory activity of circulating endothelial progenitor cells inversely correlate with risk factors for coronary artery disease. Circ Res. 2001;89:E1–7.
31. Asahara T, Murohara T, Sullivan A, et al. Isolation of putative progenitor endothelial cells for angiogenesis. Science. 1997;275:964–7.
32. Timmermans F, Plum J, Yoder MC, et al. Endothelial progenitor cells: identity defined? J Cell Mol Med. 2009;13:87–102.
33. Kim JH, Jung JH, Phi JH, et al. Decreased level and defective function of circulating endothelial progenitor cells in children with moyamoya disease. J Neurosci Res. 2010;88:510–8.
34. Bersano A, Guey S, Bedini G, et al. Research progresses in understanding the pathophysiology of Moyamoya disease. Cerebrovasc Dis. 2016;41:105–18.
35. Psaltis PJ, Simari RD. Vascular wall progenitor cells in health and disease. Circ Res. 2015;116:1392–412.
36. Lee JY, Moon YJ, Lee HO, et al. Deregulation of Retinaldehyde dehydrogenase 2 leads to defective Angiogenic function of endothelial Colony-forming cells in pediatric Moyamoya disease. Arterioscler Thromb Vasc Biol. 2015;35:1670–7.
37. Simper D, Stalboerger PG, Panetta CJ, et al. Smooth muscle progenitor cells in human blood. Circulation. 2002;106:1199–204.
38. Urbich C, Heeschen C, Aicher A, et al. Relevance of monocytic features for neovascularization capacity of circulating endothelial progenitor cells. Circulation. 2003;108:2511–6.
39. Kang HS, Moon YJ, Kim YY, et al. Smooth-muscle progenitor cells isolated from patients with moyamoya disease: novel experimental cell model. J Neurosurg. 2014;120:415–25.
40. Phi JH, Suzuki N, Moon YJ, et al. Chemokine ligand 5 (CCL5) derived from endothelial Colony-forming cells (ECFCs) mediates recruitment of smooth muscle progenitor cells (SPCs) toward critical vascular locations in Moyamoya disease. PLoS One. 2017;12:e0169714.
41. Phi JH, Wang KC, Lee JY, et al. Moyamoya syndrome: a window of Moyamoya disease. J Korean Neurosurg Soc. 2015;57:408–14.
42. Kim SJ, Heo KG, Shin HY, et al. Association of thyroid autoantibodies with moyamoya-type cerebrovascular disease: a prospective study. Stroke. 2010;41:173–6.
43. Lanterna LA, Galliani S, Brembilla C, et al. Association of moyamoya disease with thyroid autoantibodies and thyroid function. Eur J Neurol. 2017;24:e9.
44. Hu J, Luo J, Chen Q. The susceptibility pathogenesis of Moyamoya disease. World Neurosurg. 2017;101:731–41.
45. Wang Z, Fu Z, Wang J, et al. Moyamoya syndrome with antiphospholipid antibodies: a case report and literature review. Lupus. 2014;23:1204–6.
46. Sfikakis PP, Mitsikostas DD, Manoussakis MN, et al. Headache in systemic lupus erythematosus: a controlled study. Br J Rheumatol. 1998;37:300–3.
47. Kikuta K, Takagi Y, Nozaki K, et al. Asymptomatic microbleeds in moyamoya disease: T2*-weighted gradient-echo magnetic resonance imaging study. J Neurosurg. 2005;102:470–5.

48. Kuroda S, Kashiwazaki D, Ishikawa T, et al. Incidence, locations, and longitudinal course of silent microbleeds in moyamoya disease: a prospective T2*-weighted MRI study. Stroke. 2013;44: 516–8.
49. Qin Y, Ogawa T, Fujii S, et al. High incidence of asymptomatic cerebral microbleeds in patients with hemorrhagic onset-type moyamoya disease: a phase-sensitive MRI study and meta-analysis. Acta Radiol. 2015;56:329–38.
50. Charbel FT, Misra M, Clarke ME, et al. Computer simulation of cerebral blood flow in moyamoya and the results of surgical therapies. Clin Neurol Neurosurg. 1997;99(Suppl 2):S68–73.
51. Seol HJ, Shin DC, Kim YS, et al. Computational analysis of hemodynamics using a two-dimensional model in moyamoya disease. J Neurosurg Pediatr. 2010;5:297–301.
52. Lee JY, Kim SK, Cheon JE, et al. Posterior cerebral artery involvement in moyamoya disease: initial infarction and angle between PCA and basilar artery. Childs Nerv Syst. 2013;29:2263–9.
53. Mineharu Y, Takenaka K, Yamakawa H, et al. Inheritance pattern of familial moyamoya disease: autosomal dominant mode and genomic imprinting. J Neurol Neurosurg Ps. 2006;77:1025–9.
54. Ikeda H, Sasaki T, Yoshimoto T, et al. Mapping of a familial moyamoya disease gene to chromosome 3p24.2-p26. Am J Hum Genet. 1999;64:533–7.
55. Inoue TK, Ikezaki K, Sasazuki T, et al. Linkage analysis of moyamoya disease on chromosome 6. J Child Neurol. 2000;15:179–82.
56. Sakurai K, Horiuchi Y, Ikeda H, et al. A novel susceptibility locus for moyamoya disease on chromosome 8q23. J Hum Genet. 2004;49:278–81.
57. Yamauchi T, Tada M, Houkin K, et al. Linkage of familial moyamoya disease (spontaneous occlusion of the circle of Willis) to chromosome 17q25. Stroke. 2000;31:930–5.
58. Aoyagi M, Ogami K, Matsushima Y, et al. Human leukocyte antigen in patients with moyamoya disease. Stroke. 1995;26:415–7.
59. Han H, Pyo CW, Yoo DS, et al. Associations of Moyamoya patients with HLA class I and class II alleles in the Korean population. J Korean Med Sci. 2003;18:876–80.
60. Inoue TK, Ikezaki K, Sasazuki T, et al. Analysis of class II genes of human leukocyte antigen in patients with moyamoya disease. Clin Neurol Neurosurg. 1997;99(Suppl 2):S234–7.
61. Kraemer M, Horn PA, Roder C, et al. Analysis of human leucocyte antigen genes in Caucasian patients with idiopathic moyamoya angiopathy. Acta Neurochir. 2012;154:445–54.
62. Roder C, Peters V, Kasuya H, et al. Polymorphisms in TGFB1 and PDGFRB are associated with Moyamoya disease in European patients. Acta Neurochir. 2010;152:2153–60.
63. Ye S. Polymorphism in matrix metalloproteinase gene promoters: implication in regulation of gene expression and susceptibility of various diseases. Matrix Biol. 2000;19:623–9.
64. Liu W, Morito D, Takashima S, et al. Identification of RNF213 as a susceptibility gene for moyamoya disease and its possible role in vascular development. PLoS One. 2011;6:e22542.
65. Kamada F, Aoki Y, Narisawa A, et al. A genome-wide association study identifies RNF213 as the first Moyamoya disease gene. J Hum Genet. 2011;56:34–40.
66. Miyatake S, Miyake N, Touho H et al (2012) Homozygous c.14576G>A variant of RNF213 predicts early-onset and severe form of moyamoya disease. Neurology 78:803–810.
67. Cecchi AC, Guo D, Ren Z, et al. RNF213 rare variants in an ethnically diverse population with Moyamoya disease. Stroke. 2014;45:3200–7.
68. Morito D, Nishikawa K, Hoseki J, et al. Moyamoya disease-associated protein mysterin/RNF213 is a novel AAA+ ATPase, which dynamically changes its oligomeric state. Sci Rep. 2014;4:4442.
69. Hitomi T, Habu T, Kobayashi H, et al. Downregulation of Securin by the variant RNF213 R4810K (rs112735431, G>A) reduces angiogenic activity of induced pluripotent stem cell-derived vascular endothelial cells from moyamoya patients. Biochem Biophys Res Commun. 2013;438:13–9.
70. Sonobe S, Fujimura M, Niizuma K, et al. Temporal profile of the vascular anatomy evaluated by 9.4-T magnetic resonance angiography and histopathological analysis in mice lacking RNF213: a susceptibility gene for moyamoya disease. Brain Res. 2014;1552:64–71.
71. Kanoke A, Fujimura M, Niizuma K, et al. Temporal profile of the vascular anatomy evaluated by 9.4-tesla magnetic resonance angiography and histological analysis in mice with the R4859K mutation of RNF213, the susceptibility gene for moyamoya disease. Brain Res. 2015;1624:497–505.
72. Fujimura M, Sonobe S, Nishijima Y, et al. Genetics and biomarkers of Moyamoya disease: significance of RNF213 as a susceptibility gene. J Stroke. 2014;16:65–72.
73. Guo DC, Papke CL, Tran-Fadulu V, et al. Mutations in smooth muscle alpha-actin (ACTA2) cause coronary artery disease, stroke, and Moyamoya disease, along with thoracic aortic disease. Am J Hum Genet. 2009;84:617–27.
74. Wallace S, Guo DC, Regalado E, et al. Disrupted nitric oxide signaling due to GUCY1A3 mutations increases risk for moyamoya disease, achalasia and hypertension. Clin Genet. 2016;90:351–60.

Part II

Diagnosis and Treatment of Hemorrhagic Stroke

Overview of Hemorrhagic Stroke Care in the Emergency Unit

7

Natalie Kreitzer and Daniel Woo

7.1 Introduction

Non-traumatic intracerebral hemorrhage (ICH) is defined as bleeding into the parenchyma of the brain that may extend into the ventricles and, in rare cases, the subarachnoid space [1]. Historically, the morbidity and mortality rate of ICH has been notoriously high; however, recent advances regarding the treatment of blood pressure as well as anticoagulation reversal have led to improved patient outcomes. ICH is the second most common subtype of stroke, following ischemic stroke [2]. Emergency physicians are typically the first physician contact with patients who have an ICH and, as such, can make an impactful difference in the care of these patients. Ongoing and future research is targeted both at preventing hematoma expansion and developing tools for endoscopic hematoma evacuation.

N. Kreitzer
Department of Emergency Medicine and Division of Neurocritical Care, University of Cincinnati, Cincinnati, OH, USA

D. Woo (✉)
Department of Neurology and Rehabilitation Medicine, University of Cincinnati, Cincinnati, OH, USA
e-mail: WOODL@ucmail.uc.edu

7.2 Identification and Triage of Stroke-Like Symptoms in the Emergency Department

7.2.1 Differential Diagnosis

A schematic diagram showing evaluation and management for patients with ICH is described in Fig. 7.1. The classical presenting signs and symptoms of ICH may include headache, vomiting, syncope, altered mental status, or abrupt onset of focal neurologic deficits which might include speech disturbances or weakness on half of the body. Patients with symptoms concerning for ICH have a wide differential diagnosis. Hypoglycemia should be considered in any patient with altered mental status presenting to the ED and finger-stick blood glucose performed immediately. Otherwise, the differential diagnosis should include ischemic stroke, seizure, complicated migraine, intracranial tumors, intracranial infections or encephalitis, and Todd's paralysis. Depending on the location of hemorrhage, size of hemorrhage, intraventricular extension, comorbidities, and time since onset, the presentation may differ from patient to patient in the setting of ICH.

S.-H. Lee (ed.), *Stroke Revisited: Hemorrhagic Stroke*, Stroke Revisited,
https://doi.org/10.1007/978-981-10-1427-7_7

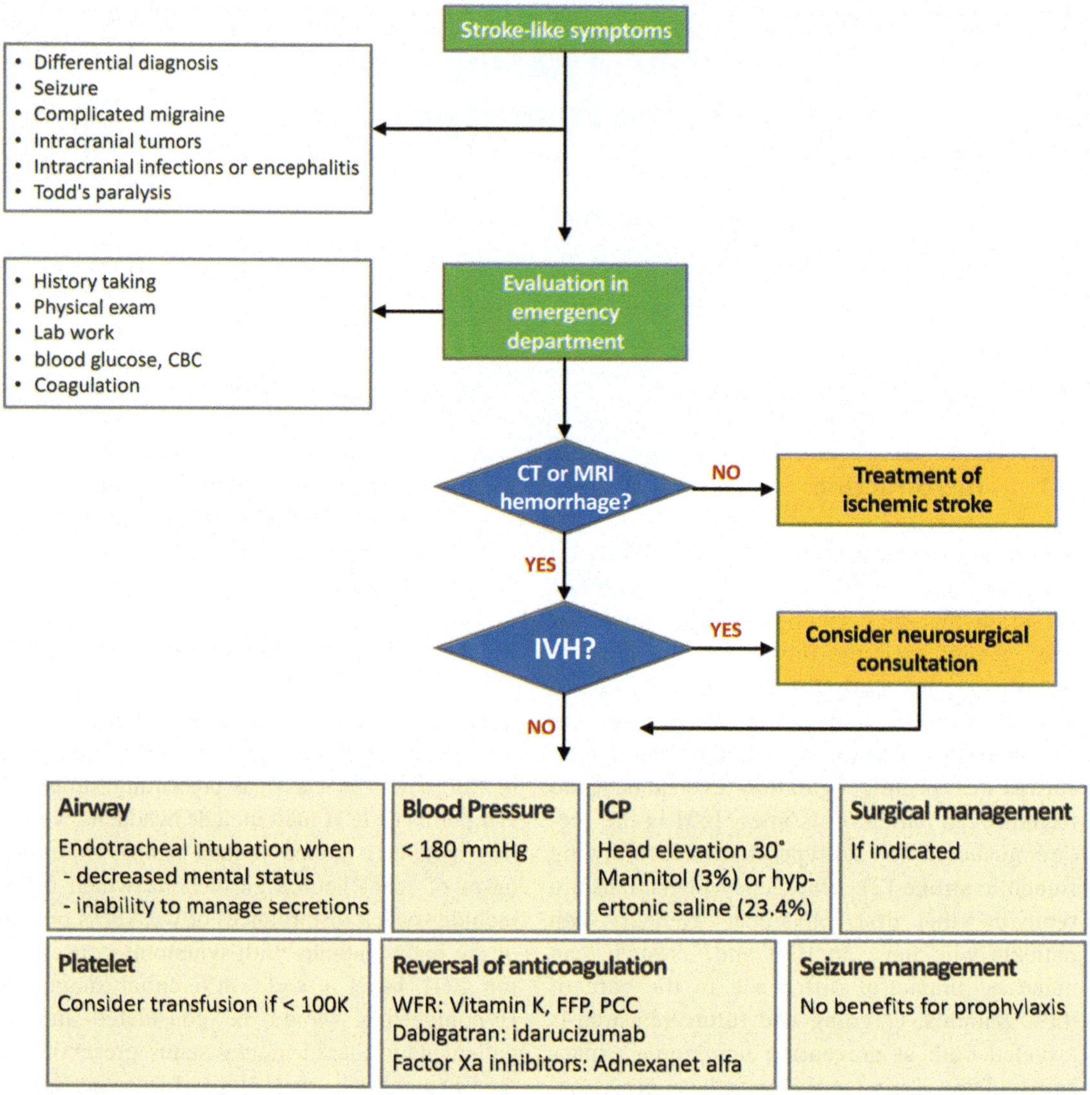

Fig. 7.1 A schematic diagram showing evaluation and management for patients with ICH. *CBC* complete blood count, *IVH* intraventricular hemorrhage, *ICP* intracranial pressure, *WFR* warfarin, *FFP* fresh frozen plasma, *PCC* prothrombin complex concentrate

7.2.2 Emergency Department Evaluation and Workup

The vast majority of patients presenting to the ED with ICH will be undifferentiated, and it will be unknown whether their symptoms are secondary to ischemic or hemorrhagic stroke. As more and more hospital systems are moving toward protocoled rapid triage and imaging of patients with stroke-like symptoms, patients with ICH symptoms may ultimately go directly to the CT scanner for immediate diagnosis of ICH. Given the time-sensitive nature of both ischemic stroke and ICH, with the need for simultaneous blood pressure control and reversal of potential anticoagulation, history and physical should be performed in concert with preparation for imaging and both diagnosis and treatment modalities pursued at the same times as the initial history and physical are performed.

7.2.3 History and Physical Exam

Depending on the patient's neurologic deficits, he or she may not be able to provide much, if any, of his or her medical history. In these instances, it is important to find family members or friends to determine history. The pertinent portions of history should include the last time the patient was without neurologic deficits and medications—especially anticoagulants and antiplatelets. If the patient uses antiplatelets or anticoagulants, it is important to determine the last time these medications were taken. The 2015 American Heart Association (AHA) guidelines also recommend that ED providers determine any vascular risk factors, recent trauma or surgery, alcohol or illicit drug use, past or current seizures, liver disease, cancer, or other hematologic disorders [3]. Additionally, it is beneficial to know if the patient has a known intracranial mass, arteriovenous malformation (AVM), recent ischemic stroke, or other intracranial pathology, as this will help in determining the cause of ICH.

The physical exam should ideally be completed at the same time the history is taken to expedite care. After assessing the patient's respiratory status, mental status, and potential need for intubation prior to imaging, the exam should be focused on the neurologic symptoms. Although an entire neurologic exam consists of level of consciousness, cranial nerve exam, vision, motor, sensory, cerebellar findings, and language, the initial physical exam may be briefer such that a timely diagnosis is made. There is no neurologic exam specific to ICH. Even though the Glasgow Coma Scale was developed for the trauma setting, it is often utilized in the emergency department for ICH, given that it is so widely recognized among healthcare providers. Although the National Institutes of Health Stroke Scale (NIHSS) was originally developed for use in ischemic stroke, it provides an additional mechanism for reporting physical exam findings in ICH [4].

7.2.4 Imaging

Until imaging has been obtained, it is unknown whether a patient has had an ischemic or hemorrhagic stroke. Thus, imaging should be performed quickly. The most efficient imaging method to diagnose ICH is with a non-contrast head CT (NCHCT). Non-contrast head CT should be performed as soon as safely possible in the ED [5]. On NCHCT, the hemorrhage has increased attenuation compared to brain parenchyma in the setting of the acute hemorrhage (Fig. 7.2a). When reviewing the NCHCT, it is important for emergency clinicians to evaluate for perihematomal edema, herniation, intraventricular hemorrhage, and midline shift, all of which can be visualized on initial head CT. Hematoma volume can easily be calculated as well on initial head CT. Since a higher hematoma volume is significantly associated with higher mortality, this information is important to evaluate. The ICH volume can be estimated using the ABC/2 formula, "where A is the greatest hemorrhage diameter by CT, B is the diameter 90° to A, and C is the approximate number of CT slices with hemorrhage multiplied by the slice thickness." [6].

ICH is frequently complicated by intraventricular hemorrhage (IVH), which occurs when blood leaks into the ventricles (Fig. 7.2b). When this happens, hydrocephalus may worsen rapidly, leading to brain herniation. One of the indications for acute neurosurgical intervention in the setting of ICH is the occurrence of IVH. An external ventricular drain (EVD) may need to be placed; thus neurosurgical consultation should be obtained immediately when IVH is recognized.

An important feature to note if vascular imaging is obtained in the ED is the significance of the "spot sign." The spot sign, which is one or more areas of enhancement noted on contrasted images within the ICH, has been recognized as a marker of hemorrhagic expansion (Fig. 7.2c). It is demonstrative of active contrast extravasation occurring during the study, meaning that the hemorrhage is increasing in real time. The spot sign has been described in several prospective studies, including in a multicenter prospective observational cohort study of 268 patients with ICH. In this study, patients who were spot sign positive had a significantly higher amount of ICH expansion, defined as growth >6 mL or 33% at follow-up CT, as well as higher mortality at 3 months, and decreased functional status at 3 months [7].

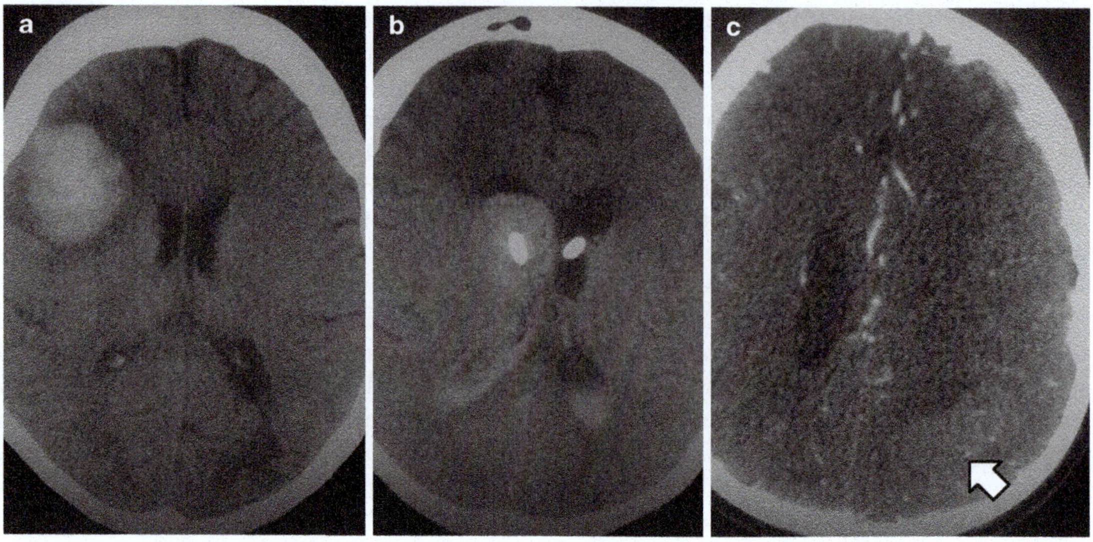

Fig. 7.2 (**a**) Demonstrates a right frontal intracerebral hemorrhage (ICH). Note the increased attenuation of hemorrhage in comparison to brain parenchyma. (**b**) Demonstrates an ICH with significant intraventricular hemorrhage (IVH). This IVH has required the placement of two external ventricular drains (EVDs). (**c**) Demonstrates a spot sign in a left parietal occipital ICH. The spot sign is noted by an arrow and demonstrates active contrast extravasation into the hemorrhage

Additionally, magnetic resonance imaging (MRI) may be necessary in certain patients with ICH. Typically, an MRI can be delayed until a patient is admitted or transferred and is generally not necessary in the ED in the setting of ICH. MRIs are time-consuming and are not safe for unstable patients or patients at risk of becoming unstable. The timing of subacute hemorrhages can be determined by MRI, as the appearance of hemorrhage changes in a predictable fashion. Gradient recalled echo (GRE) sequences may demonstrate microbleeds, assisting in the diagnosis of amyloid angiopathy, if multilobar. If microbleeds appear concentrated in deeper structures, this may be more suggestive of chronic hypertensive arteriopathy.

It is worthwhile to note that the ICH score developed in 2001, which has been derived and externally validated to predict 30-day mortality following ICH, hinges on key imaging findings from the NCHCT. Patients with higher scores on ICH score have a predicted worse outcome, and points are given for lower GCS, higher age, infratentorial location, higher ICH volume, and presence of IVH [8].

7.2.5 Lab Work

Patients with ICH should undergo a comprehensive lab workup in the ED. Any patient with a presentation of altered mental status should have an immediate finger-stick blood glucose obtained. Hypoglycemia is a rapidly treatable and correctable condition and should be diagnosed, ideally, in the prehospital setting. A complete blood count (CBC) should be performed, with particular attention to platelet count. Platelets should be transfused if under 100 K in the acute setting. Platelets should not be if patients are taking an antiplatelet drug and platelet count is normal. The recently published platelet transfusion in cerebral hemorrhage (PATCH) trial, a randomized controlled trial in which patients on antiplatelet medications were randomized to receive either standard care or standard care plus platelet transfusion, did not find a difference in patients who received platelet transfusions [9]. Coagulation status, measured by protime (PT) and activated prothrombin time (aPTT), should be obtained as well. Although the PT with conversion to the INR is an excellent measurement of the effects of warfarin, there is more ambiguity in the setting of novel oral anticoagulants [10]. A serum chemistry panel should be performed, in addition to a toxicology screen if concern for illicit drugs as an etiology for the hemorrhage. Women of childbearing age should also have a pregnancy test obtained. American Heart Association (AHA) guidelines also recommend a chest x-ray (CXR) and electrocardiogram (EKG) initially [3]. If possible, lab work should be completed point of care (POC), such that the results of coagulation status are available so that coagulopathy can be rapidly managed.

7.3 Organization of Care of Hemorrhagic Stroke

7.3.1 Emergency Department Management

Unlike the treatment of ischemic stroke, which may be treated with IV tPA and endovascular reperfusion in certain patients [11–16], there are no well-defined, targeted treatment modalities for ICH. Priorities for ED management are airway and hemodynamic stabilization, diagnosis, blood pressure treatment, anticoagulation reversal, and timely disposition.

7.3.2 Airway

Depending on the size and location of the hemorrhage, patients with ICH may require endotracheal intubation upon arrival to the ED secondary to decreased mental status and inability to manage secretions safely. In a prospective cohort study of 574 patients, 33% of patients with ICH required intubation either prior to arrival, during their ED stay, or within the first 24 h of admission [17]. In patients who do require intubation, both etomidate and ketamine are safe drug choices for induction during rapid sequence intubation (RSI). A 2009 randomized controlled trial demonstrated no difference between the two in critically ill ED patients requiring intubation [18]. Ideally, if neuromuscular blockade is performed, a short-acting paralytic agent, such as succinylcholine, should be used, so that the neurologic exam is not obscured for a lengthy period of time. Adequate analgesia and sedation should be given to intubated patients to prevent ICP elevation. In patients who do not require intubation initially, it is critical to monitor the patient's airway status with serial exams, as the neurologic exam may deteriorate while the patient is in the ED, as 9.8% of patients in the previously described prospective cohort required intubation while in the ED [17]. Following intubation, providers should maintain eucapnia. Patients should not be artificially hyperventilated, as hyperventilation is a temporizing measure, meant only for patients who are about to receive definitive operative therapy. Although hyperventilation does decrease intracranial pressure for a short period of time, patients who are artificially hyperventilated for a longer time course have worse outcomes compared to patients maintained with eucapnia. This association has been well-demonstrated previously in the TBI literature and has even led to long-term poor outcomes in this patient population [19]. Patients with ICH who are not intubated should not eat or drink initially until further formal evaluation, as they are at risk of aspiration. Of patients who initially survive an ICH, approximately 9% will ultimately require percutaneous endoscopic gastrostomy (PEG) placement [20].

7.3.3 Blood Pressure

Once the patient's airway has been assessed and managed and the diagnosis of ICH has been made, it is important for the emergency medicine physician to direct his or her attention to blood pressure management. If hypotension is noted or intravenous fluids are required, it is imperative to avoid hypotonic or dextrose containing fluids, as these may worsen cerebral edema. However, hypertension is significantly more common in patients with acute ICH.

Acute hypertension management in the setting of ICH has been the subject of several large recently published and ongoing studies. Elevated blood pressure in the setting of acute ICH is an independently associated measure of neurologic deterioration, hematoma expansion, and unfavorable long-term outcome in the setting of acute ICH; thus, controlling hypertension in acute ICH is important [21]. Unlike in ischemic stroke, where rapid substantial blood pressure reduction is unsafe and leads to decreased penumbra perfusion, it is generally well tolerated in patients with ICH, and aggressive blood pressure management does not lead to additional brain ischemia [22, 23]. Both the acute cerebral hemorrhage study (ATACH 1) and the intensive blood pressure reduction in acute cerebral hemorrhage trial (INTERACT-1) did not note a difference in the safety when lowering systolic blood pressure (SBP) to <140 mmHg [21, 22]. Current American Heart Association (AHA) guidelines have given a Class 1; level of evidence A for acutely lowering blood pressure to 140 mmHg if SBP on arrival is between 150 and 220 mg as being safe [3]. INTERACT-2 randomized 2839 patients to either intensive blood pressure management, defined as SBP < 140 mmHg within 1 h, or standard blood pressure management, defined as a SBP < 180 mmHg. The endpoints of INTERACT-2 were 90-day death or disability. Fifty-two percent of patients in the treatment arm compared to 56% in the standard arm experienced the primary outcome (odds ratio 0.87; 95% CI 0.75–1.01, P = 0.06). INTERACT-2 demonstrated that the intensive blood pressure management was safe but did not overall reduce likelihood of death, improve functional outcome, or significantly reduce hematoma expansion [24]. ATACH II, currently ongoing, is comparing blood pressure management in ICH patients to a goal of <140 mmHg SBP versus <180 mmHg SBP [25]. With the results of INTERACT-2, the AHA has given a Class IIa, level of evidence B guideline that lowering SBP to 140 mmHg in the setting of acute ICH is effective for improving functional outcomes [3].

7.3.4 Anticoagulation/Antiplatelet Considerations/Reversal

Patients who are anticoagulated for any reason and found to have an ICH in the ED should have the anticoagulation reversed promptly. Indeed, emergency physicians need to be well-prepared for anticoagulation reversal. Anticoagulation is common in this patient population, with approximately one in five cases of ICH associated with anticoagulation use [26]. This particular knowledge basis has become much more complicated since the addition of novel oral anticoagulants (NOACS). Anticoagulant reversal and blood pressure management are the two most critical actions that must be taken in treating patients with ICH. For instance, when FFP is utilized to reverse warfarin, each 30-min delay in the start of FFP is associated with a 20% reduction in INR correction within the first 24 h [27]. Indeed, a 2015 retrospective study of 1176 anticoagulated patients with ICH demonstrated a substantial mortality reduction to patients who had both INR reversal to <1.3 and SBP controlled to <160 mmHg within 4 h of ED presentation [28].

Warfarin, a vitamin K antagonist (VKA), is the most commonly used anticoagulant, has been on the market for decades, and, thus, has the most data regarding its reversal in the setting of ICH. All patients on warfarin must receive vitamin K. It should be given intravenously in the ED for the most rapid absorption [29]. Vitamin K allows the patient to generate new clotting factors, but this may take hours to days. For immediate reversal, fresh frozen plasma (FFP) to replace all factors, or prothrombin complex concentrates (PCCs) which contain either three or four factors only, must be given as well to patients. PCCs may be preferable, given that there is less volume to infuse, are able to be stored at room temperature, and result in faster INR correction compared to FFP for the reversal of warfarin-associated ICH [30]. However, they are more expensive in many institutions and, as such, more restricted. PCCs have been in use in Europe for over 20 years but were only recently FDA approved in the United States. PCCs generally contain factors II, VII, IX, X, C, S, Z, and antithrombin 3, whereas FFP contains all plasma factors [31, 32]. When compared to one another, 62% of patients given PCCs achieve INR correction by 0.5 h after the end of the infusion, compared to 9.6% of patients who are given FFP, with similar safety events [30].

Frontera et al. conducted a prospective observational study of PCC vs. FFP vs. PCC + FFP in the setting of VKA-associated ICH. Patients who received PCCs had a significantly lower risk of death and severe disability at 3 months compared to FFP alone, without an increase of adverse events [33]. The fresh frozen plasma versus prothrombin complex concentrate in patients with intracranial hemorrhage related to vitamin K antagonists trial (INCH trial) enrolled 54 patients but was terminated early due to safety concerns. Prior to termination, they found that PCCs were superior in normalizing INR and stated that the faster INR normalization was associated with smaller hematoma expansion [34]. Ultimately, current CHEST and AHA guidelines recommend that patients with VKA-associated major hemorrhage or ICH receive 4-factor PCC instead of FFP (Grade 2C—CHEST; Class IIb, level of evidence B—AHA) [3, 5, 10].

Newer anticoagulant classes have been approved for the management of non-valvular atrial fibrillation and thromboembolic disease. These classes of medications include direct thrombin inhibitors and factor Xa inhibitors and, as such, utilize different mechanisms within the clotting cascade to provide anticoagulant benefit. In patients who are taking direct thrombin inhibitors, first-line therapy for reversal should be idarucizumab, which is able to completely reverse the drug within minutes [35]. Direct thrombin inhibitors are cleared by the kidneys and, as such, can also be removed by hemodialysis [36]. However, starting hemodialysis in the ED poses many challenges, including the need for dialysis access, equipment, and hemodialysis monitoring capabilities. Factor eight inhibitor bypassing activity (FEIBA), also known as activated 4-factor PCC, may be another option for dabigatran reversal based on in vitro testing [37]. Factor Xa inhibitors may be best reversed with andexanet alfa. Andexanet alfa is a modified recombinant form of factor Xa, and thus it binds to factor Xa inhibitors [38]. It currently is in phase III trials for the reversal of factor Xa inhibitors but showed promise in a single-arm study of patients with acute bleeding [39]. In vitro testing has shown that 4-factor PCCs are appropriate for the reversal of factor Xa inhibitors, given that these drugs are protein bound and cannot be removed with hemodialysis [40, 41]. Recombinant factor VIIa may also be an option for reversal of NOACs, also based on in vitro animal testing [42–44].

Patients receiving antiplatelet therapy may also develop ICH, and the optimal treatment and reversal mechanisms for this class of patients are still under study. The recently published platelet transfusion in cerebral hemorrhage (PATCH) trial, a randomized controlled trial in which patients on antiplatelet medications were randomized to receive standard care or standard care plus platelet transfusion, failed to find a difference in patients who received platelet transfusions and even trended toward harm with platelet transfusion [9]. Desmopressin, or DDAVP, may be an option for reversal of antiplatelets. A small study of 14 patients who were on antiplatelets and had sustained an ICH showed that the drug was well tolerated and improved platelet function [45]. However, larger studies are necessary to determine if this will provide more clinically meaningful endpoints in ICH patients. More details about antithrombotic-induced bleeding will be discussed as a main topic in Chap. 14.

7.3.5 Hemostatic Agents

Hemostatic agents, such as recombinant factor VIIa, have been explored as a treatment for ICH both in anticoagulated patients and non-anticoagulated patients. The efficacy and safety of recombinant-activated factor VIIa for acute intracerebral hemorrhage (FAST) study was a randomized controlled trial of 841 patients with ICH. Although there was a significant difference in the size of hematoma growth, with the treatment group demonstrating less hematoma group, there was no difference in clinical outcomes [46]. Further data suggested that rFVIIa may be most beneficial in patients with spot sign noted on CT angiogram. There are two ongoing randomized placebo-controlled trials to test rFVIIa—the Spot Sign for Predicting and Treating ICH (STOP-IT) trial and the Spot Sign Selection of Intracerebral Hemorrhage to Guide Hemostatic Therapy

(SPOTLIGHT) trial. Tranexamic acid (TXA) is another promising hemostatic agent. This drug has not yet been tested in ICH, but two randomized controlled trials in the TBI literature demonstrated statistically significant reduction of hemorrhage progression without clinically meaningful differences [47].

7.3.6 Seizure Management and Prophylaxis

Patients with clinical seizure-like activity after ICH should be treated with anti-seizure medications while in the ED and should be managed similar to any other patient with seizures [3]. The incidence of seizures following ICH in the immediate period is unknown; is likely dependent on ICH location, comorbidities, and size of hemorrhage; but may be as low as 1.7% in one series and as high as 17% in patients with supratentorial ICH [48, 49]. Seizure prophylaxis is not recommended and has been associated with poor outcomes when adjusted for age, initial hematoma volume, presence of intraventricular blood, initial GCS, and previous warfarin use [49]. However these studies demonstrating harm predominately utilized phenytoin for seizure prophylaxis. Newer data report that levetiracetam may be a safer option for seizure prophylaxis [50].

7.3.7 Management of Increased Intracranial Pressure

After ICH, patients may experience increased intracranial pressure. Much of the literature from traumatic brain injury has been extrapolated into the realm of ICH, especially for the role of ICP management. There is an association between elevated ICP and outcome in ICH however. In a study of 121 patients with ICH and ICP monitoring in place, there was a significant association with both poor functional outcome and mortality with ICP greater than 20 [51]. Simple maneuvers, such as raising the head of the bed to 30°, have previously demonstrated a decrease in intracranial pressure and improved cerebral perfusion pressure, without compromising cardiac output in other types of intracranial hemorrhages, although less specifically in ICH [52]. As long as there is no concern for concomitant spinal cord injury, the head of the bed should be raised to 30–45° as a basic maneuver to prevent elevated intracranial pressure. Both mannitol and hypertonic saline (3% or 23.4%) are used to manage increased intracranial pressure [53]. It is important to note that mannitol's mechanism of action is via osmotic diuresis, so clinicians must be careful to monitor urine output and guard against hypotension. Hypertonic saline can be used as 3% or 23.4%; however, 23.4% cannot be used with a peripheral IV, and patients must have central venous access. 23.4% hypertonic saline provides an osmolar load in the serum with lower volume and shorter infusion time.

7.3.8 Role of Surgical Management

Two multicenter randomized controlled trials have been conducted to determine if there is a potential benefit of surgical intervention in supratentorial ICH—the STICH I and STICH II trials. Neither the STICH I nor STICH II trial demonstrated benefit in surgical management of ICH [54, 55]. However, these trials had high numbers of crossover from medical management into surgical management groups, so neurosurgeons may decompress some ICHs, depending on the indications. On the other hand, posterior fossa ICHs require surgical intervention much more frequently. Although there is no randomized controlled trial data, case series describe the benefit of posterior fossa decompression [56]. Due to the proximity of the fourth ventricle and brainstem, patients with posterior fossa ICH should have surgical decompression if they have any signs of deterioration, brainstem compression, or hydrocephalus. Since there is no equipoise regarding this topic, there is unlikely to be a trial conducted evaluating the utility of posterior fossa decompression [3]. Emergency medicine physicians should recognize this surgical indication and be able to communicate the findings of posterior fossa ICH to neurosurgical colleagues, as well as any signs of early deterioration that might mandate surgical intervention.

7.3.9 Prognostic Factors Associated with ICH

Prognosis following ICH is dependent on many factors. The ICH score, derived and externally validated, is the most common tool to determine prognosis [8]. However, the ICH score should not be the only factor used in determining prognosis. Recently, Morgenstern et al. described that a cohort of patients who were predetermined to have poor prognosis based on ICH score had a much lower mortality than expected (20% compared to 50% expected prognosis) simply by the avoidance of early DNR orders [57]. The ICH score ranges from 0 to 6, with higher score indicating worse prognosis. A score of 5 or 6 indicates 100% mortality, for instance. The ICH score factors in GCS, ICH volume, IVH, location of hemorrhage, and age [8]. Overall, the volume of ICH on head CT is the most important of these factors and weighs the heaviest in determining mortality [58]. Patients with brainstem hemorrhages and those with hematoma expansion also tend to have poorer prognosis [59, 60]. More details will be discussed as a main topic in Chap. 15.

7.3.10 Disposition

All patients with spontaneous ICH require admission to the hospital and in nearly all cases require admission to the intensive care unit (ICU). The ICU disposition is usually institution specific and may be managed by an internist, intensivist, neuro-intensivist, neurologist, or neurosurgeon. Interestingly, in a study of 13 ICUs, it was noted that after controlling for demographics, ICH severity, and institutional and ICU characteristics, patients admitted to a neuro ICU demonstrated an improvement in mortality rate when compared to general ICUs (odds ratio 3.4; 95% CI 1.65–7.6). A dedicated full-time neuro-intensivist also was associated with lower mortality rate (OR 0.388; 95% CI 0.22–0.67) [61].

7.3.11 DNR Status/Physician Pessimism

Early withdrawal of care is independently associated with mortality in ICH [62]. An early DNR, defined as <24 h after arrival, was associated with doubling in hazard ratio of death at 30 days (hazard ratio [HR] 2.17, 95% CI 1.38, 3.41) with adjustment made for age, gender, ethnicity, presenting Glasgow Coma Scale, ICH volume, intraventricular hemorrhage, and infratentorial hemorrhage [62]. Factors that have been notable for an association with DNR orders signed in the ED include increased age, ambulatory status before the event, CT findings with midline shift, intraventricular extension, larger hematoma size, and arrival to the ED with GCS ≤8 [63]. This has been described in the literature as the "self-fulfilling prophecy," such that patients have care withdrawn when they may have otherwise had a potentially good outcome if exposed to aggressive care early in their course. Recent data also suggests that patients with ICH continue to have neurologic improvements beyond 6 months [64]. These studies have led to changes in the AHA guidelines, now giving a Class IIa recommendation to avoid signing a DNR order until the second full day of hospitalization. Thus, emergency physicians should provide maximal care to patients with ICH in the immediate period.

References

1. Qureshi AI, Tuhrim S, Broderick JP, et al. Spontaneous intracerebral hemorrhage. N Engl J Med. 2001;344:1450–60.
2. Van Asch CJ, Luitse MJ, Rinkel GJ, et al. Incidence, case fatality, and functional outcome of intracerebral haemorrhage over time, according to age, sex, and ethnic origin: a systematic review and meta-analysis. Lancet Neurol. 2010;9:167–76.
3. Hemphill JC, Greenberg SM, Anderson CS, et al. Guidelines for the management of spontaneous intracerebral hemorrhage a guideline for healthcare professionals from the American Heart Association/American Stroke Association. Stroke. 2015;46:2032–60.
4. Brott T, Adams HP Jr, Olinger CP, et al. Measurements of acute cerebral infarction: a clinical examination scale. Stroke. 1989;20:864–70.

5. Morgenstern LB, Hemphill JC 3rd, Anderson C, et al. Guidelines for the management of spontaneous intracerebral hemorrhage: a guideline for healthcare professionals from the American Heart Association/American Stroke Association. Stroke. 2010;41:2108–29.
6. Kothari RU, Brott T, Broderick JP, et al. The ABCs of measuring intracerebral hemorrhage volumes. Stroke. 1996;27:1304–5.
7. Demchuk AM, Dowlatshahi D, Rodriguez-Luna D, et al. Prediction of haematoma growth and outcome in patients with intracerebral haemorrhage using the CT-angiography spot sign (PREDICT): a prospective observational study. Lancet Neurol. 2012;11:307–14.
8. Hemphill JC 3rd, Bonovich DC, Besmertis L, et al. The ICH score: a simple, reliable grading scale for intracerebral hemorrhage. Stroke. 2001;32:891–7.
9. Baharoglu MI, Cordonnier C, Al-Shahi Salman R, et al. Platelet transfusion versus standard care after acute stroke due to spontaneous cerebral haemorrhage associated with antiplatelet therapy (PATCH): a randomised, open-label, phase 3 trial. Lancet. 2016;387:2605–13.
10. Samama MM, Guinet C. Laboratory assessment of new anticoagulants. Clin Chem Lab Med. 2011;49:761–72.
11. The National Institute of Neurological Disorders and Stroke rt-PA Stroke Study Group. Tissue plasminogen activator for acute ischemic stroke. N Engl J Med. 1995;333:1581–7.
12. Hacke W, Kaste M, Bluhmki E, et al. Thrombolysis with alteplase 3 to 4.5 hours after acute ischemic stroke. N Engl J Med. 2008;359:1317–29.
13. Berkhemer OA, Majoie CB, Dippel DW. Endovascular therapy for ischemic stroke. N Engl J Med. 2015;372:2363.
14. Goyal M, Demchuk AM, Menon BK, et al. Randomized assessment of rapid endovascular treatment of ischemic stroke. N Engl J Med. 2015;372:1019–30.
15. Campbell BC, Mitchell PJ. Endovascular therapy for ischemic stroke. N Engl J Med. 2015;372:2365–6.
16. Saver JL, Goyal M, Bonafe A, et al. Stent-retriever thrombectomy after intravenous t-PA vs. t-PA alone in stroke. N Engl J Med. 2015;372:2285–95.
17. Elmer J, Pallin DJ, Liu S, et al. Prolonged emergency department length of stay is not associated with worse outcomes in patients with intracerebral hemorrhage. Neurocrit Care. 2012;17:334–42.
18. Jabre P, Combes X, Lapostolle F, et al. Etomidate versus ketamine for rapid sequence intubation in acutely ill patients: a multicentre randomised controlled trial. Lancet. 2009;374:293–300.
19. Muizelaar JP, Marmarou A, Ward JD, et al. Adverse effects of prolonged hyperventilation in patients with severe head injury: a randomized clinical trial. J Neurosurg. 1991;75:731–9.
20. Faigle R, Bahouth MN, Urrutia VC, et al. Racial and socioeconomic disparities in gastrostomy tube placement after intracerebral hemorrhage in the United States. Stroke. 2016;47:964–70.
21. Sakamoto Y, Koga M, Yamagami H, et al. Systolic blood pressure after intravenous antihypertensive treatment and clinical outcomes in hyperacute intracerebral hemorrhage: the stroke acute management with urgent risk-factor assessment and improvement-intracerebral hemorrhage study. Stroke. 2013;44:1846–51.
22. Zazulia AR, Diringer MN, Videen TO, et al. Hypoperfusion without ischemia surrounding acute intracerebral hemorrhage. J Cereb Blood Flow Metab. 2001;21:804–10.
23. Koch S, Romano JG, Forteza AM, et al. Rapid blood pressure reduction in acute intracerebral hemorrhage: feasibility and safety. Neurocrit Care. 2008;8:316–21.
24. Anderson CS, Heeley E, Huang Y, et al. Rapid blood-pressure lowering in patients with acute intracerebral hemorrhage. N Engl J Med. 2013;368:2355–65.
25. Qureshi AI, Palesch YY. Antihypertensive treatment of acute cerebral hemorrhage (ATACH) II: design, methods, and rationale. Neurocrit Care. 2011;15:559–76.
26. Flaherty ML, Kissela B, Woo D, et al. The increasing incidence of anticoagulant-associated intracerebral hemorrhage. Neurology. 2007;68:116–21.
27. Goldstein JN, Thomas SH, Frontiero V, et al. Timing of fresh frozen plasma administration and rapid correction of coagulopathy in warfarin-related intracerebral hemorrhage. Stroke. 2006;37:151–5.
28. Kuramatsu JB, Gerner ST, Schellinger PD, et al. Anticoagulant reversal, blood pressure levels, and anticoagulant resumption in patients with anticoagulation-related intracerebral hemorrhage. JAMA. 2015;313:824–36.
29. Nee R, Doppenschmidt D, Donovan DJ, et al. Intravenous versus subcutaneous vitamin K1 in reversing excessive oral anticoagulation. Am J Cardiol. 1999;83:286–8.
30. Sarode R, Milling TJ Jr, Refaai MA, et al. Efficacy and safety of a 4-factor prothrombin complex concentrate in patients on vitamin K antagonists presenting with major bleeding: a randomized, plasma-controlled, phase IIIb study. Circulation. 2013;128:1234–43.
31. Levy J, Tanaka K, Dietrich W. Perioperative hemostatic management of patients treated with vitamin K antagonists. Anesthesiology. 2008;109:918.
32. Dusel CH, Grundmann C, Eich S, et al. Identification of prothrombin as a major thrombogenic agent in prothrombin complex concentrates. Blood Coagul Fibrinolysis. 2004;15:405–11.
33. Frontera JA, Gordon E, Zach V, et al. Reversal of coagulopathy using prothrombin complex concentrates is associated with improved outcome compared to fresh frozen plasma in warfarin-associated intracranial hemorrhage. Neurocrit Care. 2014;21:397–406.
34. Steiner T, Poli S, Griebe M, et al. Fresh frozen plasma versus prothrombin complex concentrate in patients with intracranial haemorrhage related to vitamin K antagonists (INCH): a randomised trial. Lancet Neurol. 2016;15:566–73.
35. Pollack CV Jr, Reilly PA, Eikelboom J, et al. Idarucizumab for Dabigatran Reversal. N Engl J Med. 2015;373:511–20.

36. Garcia DA, Baglin TP, Weitz JI, et al. Parenteral anticoagulants: antithrombotic therapy and prevention of thrombosis, 9th ed: American College of Chest Physicians. Evidence-based clinical practice guidelines. Chest. 2012;141:e24S–43S.
37. Khoo TL, Weatherburn C, Kershaw G, et al. The use of FEIBA(R) in the correction of coagulation abnormalities induced by dabigatran. Int J Lab Hematol. 2013;35:222–4.
38. Yates SW. Interrupting anticoagulation in patients with nonvalvular atrial fibrillation. P T. 2014;39:858–80.
39. Connolly SJ, Milling TJ Jr, Eikelboom JW, et al. Andexanet alfa for acute major bleeding associated with factor Xa inhibitors. N Engl J Med. 2016;375:1131–41.
40. Perzborn E, Heitmeier S, Laux V, et al. Reversal of rivaroxaban-induced anticoagulation with prothrombin complex concentrate, activated prothrombin complex concentrate and recombinant activated factor VII in vitro. Thromb Res. 2014;133:671–81.
41. Escolar G, Fernandez-Gallego V, Arellano-Rodrigo E, et al. Reversal of apixaban induced alterations in hemostasis by different coagulation factor concentrates: significance of studies in vitro with circulating human blood. PLoS One. 2013;8:e78696.
42. Zhou W, Schwarting S, Illanes S, et al. Hemostatic therapy in experimental intracerebral hemorrhage associated with the direct thrombin inhibitor dabigatran. Stroke. 2011;42:3594–9.
43. Godier A, Miclot A, Le Bonniec B, et al. Evaluation of prothrombin complex concentrate and recombinant activated factor VII to reverse rivaroxaban in a rabbit model. Anesthesiology. 2012;116:94–102.
44. Fukuda T, Honda Y, Kamisato C, et al. Reversal of anticoagulant effects of edoxaban, an oral, direct factor Xa inhibitor, with haemostatic agents. Thromb Haemost. 2012;107:253–9.
45. Naidech AM, Maas MB, Levasseur-Franklin KE, et al. Desmopressin improves platelet activity in acute intracerebral hemorrhage. Stroke. 2014;45:2451–3.
46. Mayer SA, Brun NC, Begtrup K, et al. Efficacy and safety of recombinant activated factor VII for acute intracerebral hemorrhage. N Engl J Med. 2008;358:2127–37.
47. Zehtabchi S, Abdel Baki SG, Falzon L, et al. Tranexamic acid for traumatic brain injury: a systematic review and meta-analysis. Am J Emerg Med. 2014;32:1503–9.
48. Berger AR, Lipton RB, Lesser ML, et al. Early seizures following intracerebral hemorrhage: implications for therapy. Neurology. 1988;38:1363–5.
49. Messe SR, Sansing LH, Cucchiara BL, et al. Prophylactic antiepileptic drug use is associated with poor outcome following ICH. Neurocrit Care. 2009;11:38–44.
50. Sheth KN, Martini SR, Moomaw CJ, et al. Prophylactic antiepileptic drug use and outcome in the ethnic/racial variations of intracerebral hemorrhage study. Stroke. 2015;46:3532–5.
51. Sykora M, Steinmacher S, Steiner T, et al. Association of intracranial pressure with outcome in comatose patients with intracerebral hemorrhage. J Neurol Sci. 2014;342:141–5.
52. Schulz-Stubner S, Thiex R. Raising the head-of-bed by 30 degrees reduces ICP and improves CPP without compromising cardiac output in euvolemic patients with traumatic brain injury and subarachnoid haemorrhage: a practice audit. Eur J Anaesthesiol. 2006;23:177–80.
53. Qureshi AI, Wilson DA, Traystman RJ. Treatment of elevated intracranial pressure in experimental intracerebral hemorrhage: comparison between mannitol and hypertonic saline. Neurosurgery. 1999;44:1055–63.
54. Mendelow AD, Gregson BA, Fernandes HM, et al. Early surgery versus initial conservative treatment in patients with spontaneous supratentorial intracerebral haematomas in the international surgical trial in intracerebral haemorrhage (STICH): a randomised trial. Lancet. 2005;365:387–97.
55. Mendelow AD, Gregson BA, Rowan EN, et al. Early surgery versus initial conservative treatment in patients with spontaneous supratentorial lobar intracerebral haematomas (STICH II): a randomised trial. Lancet. 2013;382:397–408.
56. Da Pian R, Bazzan A, Pasqualin A. Surgical versus medical treatment of spontaneous posterior fossa haematomas: a cooperative study on 205 cases. Neurol Res. 1984;6:145–51.
57. Morgenstern LB, Zahuranec DB, Sanchez BN, et al. Full medical support for intracerebral hemorrhage. Neurology. 2015;84:1739–44.
58. Broderick JP, Brott TG, Duldner JE, et al. Volume of intracerebral hemorrhage. A powerful and easy-to-use predictor of 30-day mortality. Stroke. 1993;24:987–93.
59. Broderick J, Connolly S, Feldmann E, et al. Guidelines for the management of spontaneous intracerebral hemorrhage in adults: 2007 update: a guideline from the American Heart Association/American Stroke Association Stroke Council, High Blood Pressure Research Council, and the Quality of Care and Outcomes in Research Interdisciplinary Working Group. Stroke. 2007;38:2001–23.
60. Davis SM, Broderick J, Hennerici M, et al. Hematoma growth is a determinant of mortality and poor outcome after intracerebral hemorrhage. Neurology. 2006;66:1175–81.
61. Diringer MN, Edwards DF. Admission to a neurologic/neurosurgical intensive care unit is associated with reduced mortality rate after intracerebral hemorrhage. Crit Care Med. 2001;29:635–40.
62. Zahuranec DB, Brown DL, Lisabeth LD, et al. Early care limitations independently predict mortality after intracerebral hemorrhage. Neurology. 2007;68:1651–7.
63. Fan JS, Huang HH, Chen YC, et al. Emergency department do-not-resuscitate order in patients with spontaneous intracerebral hemorrhage. Am J Emerg Med. 2017;35:1850–4.
64. Hanley DF, Awad IA, Vespa PM, et al. Hemorrhagic stroke: introduction. Stroke. 2013;44:S65–6.

Symptoms and Signs of Hemorrhagic Stroke

8

Seung-Hoon Lee

A patient with acute hemorrhagic stroke (HS) may present with a sudden onset of focal neurologic deficits and other symptoms due to increased intracranial pressure. Most HS patients visit an emergency center through a prehospital delivery system instead of an outpatient clinic. Because HS is very likely to worsen during the first 24 h, the physician in the emergency center who is in charge of such a patient should promptly suspect the possibility of HS on the basis of the patient's medical history and symptoms and immediately perform a brain computed tomography (CT). HS, which mainly presents as intracerebral hemorrhage (ICH) or subarachnoid hemorrhage (SAH), is caused by a rupture of cerebral arteries. Because the brain has the lowest tissue pressure in the human body, bleeding into the brain is likely to persist for more than several hours, which increases the risk of a poorer outcome. Therefore, the process of diagnosis and treatment for HS should begin as early as possible. The first step to a quicker HS diagnosis is an understanding of its symptoms and signs.

In fact, within emergency centers, the symptoms of HS that duty doctors should pay attention to are easily identifiable. In any case, the possibility of a stroke should be promptly taken into consideration, if a focal neurologic deficit develops suddenly, and brain CT should be performed immediately. If a headache is accompanied by other neurologic symptoms, the probability of HS is greatly increased. This chapter lists various symptoms and signs of HS and categorizes them for better understanding. It is true that, compared to the past, the necessity for understanding symptoms and signs of stroke is reduced, because of the remarkable developments in brain imaging. However, we should keep in mind that the more we know, the more likely it is that the patient will get faster and more appropriate care.

8.1 Symptoms and Signs of Intracerebral Hemorrhage

ICH is caused by a rupture of small penetrating or leptomeningeal arteries branching from the large intracranial arteries that run through the subarachnoid space. This rupture results in extravasation of blood, leading to brain tissue damage.

Two important facts help in understanding the symptoms of ICH. Firstly, the mass effect of the hematoma itself causes symptoms. Extravasated blood creates a space-occupying lesion in the limited space within the cranial cavity and subsequently increases intracranial pressure (ICP). This increased ICP typically causes headache, nausea, and vomiting. Secondly, most ICHs

S.-H. Lee
Department of Neurology, Seoul National University Hospital, Seoul, South Korea

Korean Cerebrovascular Research Institute, Seoul, South Korea
e-mail: sb0516@snu.ac.kr

S.-H. Lee (ed.), *Stroke Revisited: Hemorrhagic Stroke*, Stroke Revisited,
https://doi.org/10.1007/978-981-10-1427-7_8

develop from "cerebral arteriolosclerosis," which is caused by vascular risk factors such as long-standing hypertension. Lacunar infarction, a subtype of ischemic stroke, is caused by small vessel occlusions, whose underlying pathological findings are almost identical to those of ICH. Simply stated, if cerebral arteriolosclerotic lesions suddenly block blood vessels, lacunar infarction will occur, and if they rupture, ICH will develop. In patients with small-sized ICHs, symptoms may not be indistinguishable from those of lacunar infarctions. Since ICH generally has a progressive nature, most ICH cases are more severe than lacunar infarctions. Cerebral amyloid angiopathy (one of the main causes of ICH, especially lobar hemorrhage) is pathophysiologically unlikely to cause lacunar infarctions. In lobar hemorrhages, symptoms may appear to be similar to those in territorial rather than in lacunar infarctions.

In summary, ICH can present with i) general symptoms such as decreased level of consciousness, nausea, vomiting, and headache, and ii) focal neurologic impairments according to the ICH location (Fig. 8.1). If the size of the hematoma is larger, symptoms such as loss of consciousness or seizures appear more frequently, neurological damage becomes more aggravated, and consequently, the prognosis of the patient may be worse.

8.1.1 Lobar Hemorrhage

Headache is the most common symptom in patients with lobar hemorrhage and is found in about 60–70% of the patients [1]. Nausea and/or vomiting is the second most common with about 30%, followed by seizures with about 20% [1]. Seizures occur more frequently in lobar hemorrhage than in other types of hemorrhage, which is directly related to the involvement of the cerebral cortex. At the initial stage, a serious depression in mental functions such as semicoma or coma is not common, but 10% of the patients show a decreased level of consciousness [1]. Lobar hemorrhages occur most frequently in the parieto-occipital area, and accordingly, hemisensory dysfunction, hemibody neglect, and visual field defects are frequently observed in these cases. Temporal lobar hemorrhage in the left side may cause sensory-dominant aphasia (Wernicke type) whereas that in the right side may arouse acute confusional states or agitated confusion. Frontal hemorrhage may cause hemibody weakness on the opposite side and may rarely induce mental status dysfunction such as abulia or apathy.

8.1.2 Basal Ganglia Hemorrhage

Basal ganglia hemorrhage, which occurs mainly in the putamen or the internal capsule, is the most common type of ICH. This is because of the anatomy of the lenticulostriate arteries, which supply the basal ganglia. As penetrating arteries, which directly branch from the internal carotid artery, they are vulnerable to high blood pressure. Basal ganglia hemorrhage can be asymptomatic if the hemorrhage is small in size and remains within the putamen. A hemorrhage, which expands into the surrounding area, especially the posterior limb of the internal capsule, causes in most cases hemibody weakness in the contralateral side. Hemisensory loss in the contralateral side may be seen in case of an expansion into the thalamus. Depending on the degree of involvement of the thalamus, eyeball gaze abnormalities, altered consciousness, and visual field defects may be present. When an intraventricular hemorrhage (IVH) or midline shift due to mass effect occurs, the patient's consciousness level may deteriorate, and the patient may even become comatose. Involvement of a lobar area can be accompanied by various forms of aphasia and mental state dysfunction. Taken together, the most common symptoms of basal ganglia hemorrhage are headache and contralateral weakness, but patients may present various neurological symptoms depending on the extent of expansion into the surrounding tissue.

Caudate hemorrhage usually shows very mild or even no distinct symptoms. Mild cognitive or behavioral abnormalities have been reported, but they are not common. Thus, caudate hemorrhages are usually identified as previous bleeding lesions such as slit-like lesions in magnetic resonance imaging. Because the caudate nucleus is directly in contact with the lateral ventricle, a sizable

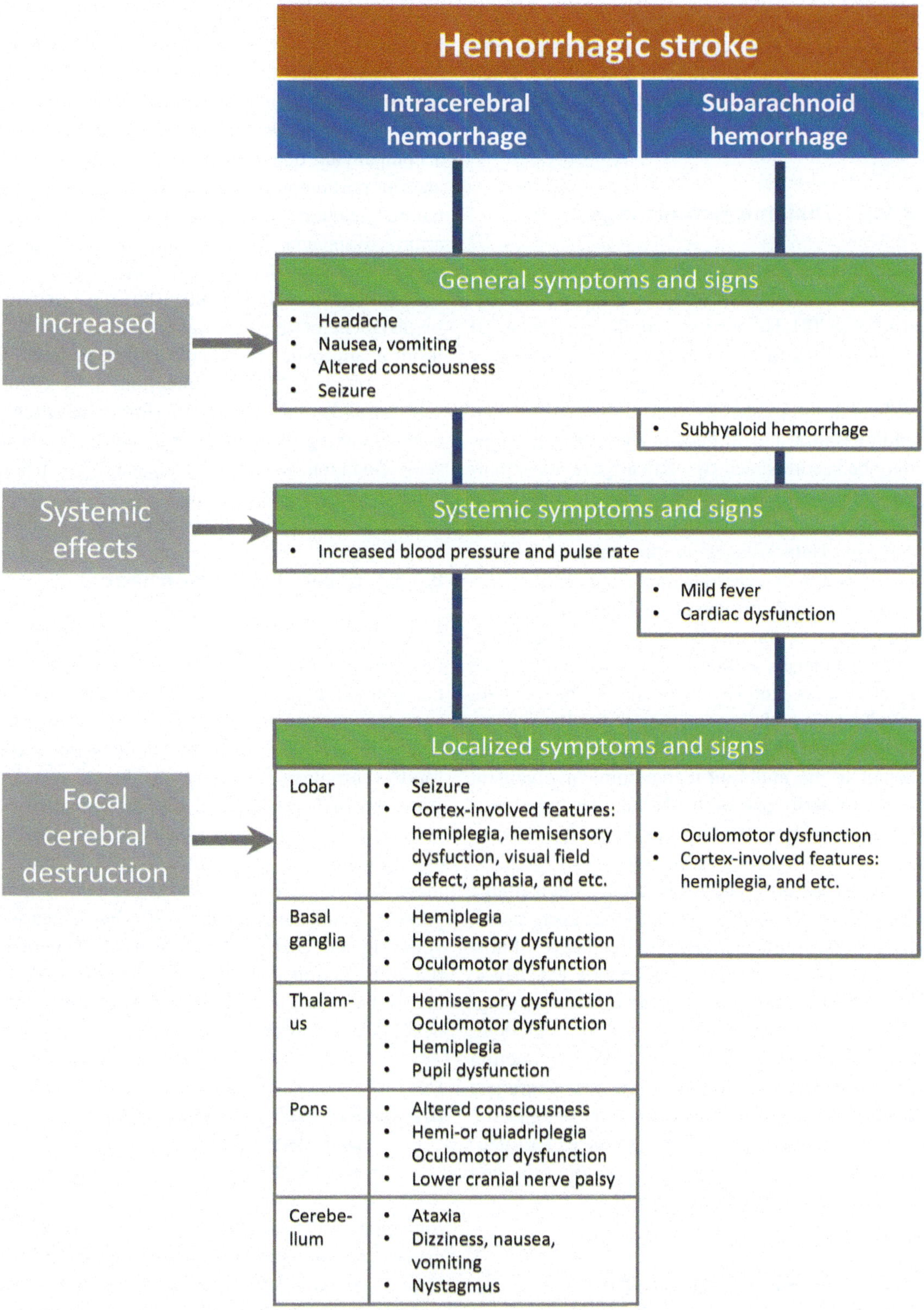

Fig. 8.1 Symptoms and signs of hemorrhagic stroke. *ICP* intracranial pressure

hemorrhage in this area is likely to cause bleeding into the lateral ventricle. The possibility of a caudate hemorrhage should be considered when primary IVH is detected without lesions of the brain parenchyma.

8.1.3 Thalamic Hemorrhage

Thalamic hemorrhages show symptoms similar to thalamic infarctions when their diameter is less than 2 cm [2]. Hemorrhages in the posterolateral portion of the thalamus are characterized mainly by hemisensory loss due to an involvement of ventral posterolateral, ventral posteromedial, and/or ventral lateral nuclei. These hemorrhages may be accompanied by vertical gaze abnormality and small, fixed pupils. The posterolateral portion is the most common site of thalamic hemorrhage. Hemorrhages in the anterior portion may result in decreased mental status and/or neuropsychiatric disturbances, and hemorrhages in the medial portion may cause vertical gaze abnormality, amnesia, and/or abulia. The vertical gaze limitation is known to occur in cases with involvement of the medial longitudinal fasciculus of the rostral interstitial nucleus, the vertical gaze center in the midbrain tegmentum. Involvement of the posterior part of the thalamus may be associated with visual field defects due to the destruction of the lateral geniculate body.

A relatively large thalamic hemorrhage (>2 cm) has four major symptoms: severe hemiparesis, hemisensory loss, vertical gaze abnormality, and constricted, fixed pupils [3]. These symptoms are not always present, but the symptoms and the prognosis worsen with an increase in the size of the bleed. Oculomotor dysfunction may present as skew deviation and conjugate eyeball deviation on the lesion side or opposite side to the lesion. Speech disturbances and neuropsychiatric symptoms such as amnesia and confusion may be present as well.

8.1.4 Pontine Hemorrhage

Pontine hemorrhage is not the most common ICH; its incidence is less than 5–10% of all cases of ICH [4]. However, it is the most severe hemorrhage type with the poorest prognosis having case fatality rate of 50% or more [4]. Patients with pontine hemorrhage often fall into deep coma due to disruption of the reticular activating system. In these cases, the prognosis is extremely poor due to the accompanying quadriplegia. Hemorrhages in the anterior portion of the pons involve the corticospinal tract leading to hemiparesis. Facial palsy, dysarthria, dysphagia, dizziness, vertigo, and deafness may be caused by the destruction of the nuclei and tracts of the 7th, 8th, 9th, and 10th cranial nerves. Involvement of the respiratory center may also result in apneustic or cluster breathing patterns. A variety of oculomotor dysfunctions may occur, such as unilateral or bilateral Horner syndrome, ocular bobbing, ocular dipping, ping-pong gaze, skew deviation, horizontal conjugate gaze palsy, and one-and-a-half syndrome.

8.1.5 Cerebellar Hemorrhage

Cerebellar hemorrhages usually develop around the dentate nucleus. In the case of expansion to the pontine tegmentum, early surgery may be needed for treatment or prevention of an obstructive hydrocephalus caused by compression of the fourth ventricle or its outlets – the lateral aperture (foramen of Luschka) and the median aperture (foramen of Magendie). Headache is relatively common in cerebellar hemorrhage, but impairment of intrinsic functions of the cerebellum may present as limb/truncal ataxia, dizziness, nausea, vomiting, and gaze-evoked nystagmus. If hemorrhage is confined to the cerebellum without involvement of the brain stem, hemibody weakness is usually absent.

8.2 Symptoms and Signs of Subarachnoid Hemorrhage

Subarachnoid hemorrhage is most commonly caused by traumatic brain injury, but about 80% of non-traumatic SAHs are due to a rupture of an intracranial aneurysm; about 10% are perimesencephalic SAHs [5]. Because non-traumatic SAHs show the poorest prognosis among the various subtypes of stroke, a better understanding of its symptoms and signs is an essential prerequisite for rapid diagnosis and treatment (Fig. 8.1).

8.2.1 Symptoms of Subarachnoid Hemorrhage

8.2.1.1 Headache and Meningeal Irritation Signs

Headache is the most common and a characteristic symptom in patients with SAH. More than 70% of SAH patients complain of headache. Because the intracranial arteries that run in the subarachnoid space anatomically belong to the large arteries, sudden rupture of these vessels leads to bleeding into the intracranial space with arterial pressure. Meningeal distension and irritation due to elevated pressure of the cerebrospinal fluid cause severe headache. SAH patients often refer to it as the most severe headache they have experienced in their lifetime – "like a hammer hit," "like a bolt out of the blue," and so on. Headaches occur suddenly and become maximally severe within a few seconds to several minutes. Patients generally report generalized headaches, but the pain is often localized near the rupture site and occasionally involves the upper neck. Increased ICP is accompanied by nausea and vomiting in many cases, leading to severe convulsions and decreased consciousness. In addition to vomiting, meningeal irritation signs such as posterior neck discomfort, photophobia, and phonophobia may also be present. SAH is the worst type of stroke, and it is reported that about 10–12% of patients die before being transferred to the emergency center. If the SAH headache is not severe, it is often difficult to distinguish from other types of headache. Headaches in SAH patients may mimic vascular headaches such as migraine and tension-type headache or pain of muscular origin in the head and neck region. When the diagnosis is based only on the nature and severity of the headache, it is often difficult to differentiate headache due to SAH from other forms of headache. Brain CT is generally recommended for patients with the following conditions: (1) sudden headache in adults, (2) headaches accompanied by seizures or other neurological symptoms, and (3) severe headache that has not been experienced before.

8.2.1.2 Warning Leaks

The prodromal symptom of SAH, called "warning leaks" or "sentinel headache," refers to a situation in which a small extravasation of the blood from an aneurysm causes headaches before the incidence of an aneurysmal SAH. It is reported that these symptoms are present in 20–40% of SAH patients [6, 7] and are generally regarded as important clinical features to prevent of SAH. However, these findings were largely from retrospectively designed studies, a typical setting in which patients are exposed to a recall bias. In a prospectively designed study, only two of the 37 SAH patients were suspected of having actual warning leaks [6]. It is very difficult to distinguish real warning leaks because similar headaches are a common complaint in normal adults. In conclusion, warning leaks need to be suspected only in patients with known intracranial unruptured aneurysms, but their general value is quite limited in clinical practice.

8.2.1.3 Decreased Levels of Consciousness

Loss of consciousness is presented in about 50–70% of SAH patients [8] and mostly caused by aneurysmal SAH – rarely in perimesencephalic SAH. Behavioral symptoms such as confusion and agitation might occur together with altered consciousness, and seizures are common. Altered consciousness occurs mainly due to decreased global cerebral perfusion caused by increased ICP, which might result from accompanying cardiac arrhythmia or seizure.

8.2.1.4 Seizures

Seizures occur in about 10–20% of all SAH patients [9]. It is caused by blood-induced irritation of the cerebral cortex, so it mostly occurs in aneurysmal SAH and rarely in perimesencephalic SAH. Compared to other subtypes of stroke, the incidence of seizures in SAH is very high.

8.2.2 Signs of Subarachnoid Hemorrhage

8.2.2.1 Vital Signs

In most cases of SAH, vital signs are altered at the time of admission. Blood pressure and pulse rate are typically increased. Body temperature may be normal or slightly elevated to about 38°C, and respiration is normal or slightly increased. High blood pressure at the time of admission may aggravate SAH status or induce rebleeding and therefore needs to be treated by parenteral administration of antihypertensive drugs. However, increased blood pressures is usually the result of a sudden increase in sympathetic tone, especially in previously normotensive patients, and continuous lowering of blood pressure may cause global cerebral ischemia. Accordingly, blood pressure control should be carefully performed in the early stages, with continuous monitoring of the blood pressure. Acute cardiac abnormality is common: troponin elevation occurs in 20–30% of SAH patients, and ECG changes including cardiac arrhythmia occur in more than 50% [10]. Left ventricular dysfunction is also common but usually transient.

8.2.2.2 Ocular Signs

A sudden increase in ICP due to SAH prevents venous outflow from the retina, resulting in venous hemorrhage, which is called subhyaloid hemorrhage. It occurs in about 10–20% of SAH survivors [11], who sometimes complain of scotoma due to retinal dysfunction at the bleeding site.

Oculomotor dysfunction, including third nerve palsy, sixth nerve palsy, and impaired vertical gaze (Parinaud's syndrome), is common in SAH patients. Third nerve palsy is the most important sign. It is indicative of an aneurysm rupture of the posterior communicating artery but is rarely caused by aneurysm ruptures of the superior cerebellar artery or the posterior cerebral artery. Third nerve palsy may occur without bleeding even in an unruptured aneurysm if the aneurysm expands rapidly. In this case, aneurysm ablation therapy should be performed immediately because it suggests an impending rupture of the aneurysm. Sixth nerve palsy may be caused by increased ICP and is often seen bilaterally. Parinaud's syndrome with vertical eye movement limitation implies a proximal dilatation of the aqueduct of Sylvius due to acute hydrocephalus, a state of pressing the vertical interstitial nucleus of the medial longitudinal fasciculus as the vertical gaze center.

8.2.2.3 Other Signs

Motor weakness may occur depending on the nature of SAH, for instance, when bleeding from an aneurysmal rupture directly destroys brain parenchyma or when SAH causes a severe, focal, chemical meningoencephalitis due to extravasated blood. Hemiparesis might be present as observed in cases of ischemic stroke, but it rarely occurs, with the exception of cases wherein an aneurysm of the middle cerebral artery ruptures. In some cases, monoparesis and paraparesis might be caused by the rupture of an aneurysm of the anterior communicating artery.

References

1. Kase CS, Williams JP, Wyatt DA, et al. Lobar intracerebral hematomas: clinical and CT analysis of 22 cases. Neurology. 1982;32:1146–50.
2. Kawahara N, Sato K, Muraki M, et al. CT classification of small thalamic hemorrhages and their clinical implications. Neurology. 1986;36:165–72.
3. Barraquer-Bordas L, Illa I, Escartin A, Ruscalleda J, et al. Thalamic hemorrhage. A study of 23 patients with diagnosis by computed tomography. Stroke. 1981;12:524–7.
4. Berlit P, Tornow K. Outcome of intracerebral hemorrhage: clinical and CT findings in 326 patients. Eur J Neurol. 1994;1:29–34.
5. Miranpuri AS, Aktüre E, Baggott CD, et al. Demographic, circadian, and climatic factors in non-aneurysmal versus aneurysmal subarachnoid hemorrhage. Clin Neurol Neurosurg. 2013;115:298–303.
6. Linn FH, Wijdicks EF, van der Graaf Y, et al. Prospective study of sentinel headache in aneurysmal subarachnoid haemorrhage. Lancet. 1994;344:590–3.
7. Hijdra A, van Gijn J. Early death from rupture of an intracranial aneurysm. J Neurosurg. 1982;57:765–8.
8. Vermeulen M, van Gijn J, Hijdra A, et al. Causes of acute deterioration in patients with a ruptured intracranial aneurysm. A prospective study with serial CT scanning. J Neurosurg. 1984;60:935–9.
9. Pinto AN, Canhao P, Ferro JM. Seizures at the onset of subarachnoid haemorrhage. J Neurol. 1996;243:161–4.
10. Liu Q, Ding YH, Zhang JH, et al. ECG change of acute subarachnoid hemorrhagic patients. Acta Neurochir Suppl. 2011;111:357–9.
11. Laun A, Tonn JC. Cranial nerve lesions following subarachnoid hemorrhage and aneurysm of the circle of Willis. Neurosurg Rev. 1988;11:137–41.

Principles of Clinical Diagnosis of Hemorrhagic Stroke

9

Max Wintermark and Tanvir Rizvi

Hemorrhagic stroke can be defined as an acute neurologic injury resulting from bleeding within the skull [1]. Traumatic epidural and subdural hemorrhage are excluded from discussion in this chapter. Intracerebral, subarachnoid, and intraventricular hemorrhage are the broad subdivisions, based upon the different anatomic compartments involved. Several different underlying vasculopathies can result in hemorrhagic stroke. In intracerebral hemorrhage (ICH), bleeding occurs directly into the brain parenchyma, from where it can extend into the ventricles, subarachnoid, or less commonly the subdural spaces. The two most frequent primary causes of ICH are hypertension-related deep perforating vasculopathy and cerebral amyloid angiopathy (CAA). The less common secondary causes include hemorrhagic infarction, arteriovenous malformation (AVM)- or dural arteriovenous fistula (dAVF)-related hemorrhage, cavernous malformations, neoplasm related, coagulopathy/ bleeding dyscrasias including iatrogenic supratherapeutic anticoagulation, thrombolytic therapy, venous sinus thrombosis, septic emboli associated, CNS infections like herpes, mycotic aneurysm, vasculitis, moyamoya disease, and vasoactive drugs (Table 9.1). Subarachnoid hemorrhage (SAH) can be both aneurysmal and non-aneurysmal.

Hemorrhagic stroke comprises 10–15% of all strokes, but the proportion may be higher in Asian and African populations [2]. Certain clues in clinical history can point to a specific cause of ICH. Younger age favors AVM as a cause, while hypertension and CAA are more frequent in older patients. Family history of ICH is more common with cavernous malformations and rare genetic familial forms of CAA. Previous history of cognitive decline may suggest CAA. Patients with a known cancer require hemorrhage into a metastasis to be considered. History of illicit drug use, especially cocaine and amphetamines, in young patients with ICH needs to be elicited. Hemorrhage during pregnancy and puerperium is potentially associated with eclampsia, cerebral venous thrombosis, and rarely choriocarcinoma.

The clinical presentation includes sudden onset of focal neurologic deficits, altered consciousness, headache, seizures, nausea, and vomiting. Progressive clinical deterioration can commonly occur. It has been described that 38% of ICH patients have more than a 33% growth in the volume of parenchymal hemorrhage during the first 20 h of baseline computed tomography (CT) after admission. Most of the ongoing bleeding occurs during the first 3–4 h after hemorrhage

M. Wintermark (✉)
Neuroradiology Division, Department of Radiology, Stanford University, Stanford, CA, USA
e-mail: Max.Wintermark@stanford.edu

T. Rizvi
Neuroradiology Division, Department of Radiology, University of Mississippi Medical Center, Jackson, MS, USA
e-mail: trizvi@umc.edu

S.-H. Lee (ed.), *Stroke Revisited: Hemorrhagic Stroke*, Stroke Revisited,
https://doi.org/10.1007/978-981-10-1427-7_9

Table 9.1 Intracerebral hemorrhage: causes

Primary causes	Secondary causes
1. Hypertension-related deep perforating vasculopathy 2. Cerebral amyloid angiopathy	1. Hemorrhagic infarction 2. Vascular malformations: (a) Arteriovenous malformations (b) Dural arteriovenous fistula (c) Cavernous malformation (d) Aneurysm rupture (ICH and SAH) 3. Neoplasms: (a) Primary (b) Secondary 4. Coagulopathy: (a) Hereditary (b) Acquired (c) Iatrogenic (anticoagulants, antiplatelets) 5. Venous sinus thrombosis 6. Infections: (a) Septic emboli (bacterial endocarditis) associated (b) CNS infections like herpes (c) Mycotic aneurysms 7. Vasculitis and collagen vascular diseases 8. Moyamoya disease 9. Reversible cerebral vasoconstriction syndrome (RCVS) 10. Vasoactive drugs like cocaine, heroin, amphetamine, and ecstasy

ICH intracerebral hemorrhage, *SAH* subarachnoid hemorrhage, *CNS* central nervous system

onset [3]. Knowledge of this fact justifies a repeat CT when there is rapid neurologic deterioration.

The symptoms are usually nonspecific, and imaging occupies a central part in all management strategies in emergent settings. Quick diagnosis of hemorrhage is essential in acute stroke care as the treatment of ischemic and hemorrhagic stroke is markedly different. Different blood tests comprise an essential component of diagnostic workup of such patients. Computed tomography (CT) remains the workhorse of hemorrhagic stroke evaluation due to its easy 24 h availability, ease of patient monitoring during scanning, and less time taken for imaging and interpretation. With technological advances, higher field and gradient strengths, and faster computing power, magnetic resonance imaging (MRI) is increasingly becoming the second most important modality for hemorrhagic stroke evaluation. It provides additional important information in entities like hemorrhagic infarction, cerebral amyloid angiopathy, and primary and secondary neoplasms. CT angiography (CTA), MR angiography (MRA), and digital subtraction angiography (DSA) also provide supplemental information in patients suspected of aneurysm, vascular malformation, and venous sinus thrombosis. Neurophysiology tests including Transcranial Doppler (TCD) remain an important diagnostic tool especially in critical care settings and follow-up of accompanying entities like vasospasm.

9.1 Blood Tests

Blood tests on their own cannot diagnose intracranial hemorrhage. But they provide indirect information, which helps in the diagnostic evaluation of hemorrhagic stroke. For example, evaluation of coagulation parameters helps in the assessment of those patients who are at an increased risk of intracranial hemorrhage. Similarly, liver function tests in alcoholics can provide an assessment of those patients who have increased proclivity for intracranial hemorrhage. The following list is a comprehensive but not exhaustive list of blood tests that provide us with this kind of information:

- Complete blood count (CBC) including platelet count: Hematocrit and platelet count can be monitored to identify hemorrhagic risk and complications. Severe bleeding usually occurs when platelet count falls below 10 × 10(9)/L [4]. Admission leukocytosis has been cited to have a strong association with intraventricular hemorrhage [5].

- Prothrombin time (PT), activated partial thromboplastin time (aPTT), and international normalized ratio (INR): PT measures how quickly blood clots. Prolonged PT can be seen with warfarin use, liver disease resulting in diminished synthesis of clotting factors, and disseminated intravascular coagulation (DIC) among other causes. aPTT is used to monitor response to heparin therapy. INR is a standardized unit that can be used to compare PT done at different labs. Increased values of all these tests are seen in patients with ICH.
- Liver enzymes: Deranged liver function tests are seen in alcoholics and patients with liver failure, which results in abnormal clotting factors increasing chances of bleeding including ICH.
- C-reactive protein and fibrinogen levels can be abnormal in patients with ICH.
- Blood cultures in suspected septicemia with ICH.
- Screening for prothrombotic conditions in cases of cerebral venous thrombosis. Factor V Leiden mutation, protein C deficiency, protein S deficiency, antithrombin C deficiency, elevated factor VIII, antiphospholipid antibody syndrome, activated protein C resistance, and hyperhomocysteinemia are some of the tests that can be run to determine the cause of hypercoagulable state in patients with unexplained cerebral venous thrombosis.
- Serum chemistries including electrolytes and osmolarity can be used to assess for metabolic derangements, such as hyponatremia, and monitor osmolarity for guidance of osmotic diuresis.
- Toxicology screen and serum alcohol level if illicit drug use or excessive alcohol intake is suspected. The association between ICH and use of amphetamine, cocaine and its freebase form crack-cocaine, and ecstasy has been reported with increased frequency [6]. Cocaine metabolites can be screened in urine within 48 h of admission. Cocaine-associated ICH has worse functional outcome and three times more likely to die during their acute hospitalization compared to cocaine-negative patients [7].
- Screening for vasculitic etiologies in select patients: Selective testing for vasculitis among the more uncommon causes of intracerebral hemorrhage can be done.

9.2 Brain Imaging

As we saw in the last section, blood tests cannot diagnose hemorrhagic stroke, and imaging is a key starting point in the evaluation of suspected hemorrhagic stroke and must be obtained on an emergent basis. Imaging helps in excluding ischemic stroke and identifies complications of hemorrhagic stroke such as intraventricular hemorrhage, brain edema, herniation, and hydrocephalus. First, we will discuss the different imaging modalities including CT and MRI for structural neuroimaging and CTA, MRA, and DSA for vascular neuroimaging. Then we shall discuss neuroimaging relevant to the common etiologies of hemorrhagic stroke.

9.2.1 Non-contrast Computed Tomography (NCCT)

High sensitivity and specificity of diagnosis of acute hemorrhage, lower cost, 24-h availability, feasibility of use for unstable patients and rapid imaging and report turnover time make CT the preferred diagnostic modality in emergent settings for evaluation of hemorrhagic stroke. Acute ICH is seen as a round or oval hyperattenuating lesion on head CT within minutes of onset of symptoms. In hyperacute settings, CT density measures 40–60 Hounsfield units (HU) and can appear heterogeneous. As the clot organizes, it becomes more homogeneous and hyperdense with CT density increasing to 60–80 HU in hours to days and then 80–100HU over a course of few days, when it is surrounded by an area of hypoattenuation representing vasogenic edema. As the hemorrhage ages, the CT density gradually decreases by an average of 0.7–1.5 HU per day [8]. It decreases in density with passage of time and becoming isodense approximately after 1 week [9]. Smaller bleeds are better seen on thin-slice imaging, and those adjacent to the calvarium are better seen with a wider (150–250 HU) window setting [1]. In extreme anemia, acute blood may appear isodense because of low hematocrit. In active extravasation, liquid blood can also appear hypodense relative to hyperdense surrounding clot, resulting in the so-called "swirl" sign [10] (Fig. 9.1). Similarly, acute blood in the setting of coagulopathy can appear isodense or may demonstrate a fluid-fluid level. If there is no rebleeding, late sequela of hemorrhages can include hypodense foci (37%), slit-like lesions (25%), calcifications (10%), or no detectable abnormalities (27%) [11].

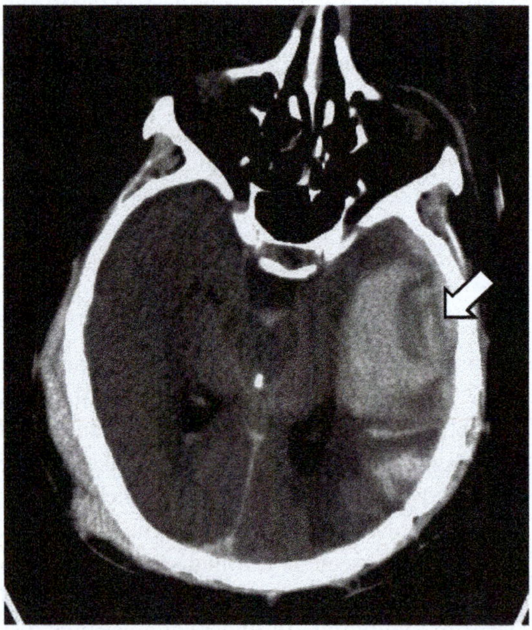

Fig. 9.1 "Swirl" sign. A 47-year-old female on anticoagulation presented with altered mental status post fall. There was a large left temporal intraparenchymal hematoma with hypodense "swirl" sign (*arrow*) suggesting active bleeding. There was surrounding edema and mass effect on left lateral ventricle. Subarachnoid and intraventricular hemorrhage was also seen

CT helps in identifying the location of the hemorrhage, any intraventricular extension, surrounding edema, mass effect, midline shift, or herniation and also estimates the hemorrhage volume. Product of three dimensions of the hematoma divided by two gives a rough volume of the hematoma. This helps in improved communication between care providers and also for prognostication, as one-third of patients will have hematoma expansion on a follow-up CT within first 3 h of symptom onset [12]. CT can also be utilized for guidance for surgical evacuation of the hematoma or for placement of external ventricular drain for those patients with ICH having an intraventricular extension and associated obstructive hydrocephalus.

9.2.2 Magnetic Resonance Imaging (MRI)

The accuracy of MRI to detect acute symptomatic ICH is equivalent to that of CT, while MRI is more sensitive in the detection of subacute and chronic hemorrhage compared to CT [13].The imaging characteristics and appearance of ICH evolve with time (Table 9.2). In the acute phase, gradient-echo T2*-weighted (T2*W) MRI is the most sensitive sequence. The paramagnetic properties of blood products induce local field inhomogeneities resulting in signal loss and hence hypointense appearance on T2*W sequences. Newer three-dimensional susceptibility-weighted imaging (SWI) sequences have been developed, which have been shown to be more sensitive than CT and even T2*W gradient recalled echo (GRE) sequences in detecting both chronic microhemorrhage and small volume hemorrhage within an acute infarct [14, 15]. Other MRI sequences such as diffusion-weighted sequence (DWI), T1, T2, and fluid-attenuated inversion recovery sequence (FLAIR) provide supportive information. DWI can show an acute or subacute infarct as an area of restricted diffusion. MRI can differentiate the primary causes of ICH, hypertension-related deep perforating vasculopathy and cerebral amyloid angiopathy. White matter T2/FLAIR hyperintensities of likely vascular origin, lacunar infarcts,

Table 9.2 Evolution of intracerebral hemorrhage with time on computed tomography (CT) and magnetic resonance imaging (MRI)

Stage	Blood product phase	Time frame	Non-contrast CT	T1W MRI	T2W MRI	T2*W MRI
Hyperacute	Oxyhemoglobin	First few hours	Hyperdense, can be heterogeneous	Isointense	Hyperintense	Marked hypointense
Acute	Deoxyhemoglobin	12–48 h	Hyperdense, more homogeneous	Isointense with thin peripheral hyperintense rim	Hypointense with hyperintense rim	Marked hypointense
Early subacute	Intracellular methemoglobin	2–7 days	Hyperdense with surrounding vasogenic edema	Hyperintense	Hypointense	Hypointense
Late subacute	Extracellular methemoglobin	7 days –1 month	Isodense	Hyperintense	Hyperintense	Hypointense
Chronic	Hemosiderin and ferritin	>1 month	Iso or hypodense	Hypointense	Hypointense	Hyper/isointense rim surrounded by hypointense rim

T1W T1-weighted, *T2W* T2-weighted, *T2*W* T2*-weighted

deep cerebral microbleeds, and brain atrophy are suggestive of deep perforating vasculopathy [16]. Lobar chronic microbleeds, superficial siderosis related to repeated bleeding in subarachnoid and subpial spaces, and white matter hyperintensities representing silent ischemic areas are known manifestations of CAA. Limitations of MRI include increased time to perform the study compared to CT, difficulty in monitoring unstable patients for the length of the study, contraindication for patients with metallic implants or foreign bodies, large body habitus, and claustrophobia.

9.2.3 Computed Tomography Angiography (CTA)

CTA is performed after intravenous administration of iodinated contrast material, tracking the contrast passage and CT scanning in arterial phase to image the arteries of the head and neck. The most common indications include evaluation for any aneurysm as a cause of SAH and evaluation of stenosis or occlusion of arteries of the neck and intracerebral arteries. A spot sign on CT angiogram is seen as a 1–2 mm focus of intense enhancement within a hematoma and represents active contrast extravasation in a bleeding focus or a small pseudoaneurysm [10] (Fig. 9.2). This sign is predictive of hematoma expansion and poorer prognosis. Besides these, entities like AVMs and dAVFs, moyamoya disease, vasculitis, and vasospasm related to drug use can be diagnosed by CTA. A variant on the same theme, CT venography (CTV), can be performed by imaging in venous phase to diagnose dural venous sinus or cortical venous thrombosis as a cause of venous infarct and associated hemorrhage. With increasing availability of multislice CT and fast scanning time, CTA has largely replaced the invasive DSA for diagnostic evaluation of the vasculature. Disadvantages include radiation exposure, risk of contrast-induced nephropathy, and allergic reactions.

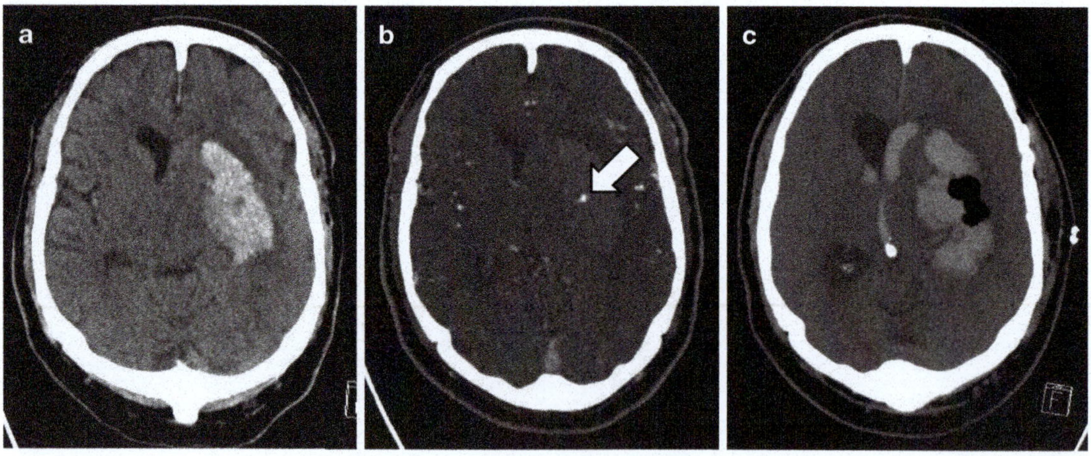

Fig. 9.2 "Spot" sign. A 59-year-old male presented with postcoital altered mental status, right hemiparesis, and aphasia. Blood pressure (BP) 223/145 mmHg at arrival. Non-contrast computed tomography (NCCT) head (**a**) showed a large 6 cm left basal ganglia/putamen intraparenchymal hemorrhage with surrounding vasogenic edema and left to right midline shift. Computed tomography (CT) angiogram head and neck showed a "spot" sign (*arrow*) corresponding to an area of active hemorrhage (**b**). Note this corresponds to a hypodense area on corresponding non-contrast CT. A left frontal craniotomy was done to evacuate the hematoma. There was increased intraventricular extension and midline shift despite evacuation (**c**). Patient died a day later due to continued bleeding

9.2.4 Magnetic Resonance Angiography (MRA)

MRA provides the same information which CTA does. However, MRA of the head utilizing time-of-flight technique does not require contrast administration and can be performed in those patients with renal insufficiency or previous serious allergic reaction to contrast. The sensitivity and specificity of 1.5T MRA are lower than that of modern multislice CTA studies [17].

9.2.5 Digital Subtraction Cerebral Angiography (DSA)

Conventional angiography or DSA is a minimally invasive neuroimaging technique involving femoral sheath introducer placement in common femoral artery followed by advancement of catheter into the common, internal carotid or vertebral artery under fluoroscopic guidance and then imaging the flow of contrast in real time to obtain dynamic images of the artery of interest. As this is a real-time imaging, arterial, capillary, and venous phases can be obtained. It remains the gold standard to evaluate underlying AVMs or dAVFs in patients with ICH. In less than 1% of patients, there is a risk of complications including stroke, vessel dissection, vessel perforation, contrast allergic reaction, contrast-induced nephropathy, and groin hematoma. DSA is also utilized for treatment in form of aneurysm coiling, stent placement, AVM obliteration, and tumor embolization, among others.

9.2.6 Evidence-Based Recommendations of Modality Usage in ICH

The American Heart Association/American Stroke Association recommends rapid neuroimaging with CT or MRI to distinguish ischemic stroke from ICH (level A of evidence) [12]. CTA or contrast-enhanced CT may be considered to help identify patients at risk for hematoma expansion (level B of evidence). Vessel examination can be useful to screen for underlying structural lesions, including vascular malformations and tumors when there is a clinical or neurologic suspicion (level B of evidence) [18].

9.3 Neuroimaging Relevant to Common Etiologies

9.3.1 Hypertension-Related Deep Perforating Vasculopathy

The most common cause of nontraumatic spontaneous ICH is arterial hypertensive vasculopathy and is associated with long-standing hypertension [19]. It commonly affects the lenticulostriate arteries arising from the middle cerebral arteries, thalamoperforating and thalamogeniculate arteries arising from the posterior cerebral arteries, and the pontine and brainstem perforators arising from the basilar artery. In patients with hypertension, these small vessels can undergo intimal hyperplasia, intimal hyalinization, and medial degeneration, which predispose them to focal necrosis and rupture. The classic location of macroscopic hypertensive hemorrhage reflects the areas supplied by these small perforators. Forty to fifty percent bleeds occur in the putamen and internal capsule, 20–30% in the thalamus, and 8% each in the pons and cerebellum with 20–30% being lobar subcortical hemorrhage [20] (Fig. 9.3). Hypertensive hemorrhage in basal ganglia and brainstem may dissect into the ventricular system resulting in intraventricular hemorrhage (IVH), which appears hyperdense on CT, hypointense on T2*W and SWI sequence, and hyperintense on FLAIR sequence relative to adjacent dark CSF. Chronic multifocal microhemorrhages can be seen in the distribution of small perforating vessels not typically detected on CT but best seen on MRI T2* or SWI sequences. The other MR imaging findings include white matter T2/FLAIR hyperintensities, lacunar infarcts, and brain atrophy.

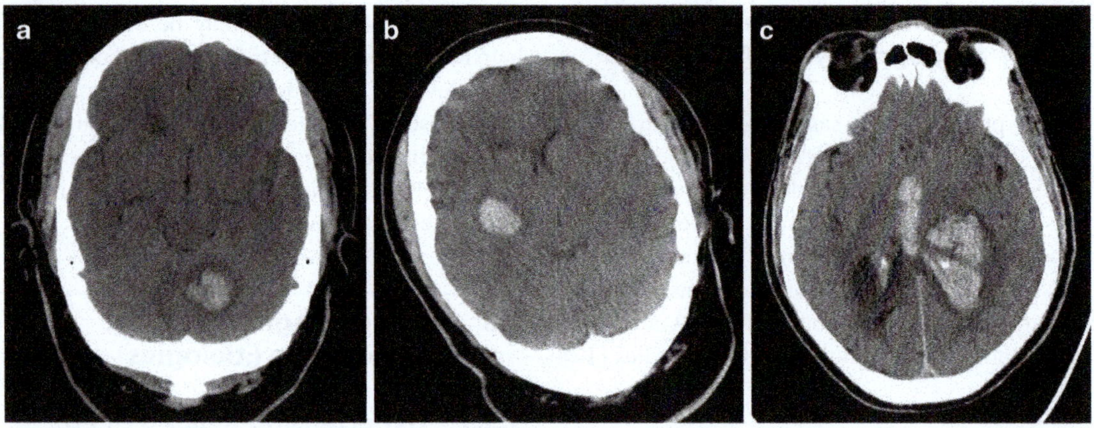

Hypertensive ICH

Fig. 9.3 Hypertensive intraparenchymal hemorrhage in two different patients. A 46-year-old female with history of hypertension and congestive heart failure presented with sudden onset headache, sweating, and nausea. Noncontrast computed tomography (NCCT) showed a left superior cerebellar intraparenchymal hematoma with surrounding edema (**a**). A CT done 2 years before on the same patient had shown a right putamen intraparenchymal hematoma (**b**). Both these are common locations for hypertensive intracerebral hemorrhage (ICH). A 64-year-old male presenting with right hemiplegia and unresponsiveness showed a left thalamic hemorrhage with intraventricular extension (**c**). The thalamus is another common location of hypertensive ICH

9.3.2 Cerebral Amyloid Angiopathy (CAA)

Lobar ICH in the settings of advanced age and history of cognitive decline is the classic picture of CAA. It is rarely seen below 60 years of age with increasing incidence after 65 years [1]. Deposition of amyloid beta-peptide in the small- and medium-sized vessels of the leptomeninges and cortex with affected vessels undergoing fibrinoid degeneration, necrosis, and microaneurysm formation followed by rupture of weakened segments results in either microhemorrhage or large hematomas [21]. Neuroimaging findings include cortical-subcortical location of hematoma, presence of microbleeds in cortical regions, and superficial siderosis (Fig. 9.4), best seen on T2*W and SWI MRI sequences, and typically not visible on CT. The widely used Boston criteria for the diagnosis of CAA rely heavily on the imaging features of both macro and microhemorrhages when pathologic evidence is not available [22]. For definite diagnosis, postmortem examination findings of lobar, cortical, or cortico-subcortical hemorrhage, severe CAA, and absence of other causative lesion are needed. Probable CAA diagnosis needs all three findings of age greater than 60; multiple hemorrhages restricted to lobar, cortical, cortico-subcortical regions; and absence of other causative lesion. Possible CAA diagnosis needs age greater than 60 AND either single lobar, cortical, cortico-subcortical hemorrhage without another cause OR multiple hemorrhages with possible but not definitive cause or with some hemorrhages in atypical location.

9.3.3 Hemorrhagic Infarction

Hemorrhagic infarction refers to bleeding in a pre-existing area of ischemia. This occurs around the second week following infarct when occurring spontaneously and earlier in those undergoing IV/IA thrombolysis or mechanical clot retrieval through endovascular approach.

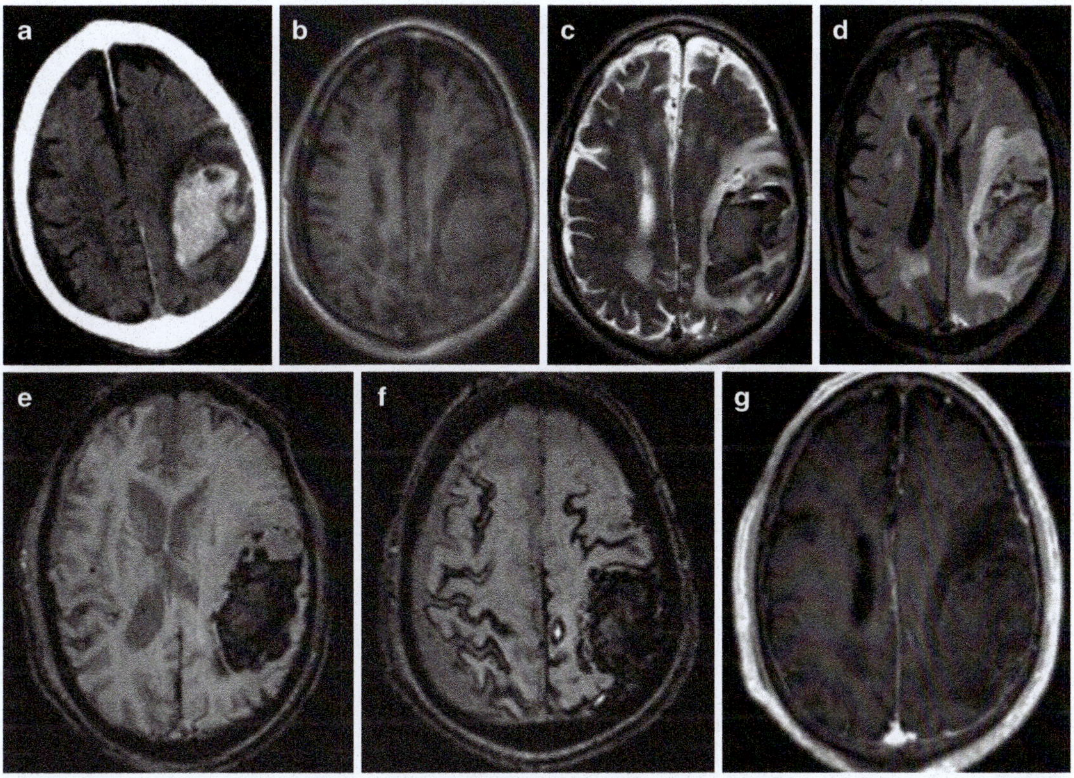

Fig. 9.4 Cerebral amyloid angiopathy (CAA)-associated lobar hemorrhage. A 84-year-old male with dementia presented with sudden onset aphasia, right facial droop, left gaze preference, and right hemiplegia. Computed tomography (CT) head showed a large left posterior frontal and parietal intracerebral hemorrhage (ICH) with surrounding edema (**a**). Magnetic resonance imaging (MRI) showed the large lobar left frontal and parietal hemorrhage isointense on T1-weighted image (T1W) (**b**) and heterogeneously hyperintense on T2-weighted image (T2W) (**c**) and fluid-attenuated inversion recovery (FLAIR) sequence (**d**) with fluid-fluid level formation and surrounding vasogenic edema. Susceptibility-weighted image (SWI) sequence showed punctate area of susceptibility in right frontal lobe representing microhemorrhage (**e**) and superficial siderosis as gyriform susceptibility along the vertex (**f**). No significant enhancement was seen on post-contrast T1W sequence (**g**). The MR findings are probable for cerebral amyloid angiopathy-associated ICH

The hemorrhage tends to occur in two patterns, petechial hemorrhage and parenchymal hematoma [23]. Petechial hemorrhage on CT appears as subtle increased density with indistinct margins, sometimes appearing speckled or punctate. On MRI, it gives characteristic signal dropout on T2*W sequence. Petechial hemorrhages are seen primarily in gray matter structures. It is of little clinical significance, and antithrombotic therapy is generally not withheld in such cases. Parenchymal hematoma can be classified as type 1 and 2, with greater than 30% infarcted area being involved and resulting mass effect in type 2, which is correlated with clinical deterioration and poor clinical outcome [24] (Figs. 9.5 and 9.6). Antithrombotic therapy is generally withheld in parenchymal hematoma. MR is more sensitive in detection of ischemia with DWI sequences and hemorrhagic transformation with T2*W and SWI sequences compared to CT.

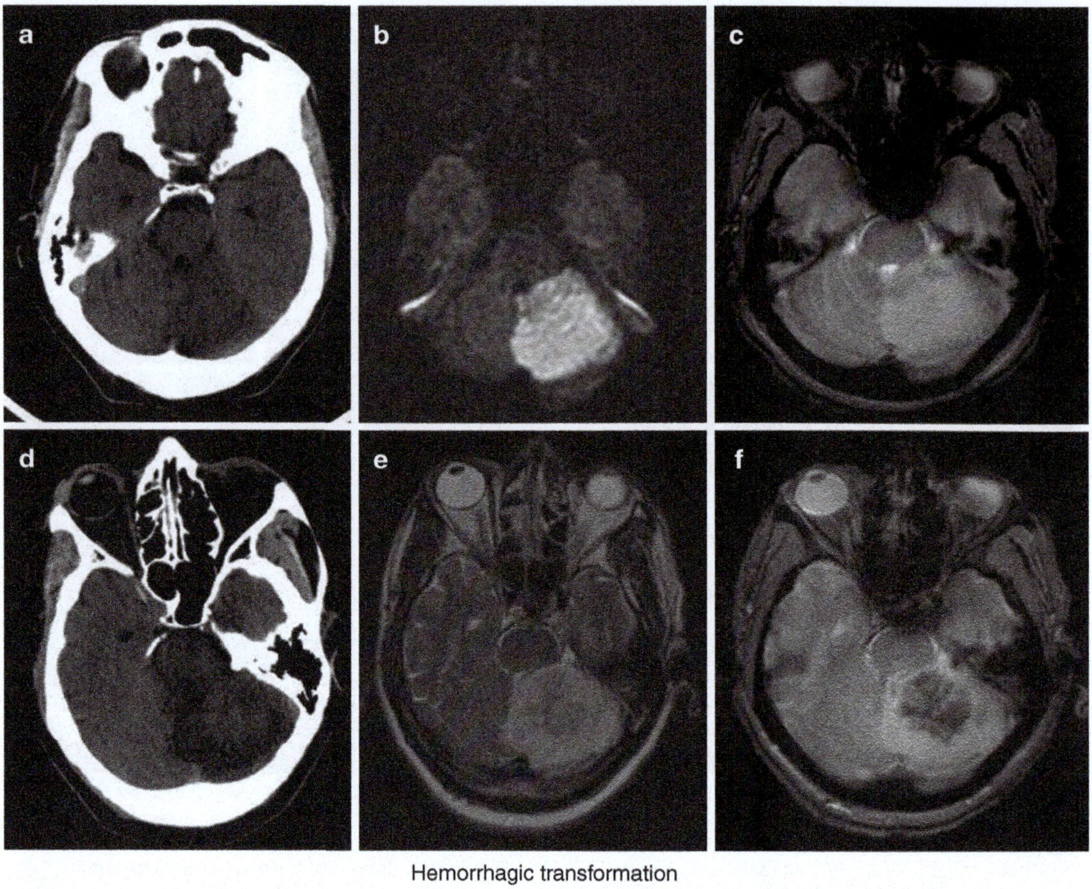

Fig. 9.5 Hemorrhagic transformation of left superior cerebellar artery (SCA) territory infarct. A 66-year-old male presented with acute onset dysarthria and vertigo. Computed tomography (CT) (**a**) and magnetic resonance imaging (MRI) (**b**) on the day of the presentation showed a large left SCA territory infarct. Gradient sequence does not show any susceptibility (**c**). Repeat MRI 2 days later after tissue plasminogen activator (tPA) administration on T2-weighted image (T2W) (**e**) and T2* gradient-echo (GRE) (**f**) sequence shows susceptibility as hypointense signal representing blood products, which is seen as hyperdensity on CT done the same day (**d**) representing hemorrhagic transformation of infarct

9.3.4 Arteriovenous Malformation (AVM)

AVMs represent a connection between arterial and venous systems through a nidus of abnormal vascular channels without an intervening capillary bed. An AVM typically consists of enlarged feeding arteries, tightly packed vascular nidus consisting of shunting vessels and gliotic intervening brain parenchyma, and enlarged draining veins. Aneurysms on feeding arteries or within the nidus serve as potential points of hemorrhage. The risk of rupture is 2% per year in an unruptured AVM [1]. Hemorrhagic arteriovenous malformation (AVM) presentation, increasing age, deep brain location, and exclusive deep venous drainage appear to be independent predictors for AVM hemorrhage during natural history follow-up [25]. On CT, AVM without hemorrhage is seen as a tangle of vessels giving a mass-like

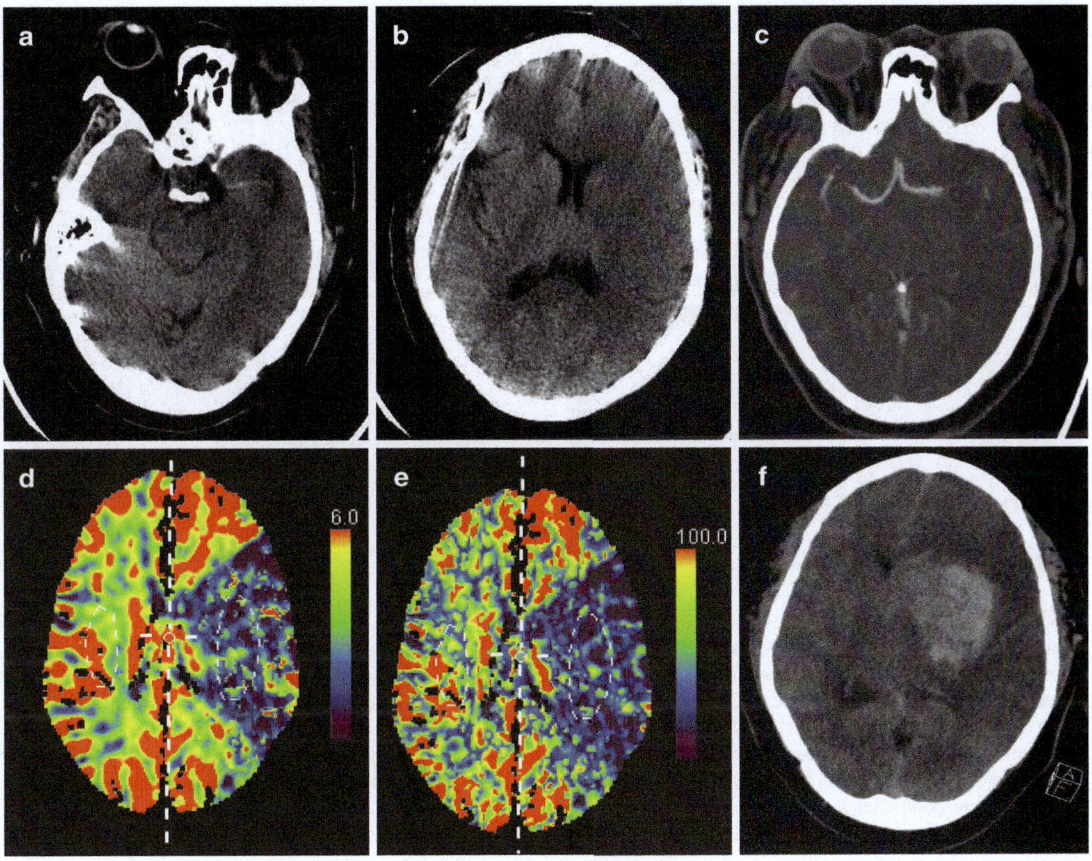

Fig. 9.6 Hemorrhagic transformation of left middle cerebral artery (MCA) territory infarct. A 62-year-old female presented with sudden onset left hemiplegia, left facial droop, and speech difficulty. Computed tomography (CT) head showed a dense left MCA (**a**) with large left MCA distribution infarct (**b**). CT angiogram axial maximum intensity projection (MIP) images showed a proximal M1 MCA cutoff (**c**). CT perfusion cerebral blood volume (CBV) (**d**) and cerebral blood flow (CBF) (**e**) maps showed matched defects in left MCA distribution representing a completed MCA territory infarct. CT done 14 h after presentation due to sudden onset deterioration showed a large hemorrhagic transformation, left to right midline shift, and subfalcine herniation (**f**)

appearance with attenuation similar to blood vessels, often accompanied by calcifications. After intracranial hemorrhage, the hematoma may obscure some or all of the AVM. Enlarged nearby vessels or calcifications can act as a clue to AVM presence. CTA typically shows vascular nidus, enlarged feeding arteries, and draining veins (Fig. 9.7). MRI may show flow voids within the nidus and along the feeding and draining vessels due to a high flow state. Small AVMs or arteriovenous fistulae may not be visible on cross-sectional imaging, and DSA remains the gold standard for detection of underlying vascular malformation in spontaneous ICH caused by these entities. In the setting of a negative initial workup in a young patient, a second evaluation is needed once the mass effect from the hematoma has subsided.

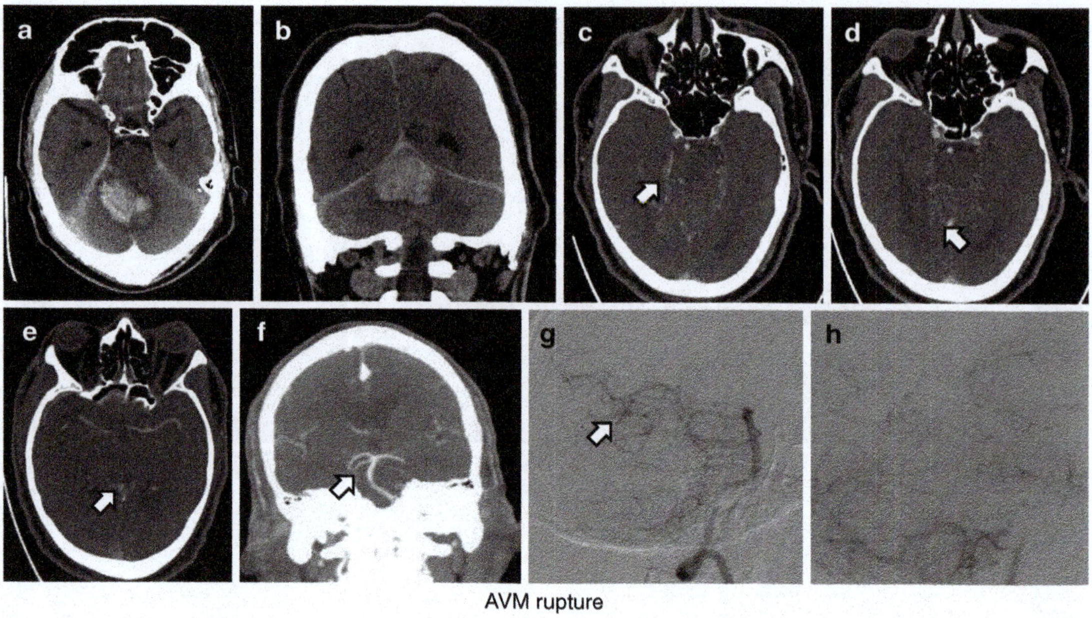

Fig. 9.7 Superior cerebellar hemorrhage due to arteriovenous malformation (AVM) rupture. A 75-year-old male found down in apartment complex. Computed tomography (CT) head (**a**, **b**) showed a right cerebellar intracerebral hemorrhage (ICH). CT angiogram showed a small prominent vascular enhancement (*arrow*, **d**) in superior aspect of right cerebellar hemisphere with enlarged right superior cerebellar artery (*arrow*, **c**) and distended veins draining into straight sinus (*arrow*, **e**). Coronal maximum intensity projection (MIP) image confirmed enlarged right superior cerebellar artery (*arrow*, **f**). Digital subtraction angiography (DSA) confirmed the right superior cerebellar AVM mainly supplied by right superior cerebellar artery (SCA) (*arrow*, **g**), which was embolized utilizing Onyx (**h**)

9.3.5 Dural Arteriovenous Fistula (dAVF)

Dural AVFs are fistulas that connect dural arterial branches to dural veins or venous sinuses. They are generally acquired. Venous sinus thrombosis appears to be a common predisposing factor. Trauma, surgery, and infections can also result in dAVFs. They can present with hemorrhage when venous hypertension becomes severe. A noncontrast CT is done to exclude intracranial hemorrhage. A CT may also show edema related to chronic venous congestion in the brain parenchyma drained by the correspondingly involved dural venous sinus. Enlarged veins or transosseous channels may be visible. On MRI, dilated cortical veins without a parenchymal nidus; thickened dural leaflet; hypertrophied pachymeningeal arteries; dilated, tortuous venous channels; and a thrombosed or stenosed dural venous sinus may be seen. Time-of-flight MRA may depict arterial feeders and fistula site. Arterial spin labeling (ASL) is a relatively new technique that can be utilized for detection of dAVFs and small AVMs. Le et al. found that identifying venous ASL signal intensity improved detection of DAVFs and small AVMs, which may improve triage to DSA in patients with suspected small vascular malformations [26]. DSA remains the gold standard for diagnosis and planning of treatment (Fig. 9.8). The common angiographic findings seen are feeders from pial and dural branches, AV shunting, venous ectasia, stenosis, calcifications, impaired drainage of cerebral parenchyma with delayed venous drainage, and cortical venous collaterals [27].

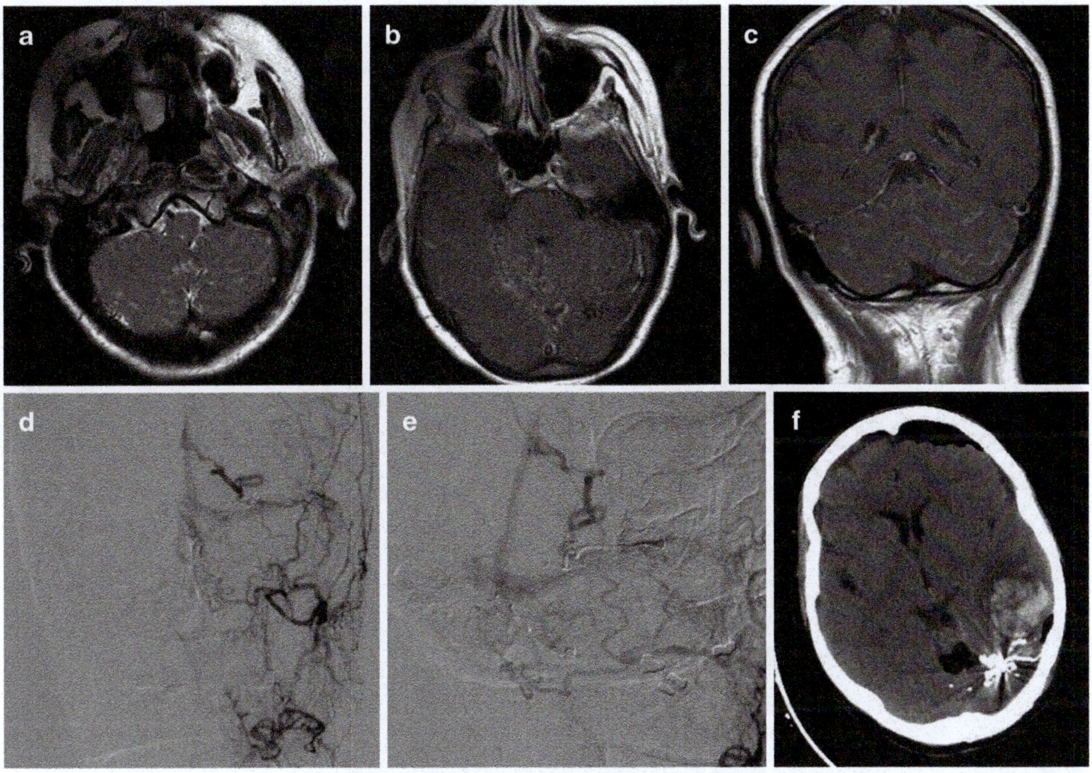

Fig. 9.8 Tentorial dural arteriovenous fistula (dAVF) with postoperative hemorrhage. A 79-year-old female presented initially with vertigo and dizziness and was found to have cerebellar edema and a complex tentorial dAVF supplied by bilateral external carotid artery (ECA) branches and cortical venous drainage in bilateral cerebellar hemispheres on magnetic resonance imaging (MRI) axial T2-weighted (T2W) (**a**), post-contrast axial (**b**) and coronal T1-weighted (T1W) (**c**) images. Digital subtraction angiography (DSA) anteroposterior (AP) (**d**) and oblique (**e**) view showed predominant arterial supply through left ECA branches. Three pedicles had previously been embolized. A right occipital craniotomy was done to disrupt the dAVF. Postoperative computed tomography (CT) (**f**) showed a left temporoparietal intracerebral hemorrhage (ICH) with surrounding edema resulting from a venous hemorrhagic infarct

9.3.6 Cavernous Malformation (CM)

Anatomically, a cavernous malformation is composed of a cluster of thin-walled vessels without elastic fibers or smooth muscles, typically with a rim of hemosiderin-laden gliotic tissue. The hemosiderin is related to chronic microhemorrhage, a hallmark of cavernous malformation. The prospective annual risk of hemorrhage is low, being around 0.6% in one study [28]. In those who have already bled, the annual risk of hemorrhage increases to around 4.5% in the same study. The most common locations are the brainstem (35%), basal ganglia/thalamus (20%), and hemispheric area (48%) [28]. The hemorrhage of CM is smaller in volume compared to that of AVM or dAVF, and so these patients present with less severe clinical symptoms when the hemorrhage is not in the brainstem or spinal cord. On CT, a CM appears iso- to slightly hyperdense with sometimes associated calcifications noted. Faint or peripheral enhancement can sometimes be seen, which is however not a reliable sign. MR imaging is the

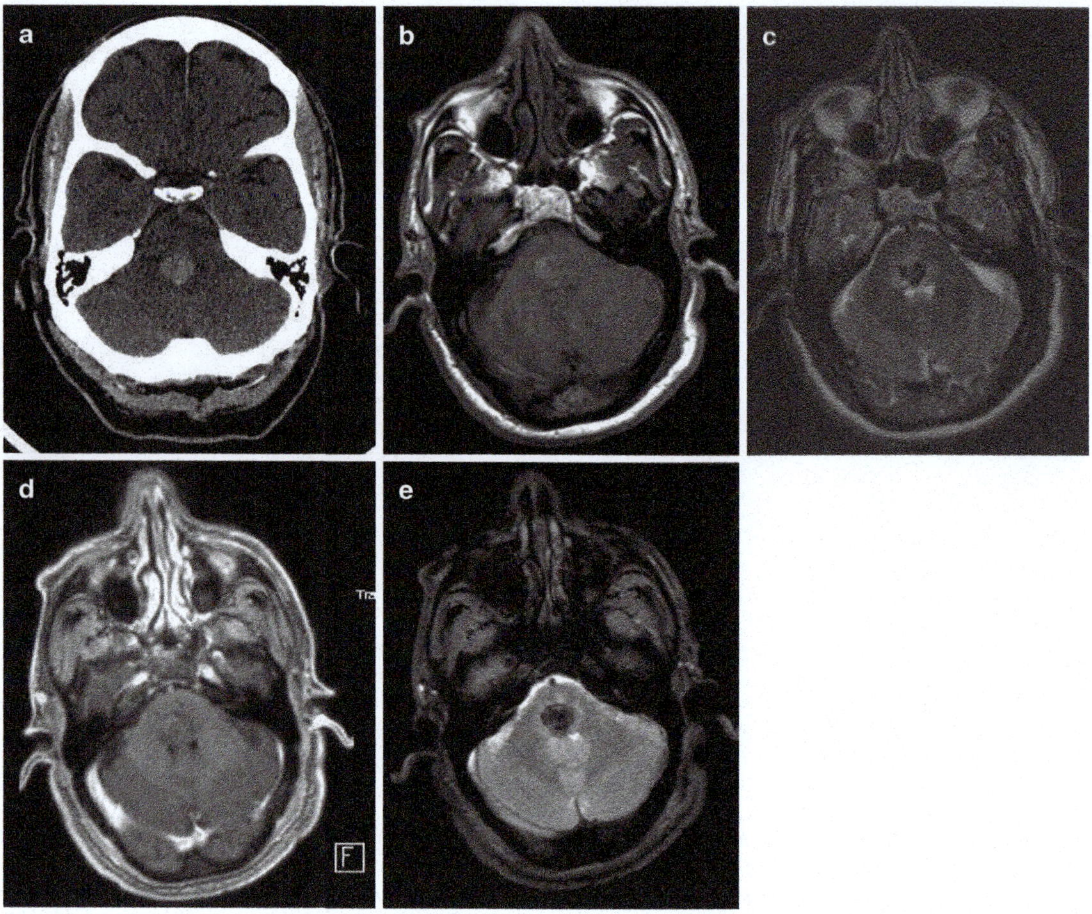

Hemorrhage associated with cavernous malformation

Fig. 9.9 Hemorrhage associated with pontine cavernous malformation. A 70-year-old male presented with horizontal gaze palsy, mild facial weakness, left side loss of proprioception, and ataxia. Computed tomography (CT) head showed a well-circumscribed hyperdensity in dorsal pons (**a**). T1-weighted (T1W) sequence (**b**) showed an area of intrinsic T1 shortening with a broken peripheral rim-like configuration. T2-weighted (T2W) sequence (**c**) showed a hypointense area corresponding to the bleed with surrounding vasogenic edema. No significant enhancement was seen on post-contrast T1W (**d**) sequence. T2*-weighted gradient-echo (GRE) sequence (**e**) showed characteristic "blooming" representing a cavernoma bleed

modality of choice with reticulated, "popcorn-like" mass of variable signal intensity (due to blood products in variable stages of evolution) on T2W sequence with a peripheral hypointense hemosiderin rim. "Blooming" is noted on T2* sequence accentuated on SWI sequence (Fig. 9.9). 3D SWI sequence detected 1.7 times as many lesions as a T2* GRE sequence and 8 times as many as spin-echo T2 sequence [29]. On digital subtraction angiography, the CMs are classically angiographically occult. They are commonly associated with developmental venous anomaly (DVA), which can be found in 8–33% of cases [30]. If resection of a CM is planned, contrast-enhanced CT or MR has to be performed to exclude an associated DVA, as inadvertent resection of all or part of DVA along with a CM can result in a venous infarct. DVA is seen as stellate arrangement of tubular veins joining at collector veins draining to a sinus or ependymal surface resulting in a "caput medusa" appearance.

9.3.7 Cerebral Aneurysm

Most aneurysm ruptures result in SAH, but about 34% are associated with ICH [31]. Such cases likely result from rupture of aneurysms that are pointed into or embedded in cerebral parenchyma (Fig. 9.13). Whenever hematoma extends from the base of the brain and is associated with SAH, rupture of berry aneurysms should be considered in the differential diagnosis and vascular evaluation by CTA or MRA should be obtained.

9.3.8 Aneurysmal and Non-aneurysmal SAH

If we exclude trauma, aneurysmal rupture is the most common cause of subarachnoid hemorrhage. The non-aneurysmal causes of SAH include AVM or AV fistula, intracranial dissection, cerebral venous sinus thrombosis, reversible cerebral vasoconstriction syndrome, vasculitis, use of sympathomimetic drugs, and perimesencephalic hemorrhage. Early diagnosis and treatment is crucial as 61% of deaths occur within 2 days of the initial event [32]. Thirty-day mortality in the same series was 45%. Non-contrast CT is highly sensitive for acute and subacute SAH. High attenuation blood is seen in subarachnoid spaces within sulci, fissures, and basal cisterns. MRI shows hyperacute blood products best on FLAIR and proton-density sequences. FLAIR sequence is sensitive for detection of SAH within 12 h of symptom onset and remains positive in first 2 weeks. But it is not specific as increased signal can be seen in infection, increased protein content in cerebrospinal fluid, and flow-related artifacts [1]. Saccular aneurysms tend to occur at branch points along cerebral vessels, at a bifurcation or the origin of a side branch. They commonly occur at the origin of anterior or posterior communicating arteries, middle cerebral artery bifurcation, basilar tip, or posterior inferior cerebellar artery origin (Fig. 9.10). Non-contrast CT sometimes may show an aneurysm as rounded or lobulated mass within a hematoma. Some aneurysms may be detected on MRI as a flow void or a mass with flow-related artifact in the phase-encoding direction. Dedicated vascular imaging including CTA or MRA is very sensitive for detection of aneurysms. DSA is the gold standard for detection of aneurysm rupture as a cause of SAH, especially for aneurysms less than 3 mm in size. An important cause of nonaneurysmal SAH is perimesencephalic SAH, in which SAH is centered immediately anterior to the midbrain in perimesencephalic cistern, which may or may not extend into ambient and Sylvain cistern. No other identifiable cause of SAH is discovered on vascular imaging, and it has a very good prognosis with low rates of recurrent hemorrhage, hydrocephalus, and vasospasm.

9.3.9 Neoplasms

Among the primary brain tumors having increased vascularity or neovascularity that have increased tendency to ICH are glioblastoma, oligodendroglioma, pituitary adenoma, ependymoma, subependymoma, peripheral neuroectodermal tumor, and epidermoid. Lung, renal and thyroid carcinoma, melanoma and choriocarcinoma are among the secondary deposits with increased chances of ICH. Resultant hemorrhage appears similar to other causes, though there a few features that favor a neoplastic process as a cause. Hematomas associated with neoplastic process have greater amount of surrounding vasogenic edema, are more heterogeneous, have slower degradation of blood products, may have an incomplete hemosiderin rim on MRI, and generally have a thick or nodular enhancement (Fig. 9.11). Like ICH associated with AVM, a small neoplasm relative to hematoma size can be obscured, and delayed imaging after resolution of hemorrhage is strongly recommended in a negative acute workup.

9.3.10 Coagulopathy

There are increased chances of ICH in patients having coagulation disorders, both hereditary

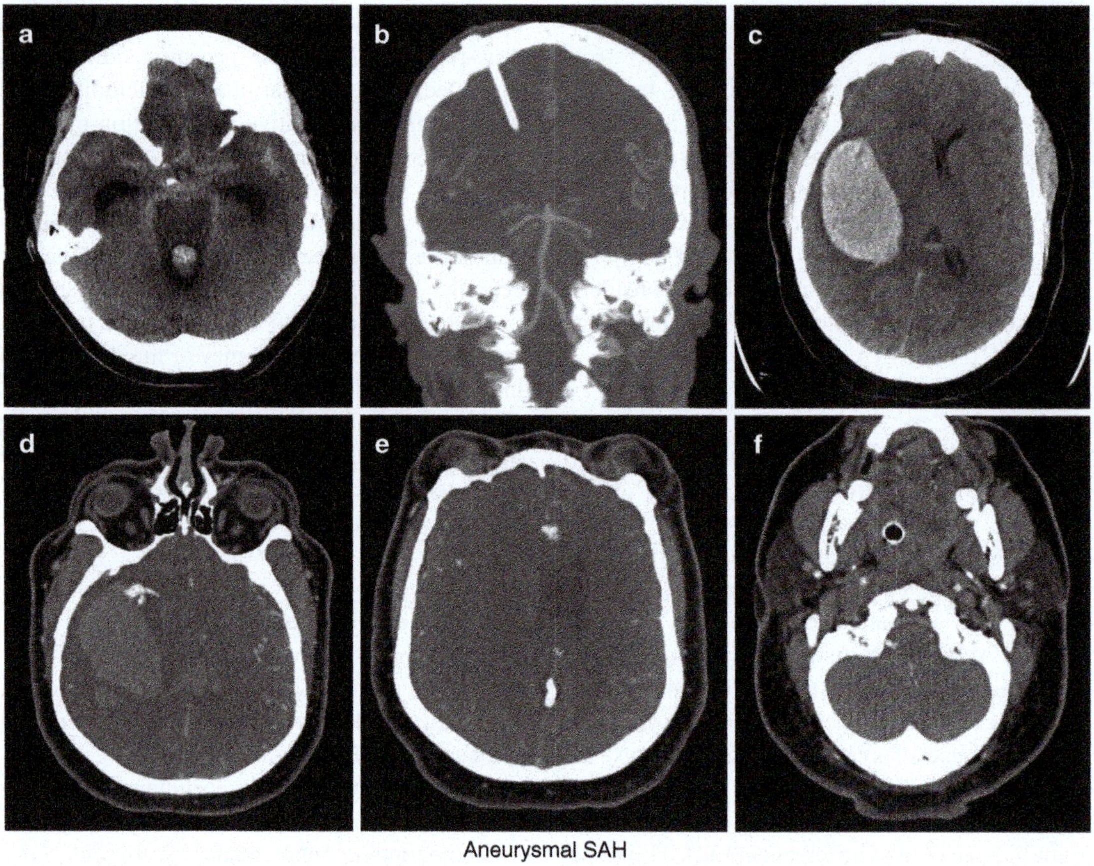

Fig. 9.10 Subarachnoid hemorrhage (SAH) related to basilar and right middle cerebral artery (MCA) bifurcation aneurysm rupture in two different patients. Computed tomography (CT) head (**a**) showed diffuse subarachnoid and intraventricular hemorrhage with hydrocephalus in a 76-year-old female. CT angiogram (CTA) head coronal maximum intensity projection (MIP) (**b**) showed a 6 mm basilar tip aneurysm projecting anterosuperiorly. CT head (**c**) in another 44-year-old hypertensive female presenting with seizures revealed a large right temporal intracerebral hemorrhage (ICH) with intraventricular extension. CTA showed a dysplastic right MCA bifurcation aneurysm (**d**) as cause of this ICH. This was subsequently clipped. Additionally, she showed multiple dysplastic aneurysms including distal anterior cerebral artery (ACA) (**e**) and right posterior inferior cerebellar artery (PICA) (**f**) aneurysm

and acquired. With aging population and increased oral anticoagulant use, there is about seven to tenfold increased risk of ICH in such patients [17]. On non-contrast CT, the ICH appears heterogeneous with tendency to fluid-fluid level formation, rapid progression, and enlargement of size with time and often "swirl" sign (Fig. 9.1) signifying active bleeding. There is overall higher mortality in patients on anticoagulants compared to other causes of ICH.

9.3.11 Venous Sinus Thrombosis

In the largest series to date, 39% of patients with thrombosis of intracerebral veins and/or dural venous sinuses were found to have associated hemorrhage [33]. This is a disease more commonly afflicting women, with 74.5% of the involved patients being female. Clinical course can be extremely insidious and variable. History of dehydration, recent childbirth/abortion, and

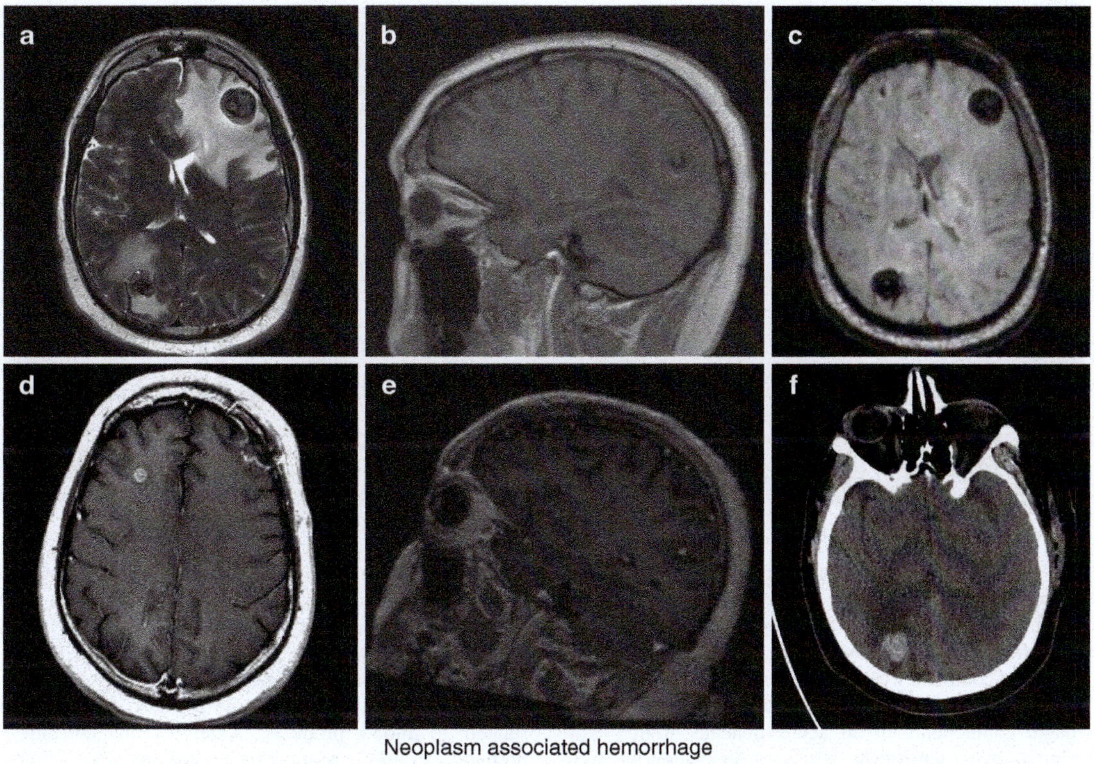

Fig. 9.11 Hemorrhagic brain parenchymal metastases from renal cell carcinoma. A 45-year-old male with renal cell carcinoma presenting with dizziness. Magnetic resonance imaging (MRI) T2-weighted (T2W) sequence (**a**) showed heterogeneously hypointense lesions with significant vasogenic edema in left frontal and right occipital lobe, which showed susceptibility on susceptibility-weighted imaging (SWI) sequence (**c**). On sagittal pre-contrast T1-weighted (T1W) sequence (**b**), the right occipital lesion is isointense with hyperintense inferior rim suggesting blood products. Post-contrast axial (**d**) and sagittal (**e**) sequence show enhancing metastasis in right frontal lobe and nodular enhancement in superior part of right occipital lesion, respectively. Computed tomography (CT) showed hyperdense hemorrhagic metastasis (**f**)

oral contraceptive use can be commonly found in patients. Neuroimaging can play a key role in early diagnosis and treatment. The imaging appearance of hematoma is nonspecific. Identification of secondary signs is essential to make this diagnosis. Associated edema resulting from venous obstruction often precedes hemorrhage and is generally greater than seen with primary ICH. The edema and hemorrhage follow a venous, rather than arterial distribution. Edema is seen as hypodense on CT. MRI can show areas of venous ischemia, and parenchymal edema is best seen on T2W and FLAIR sequences. A hyperattenuating cortical or deep vein adjacent to the hematoma can be seen on a non-contrast CT. Contrast-enhanced CT can show an "empty delta" sign representing nonenhancing thrombus in involved sinuses. Similarly, a 3D contrast-enhanced MR sequence like MPRAGE can show the thrombus as a non-enhancing area in involved sinuses. The appearance of thrombus can vary with time, being isointense on T1 and hyperintense on T2 in the acute phase, hyperintense on T1 and T2 in the subacute phase, and isointense on T1 and hyperintense on T2 in chronic phase [34]. Time-of-flight MR venography improves

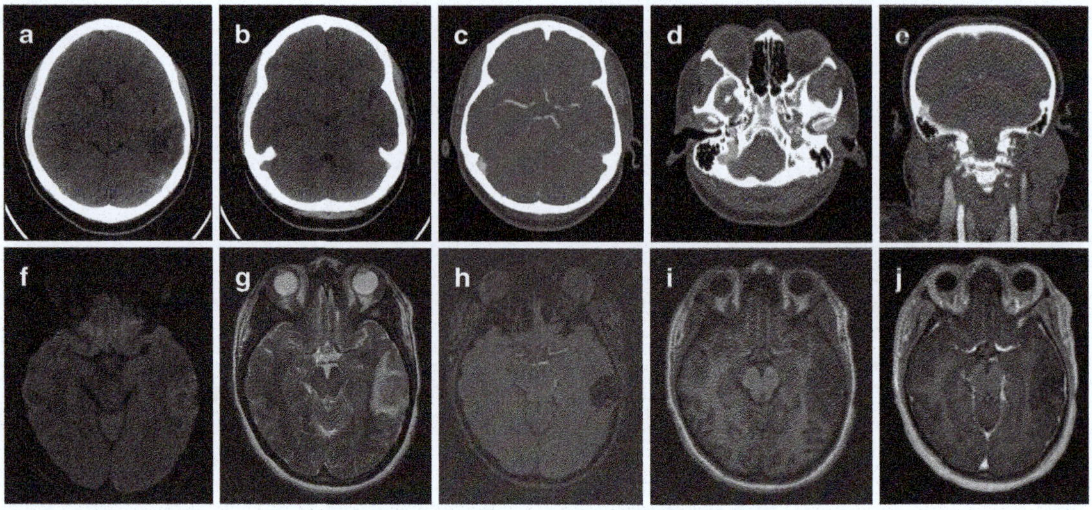

Fig. 9.12 Hemorrhagic venous infarct of left posterior temporal lobe caused by left transverse and sigmoid sinus thrombosis. A 29-year-old female presenting with intractable headache. Computed tomography (CT) head (**a**) showed a confluent hypodensity with hyperdense components in left posterior temporal lobe suggesting hemorrhagic components in an acute/subacute infarct. Note relative hyperdensity in left transverse-sigmoid sinus junction (**b**) suggesting a thrombus. CT angiogram showed thrombosis of left transverse and sigmoid sinus (**c**) as absence of contrast compared to right side, which extends into upper internal jugular vein (**d**). Coronal reconstruction (**e**) shows thrombosed left transverse and sigmoid sinus. Magnetic resonance imaging (MRI) axial diffusion-weighted image (DWI) (**f**) and T2-weighted image (T2W) (**g**) sequence show left temporal hemorrhage with surrounding vasogenic edema. Susceptibility-weighted imaging (SWI) sequence (**h**) shows susceptibility related to blood products. Axial T1 magnetization-prepared rapid acquisition gradient-echo image (MPRAGE) pre- (**i**) and post-contrast (**j**) sequence show hemorrhage with surrounding vasogenic edema and no significant enhancement

detection of sinus thrombosis (Fig. 9.12). There are pitfalls in interpretation, when in-plane signal dropout can mimic thrombosis and T1 bright thrombus can mimic flow. Also awareness of normal variations like hypoplastic/atretic sinuses or arachnoid granulations mimicking thrombus can help differentiate from true pathology. Contrast-enhanced MR and CT venography can further improve diagnostic accuracy.

9.3.12 Infections

Hemorrhage from infectious processes is relatively rare. Cerebral edema disproportionate to the size of ICH on non-contrast CT usually indicates an underlying infective or neoplastic process. Clinical history generally helps differentiate an infective from a neoplastic process as the underlying cause. On MRI, findings which suggest an underlying infective process include hypointense T2 rim surrounding the lesion, leptomeningeal enhancement, and diffusion restriction suggesting an underlying cerebral abscess, presence of subdural empyema, or mycotic aneurysm. A mycotic aneurysm is an aneurysm arising from infection of the arterial wall. Though rare, this can result in an intraparenchymal hemorrhage. Intracranial bleeding, although infrequent, can complicate the evolution of herpes simplex encephalitis and should be borne in mind since its presence may require neurosurgery. Although its presentation may overlap the encephalitic features, the lack of improvement or the worsening of initial symptoms, particularly during the second week of admission, should lead to this suspicion and to perform a neuroimaging study [35]. The hemorrhage is generally in frontal/temporal lobe, insula, and limbic system, common sites of encephalitic involvement (Fig. 9.13). Bacterial endocarditis and human immunodeficiency virus (HIV) infection have also been known to be associated with ICH. Fungal vasculitis resulting from *Aspergillus*, *Candida*, *Coccidioides*, and *Mucorales* species can lead to CNS arterial invasion resulting in cerebral infarction, aneurysm formation, thrombosis, and cerebral hemorrhage.

9.3.13 Vasculitis and Collagen Vascular Diseases

Cerebral vasculitis is defined as the inflammation of blood vessel walls with or without necrosis, leading to luminal obstruction, increased coagulation due to effects of proinflammatory cytokines, alteration of vascular tone, and wide variety of neurologic manifestations. Imaging signs of cerebral vasculitis may be direct (vessel

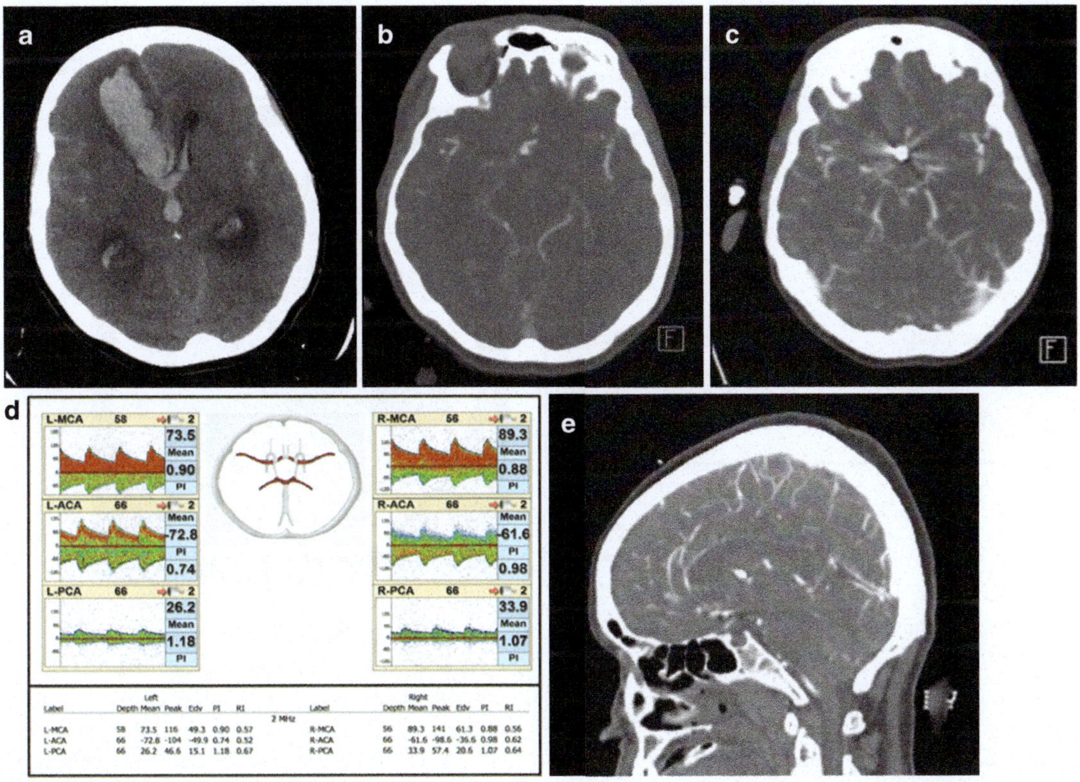

Fig. 9.13 Right frontal lobe intraparenchymal hemorrhage from anterior communicating artery aneurysm rupture followed by transcranial Doppler (TCD) for vasospasm, finally resulting in right anterior cerebral artery (ACA) distribution infarct. A 53-year-old female found down in her car on the side of the road. Computed tomography (CT) head (**a**) showed a large right frontal intraparenchymal hemorrhage, intraventricular hemorrhage, hydrocephalus, and diffuse subarachnoid hemorrhage (SAH). CT angiogram (**b**) showed a 6-mm bilobed ruptured anterior communicating artery aneurysm. This was endovascularly coiled the next day (**c**). TCD done a day later showed normal peak (systolic) and mean flow velocity, waveform, and direction in the anterior cerebral artery (ACA), middle cerebral artery (MCA), and posterior cerebral artery (PCA). There was mild vasospasm in bilateral A2 ACA (**d**) on the sixth postoperative day CT angiogram. TCD on postoperative day 7 (**e**) showed mild to moderate vasospasm in bilateral ACA and MCA. TCD on day 11 (**f**) showed increased vasospasm being severe on right side and moderate on left side. TCD on postoperative day 15 (**g**) showed improved velocities but persistent mild to moderate vasospasm in bilateral ACA and MCA. The Lindegaard ratios on right side were more compared to left side on day 11 (**f**) and 15 (**g**). TCD done on day 25 (**h**) showed Lindegaard ratios having come down. CT done on post-operative day 25 (**i**) at the time of discharge showed a right ACA territory infarct

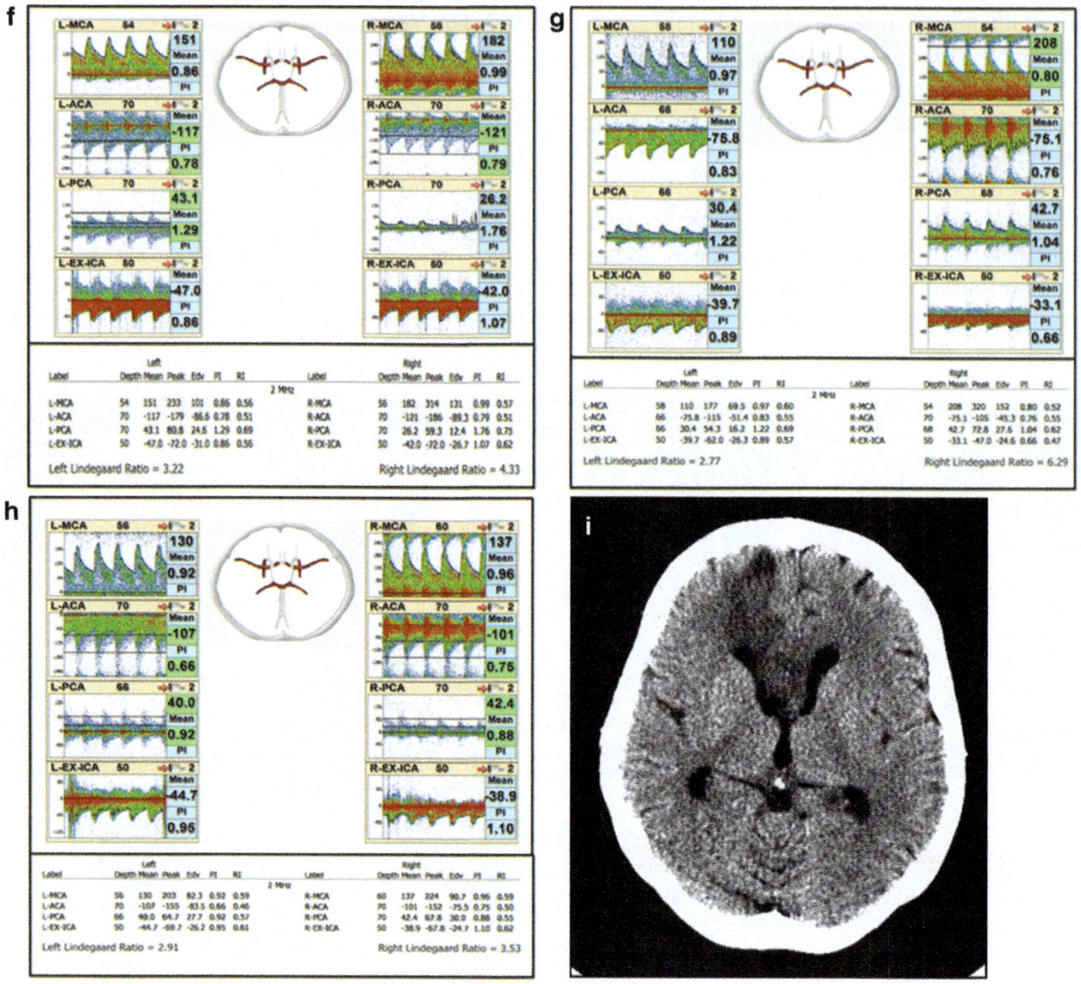

Fig. 9.13 (continued)

wall thickening and enhancement) or indirect (cerebral perfusion deficits, ischemic brain lesions, intracerebral or subarachnoid hemorrhage, vascular stenosis, and leptomeningeal and/or dural enhancement) [36]. MRI is the most commonly used imaging modality in the workup of patients with suspected cerebral vasculitis due to high tissue contrast and different available sequences for imaging. 3D high-resolution post-contrast imaging gives a good visualization of the cerebral vessel walls for diagnosis of CNS vasculitis. Diffusion sequences depict acute infarction, FLAIR sequences improve detection of subarachnoid space, and white matter lesions and SWI sequences depict microhemorrhages better. CT is less sensitive for detection of lesions associated with vasculitis. CT and MR perfusion can show areas of reduced perfusion. CT and MR angiography show vascular luminal compromise. DSA is the gold standard for depiction of vascular luminal stenosis, circumferential or eccentric vascular wall irregularities, aneurysms, collateral flow, and isolated areas of vessel narrowing or occlusion. Collagen vascular diseases like systemic lupus erythematosus (SLE), Sjogren's syndrome, rheumatoid arthritis, and scleroderma have different imaging manifestations, which are beyond the scope of discussion here. Rarely, macro- or microhemorrhages may be associated.

9.3.14 Moyamoya Disease

Moyamoya ("puff of smoke" in Japanese) disease is characterized by progressive occlusion of the terminal segments of intracranial internal carotid arteries and compensatory development of tortuous, dilated collateral networks and impairment of the cerebrovascular reserve capacity [36]. Most cases are found in East Asian countries with a bimodal age distribution, being seen in first and fourth decades. MR imaging shows stenosis or occlusion of the distal internal carotid arteries and the presence of moyamoya vessels with signal voids within the basal ganglia and thalami, as well as ischemia and infarction. SW imaging may depict microbleeding. Contrast-enhanced T1-weighted images show marked leptomeningeal enhancement along the cortical sulci corresponding to leptomeningeal collaterals as well as enhancement of moyamoya vessels. In an institutional study of moyamoya disease, 50% of patients were adults and 50% were of pediatric age group. Fourteen out of 26 patients had infarcts and 10 had hemorrhage at presentation. Of those with ICH, 50% had ICH with intraventricular extension and 30% had primary intraventricular hemorrhage [37]. In moyamoya disease, increased propensity of intraventricular hemorrhage has been proposed to be related to prominent anterior choroidal artery or posterior collateral circulation.

9.3.15 Reversible Cerebral Vasoconstriction Syndrome (RCVS)

The term RCVS refers to various disorders that are characterized by brain vasoconstriction, including Call-Fleming syndrome, postpartum angiopathy, migrainous vasospasm, and benign angiopathy of the CNS, among others [36]. RCVS can be primary or secondary to vasoactive substances like cannabis, selective serotonin reuptake inhibitors, and nasal decongestants. Transient disturbance in cerebral autoregulation is the pathologic mechanism responsible for it. Clinically, it is characterized by thunderclap headache, variable focal neurologic deficits, and multifocal segmental arterial narrowing, all of which resolve in 3 months. Major complications include brain edema (38%), localized convexity subarachnoid hemorrhage (22%), posterior reversible encephalopathy syndrome (PRES 9–14%), and less frequently ischemic or hemorrhagic stroke [38].

9.3.16 Vasoactive Drugs

MR imaging pattern in drug-induced vasculitis is inconsistent and depends on the vessels involved. Cocaine may lead to vasculitis, vasospasm, and increased platelet aggregation, resulting in infarction, leukoencephalopathy, and hemorrhage [36]. Cocaine-induced cerebral hemorrhage includes both intraparenchymal and subarachnoid hemorrhage. Intranasal administration results in hemorrhage being twice as common as ischemic stroke [39]. Chronic cocaine dependency has been linked to a moyamoya- like vasculitis with obstructed vessels and extensive collateral circulation. DSA and MRA may show vasculitis and vasospasm. Stroke and hemorrhage are seen less frequently in heroin users than in cocaine users. Spongiform leukoencephalopathy is far more common in heroin users [39] but has been described in cocaine users. Heroin-associated infarcts often include globus pallidus. Vasospasm and arteritis are described with amphetamine use resulting in ischemia and infarcts. MDMA (3,4 methylenedioxymethamphetamine), also known as ecstasy, results in ischemia and strokes [39]. Stimulation of 5 hydroxytryptamine (5HT-2A) receptors results in prolonged vasospasm and necrosis of the areas with high concentration of these receptors, including occipital cortex and globus pallidus. Cannabis use can result in ischemic infarcts related to vasospasm and vasculitis in areas of CB1 cannabinoid receptor distribution in basal ganglia, substantia nigra, dentate gyrus of hippocampus, limbic cortices, and cerebellum [39].

9.4 Neurophysiology Tests Including Transcranial Doppler

Transcranial Doppler (TCD) ultrasound is a noninvasive means of monitoring of physiologic hemodynamic variables. It is a portable technique for evaluating the intracranial vasculature. Its most useful clinical application is in the detection of vasospasm involving the cerebral vessels following subarachnoid hemorrhage due to aneurysm rupture. It has become an integral part of monitoring and managing patients with subarachnoid hemorrhage in the neurologic intensive care unit. Transcranial ultrasound originated as a "blind" nonimaging study in which pulsed Doppler technology was used [40]. Spectral waveforms were utilized for identification of major intracranial vessels with the depth of the vessel from the skull, direction of blood flow, and orientation of transducer aiding in identification of the individual vessels. Presently, the use of gray-scale imaging, color Doppler flow imaging, and spectral Doppler (sometimes together referred to as Triplex imaging) allows direct visualization of blood vessels, simplifies flow velocity measurements, and increases accuracy for vasospasm detection. TCD allows measurement of systolic and diastolic velocities, allowing the calculation of mean flow velocities (MFV) and Lindegaard ratio, which when elevated correlate with the severity of vasospasm. It also helps differentiate vasospasm from physiologic conditions like hyperemia and autoregulation. Radiographically, detectable vasospasm has been estimated to occur in 50–70% of patients after aneurysm rupture, with approximately half of those affected manifesting signs and symptoms usually within 5–15 days after onset of hemorrhage [41]. Medical treatment of these patients consists of triple H therapy consisting of induced hypertension, hemodilution, and hypervolemia to increase cerebral perfusion. If this is ineffective, vasodilator can be injected intra-arterially. Careful monitoring of patients with subarachnoid hemorrhage is necessary to detect vasospasm early before clinical manifestations of ischemia are seen and institute prophylactic treatment accordingly.

Institutional protocols may vary. But generally, spectral waveforms are obtained bilaterally from the proximal, mid, and distal middle cerebral arteries (MCA), and single measurements are obtained bilaterally in the visualized anterior cerebral (ACA), posterior cerebral (PCA), and terminal portion of the internal carotid arteries (ICA). Generally speaking, the narrower the vessel diameter and the greater the severity of vasospasm, the higher is the flow velocity. Generally, for MCA, peak systolic velocity (PSV) <200 cm/s and MFV <120 cm/s are considered reliable predictor of absence of vasospasm. PSV of 200–300 cm/s and MFV 120–200 cm/s indicate mild to moderate vasospasm and PSV >300 cm/s and MFV >200 cm/s indicate severe vasospasm [40]. For PCA, PSV >120 cm/s and MFV >85 cm/s indicate vasospasm, while for ACA, PSV >120 cm/s and MFV >80 cm/s are indicative of vasospasm [40]. Increase in flow velocities can be seen in physiologic conditions like hyperemia and autoregulation. To correct for and distinguish between these dynamic states, Lindegaard et al. [42] proposed the use of a ratio derived from MFV in the MCA to MFV in ipsilateral extracranial ICA. A Lindegaard ratio of 3–6 is indicative of mild to moderate vasospasm and a ratio of greater than 6 is indicative of severe vasospasm. Elevated flow velocities with Lindegaard ratio less than 3 are suggestive of hyperemia or another physiologic or induced state. Serial Doppler studies (Fig. 9.13) are needed to monitor vasospasm, as vasospasm is not immediately evident, but manifests later, usually in first 2 weeks after hemorrhage.

Utilizing gray scale and B-mode imaging of triplex ultrasound, size and volume of hematoma, presence or absence of intraventricular extension of ICH, and midline shift can also be assessed. To conclude, the chief benefits of TCD are non-exposure of ionizing radiations and nephrotoxic contrast agents, portability, and noninvasive nature of the examination. However, the study quality is operator dependent and can vary according to institutional protocol. False-positive results can lead to morbidity from unnecessary hemodynamic augmentation or neurointerventional procedures, and false-negative results can lead to missed window of opportunity to prevent the patient from delayed cerebral ischemia.

Vasospasm can also be assessed by CTA and DSA. DSA has the added advantage of the ability to administer vasodilator drugs intra-arterially for relief of vasospasm. Specific vessels showing reduced luminal caliber can be identified by CTA and DSA, commonly arteries in proximity to SAH or ICH. Both these techniques are invasive and require administration of contrast.

Other neurophysiological parameters that can be monitored include measurement of intracranial pressure (ICP) and mean arterial pressure (MAP), both of which can be used to derive cerebral perfusion pressure (CPP). Continuous EEG monitoring following SAH can detect increased number of subclinical seizures and may predict delayed cerebral ischemia many hours in advance [43]. Other less commonly used neurophysiology monitoring methods include near-infrared spectroscopy, brain tissue monitoring, and jugular venous oxygen saturation.

Conclusions

The timely and accurate identification of hemorrhagic stroke is essential in the clinical management of patients presenting with acute stroke symptoms. Besides the routine blood tests, neuroimaging plays a key role in diagnosis, treatment, and prognostication of patients with ICH. Cross-sectional imaging including non-contrast CT is the initial investigation modality with MRI including blood-sensitive T2* and SWI, DWI, FLAIR, and post-contrast T1W sequences providing additional information to narrow down the differential diagnosis. Vascular imaging utilizing CTA, MRA, and DSA provides additional information about vascular status including ruptured aneurysms, vasculitis, and venous sinus thrombosis. Transcranial Doppler is a noninvasive effective diagnostic tool to detect and monitor vasospasm in patients with subarachnoid hemorrhage due to ruptured aneurysms in critical carc settings.

References

1. Smith SD, Eskey CJ. Hemorrhagic stroke. Radiol Clin N Am. 2011;49:27–45.
2. Van Asch CJ, Luitse MJ, Rinkel GJ, et al. Incidence, case fatality, and functional outcome of intracerebral haemorrhage over time, according to age, sex, and ethnic origin: a systematic review and meta-analysis. Lancet Neurol. 2010;9:167–76.
3. Brott T, Broderick J, Kothari R, et al. Early hemorrhage growth in patients with intracerebral hemorrhage. Stroke. 1997;28:1–5.
4. Arnold DM. Bleeding complications in immune thrombocytopenia. Hematology Am Soc Hematol Educ Program. 2015;2015:237–42.
5. Behrouz R, Hafeez S, Miller CM. Admission leukocytosis admission leukocytosis in intracerebral hemorrhage: associated factors and prognostic implications. Neurocrit Care. 2015;23:370–3.
6. McEvoy AW, Kitchen ND, Thomas DG. Lesson of the week: intracerebral hemorrhage in young adults: the emerging importance of drug misuse. BMJ. 2000;320:1322–4.
7. Martin-Schild S, Albright KC, Hallevi H, et al. Intracerebral hemorrhage in cocaine users. Stroke. 2010;41:680–4.
8. Parizel PM, Makkat S, Van Miert E, et al. Intracranial hemorrhage: principles of CT and MRI interpretation. Eur Radiol. 2001;11:1770–83.
9. Domingues R, Rossi C, Cordonnier C. Diagnostic evaluation for nontraumatic intracerebral hemorrhage. Neurol Clin. 2015;33:315–28.
10. Wagemans BA, Klinkenberg S, Postma AA. Teaching neuroImages: swirl sign and spot sign in intraparenchymal hematoma. Neurology. 2016;87:e225–6.
11. Kreel L, Kay R, Woo J, Wong HY, et al. The radiological (CT) and clinical sequelae of primary intracerebral haemorrhage. Br J Radiol. 1991;64:1096–100.
12. Hemphill JC III, Greenberg SM, Anderson CS, et al. Guidelines for the management of spontaneous intracerebral hemorrhage: a guideline for healthcare professionals from the American Heart Association/American Stroke Association. Stroke. 2015;46:2032–60.
13. Kidwell CS, Chalela JA, Saver JL, et al. Comparison of MRI and CT for detection of acute intracerebral hemorrhage. JAMA. 2004;292:1823–30.
14. Nandigram RN, Viswanathan A, Delgado P, et al. MR imaging detection of cerebral microbleeds: effect of susceptibility-weighted imaging, section thickness, and field strength. AJNR. 2009;30:338–43.
15. Wycliffe ND, Choe J, Holshouser B, et al. Reliability in detection of hemorrhage in acute stroke by a new three-dimensional gradient recalled echo susceptibility-weighted imaging technique compared to computed tomography: a retrospective study. J Magn Reson Imaging. 2004;20:372–7.
16. Wardlaw JM, Smith C, Dichgans M. Mechanisms of sporadic cerebral small vessel disease: insights from neuroimaging. Lancet Neurol. 2013;12:483–97.
17. Hakimi R, Garg A. Imaging of hemorrhagic stroke. Continuum (Minneap Minn). 2016;22:1424–50.
18. Morgenstern LB, Hemphill JC III, Anderson C, et al. Guidelines for the management of spontaneous intracerebral hemorrhage: a guideline for healthcare professionals from the American Heart Association/American Stroke Association. Stroke. 2010;41:2108–29.

19. Sacco RL, Kasner SE, Broderick JP, et al. An updated definition of stroke for the 21st century: a statement for healthcare professionals from the American Heart Association/American Stroke Association. Stroke. 2013;44:2064–89.
20. Qureshi AI, Tuhrim S, Broderick JP, et al. Spontaneous intracerebral hemorrhage. N Engl J Med. 2001;344:1450–60.
21. Vinters HV. Cerebral amyloid angiopathy. A critical review. Stroke. 1987;18:311–24.
22. Smith EE, Greenberg SM. Clinical diagnosis of cerebral amyloid angiopathy: validation of the Boston criteria. Curr Atheroscler Rep. 2003;5:260–6.
23. Wolpert SM, Bruckmann H, Greenlee R, et al. Neuroradiologic evaluation of patients with acute stroke treated with recombinant tissue plasminogen activator. The rt-PA Acute Stroke Study Group. AJNR. 1993;14:3–13.
24. Berger C, Fiorelli M, Steiner T, et al. Hemorrhagic transformation of ischemic brain tissue: asymptomatic or symptomatic? Stroke. 2001;32:1330–5.
25. Stapf C, Mast H, Sciacca RR, et al. Predictors of hemorrhage in patients with untreated brain arteriovenous malformation. Neurology. 2006;66:1350–5.
26. Le TT, Fischbein NJ, Andre JB, et al. Identification of venous signal on arterial spin labeling improves diagnosis of dural arteriovenous fistulas and small arteriovenous malformations. AJNR. 2012;33: 61–8.
27. Gupta A, Periakaruppan A. Intracranial dural arteriovenous fistulas: a review. Indian J Radiol Imaging. 2009;19:43–8.
28. Kondziolka D, Lunsford LD, Kestle JR. The natural history of cerebral cavernous malformations. J Neurosurg. 1995;83:820–4.
29. deSouza JM, Domingues RC, Cruz LC Jr, et al. Susceptibility-weighted imaging for the evaluation of patients with familial cerebral cavernous malformations: a comparison with T2-weighted fast spin-echo and gradient-echo sequences. AJNR. 2008;29: 154–8.
30. Rammos SK, Maina R, Lanzino G. Developmental venous anomalies: current concepts and implications for management. Neurosurgery. 2009;65: 20–9.
31. Pasqualin A, Bazzan A, Cavazzani P, et al. Intracranial hematomas following aneurysmal rupture: experience with 309 cases. Surg Neurol. 1986;25:6–17.
32. Broderick JP, Brott TG, Duldner JE, et al. Initial and recurrent bleeding are the major causes of death following subarachnoid hemorrhage. Stroke. 1994;25:1342–7.
33. Ferro JM, Canhao P, STam J, et al. Prognosis of cerebral vein and dural sinus thrombosis: results of the international study on cerebral vein and dural sinus thrombosis (ISCVT). Stroke. 2004;35:664–70.
34. Walecki J, Mruk B, Nawrocka-Laskus E, et al. Neuroimaging of cerebral venous thrombosis (CVT)—old dilemma and the new diagnostic methods. Pol J Radiol. 2015;80:368–73.
35. Rodriguez-Sainz A, Escalza-Cortina I, Guio-Carrion L, et al. Intracerebral hematoma complicating herpes simplex encephalitis. Clin Neurol Neurosurg. 2013;115:2041–5.
36. Abdel Razek AA, Alvarez H, Bagg S, et al. Imaging spectrum of CNS vasculitis. Radiographics. 2014;34:873–94.
37. Srivastava T, Sannegowda RB, Mittal RS, et al. An institutional experience of 26 patients with Moyamoya disease: a study from Northwest India. Ann Indian Acad Neurol. 2014;17:182–6.
38. Ducros A. Reversible cerebral vasoconstriction syndrome. Lancet Neurol. 2012;11:906–17.
39. Tamrazi B, Almast J. Your brain on drugs: imaging of drug-related changes in the central nervous system. Radiographics. 2012;32:701–19.
40. Kirsch JD, Mathur M, Johnson MH, et al. Advances in transcranial Doppler US: imaging ahead. Radiographics. 2013;33:E1–E14.
41. Keyrouz SG, Diringer MN. Clinical review: prevention and therapy of vasospasm in subarachnoid hemorrhage. Crit Care. 2007;11:220.
42. Lindegaard KF, Nornes H, Bakke SJ, et al. Cerebral vasospasm diagnosis by means of angiography and blood velocity measurements. Acta Neurochir. 1989;100:12–24.
43. Kondziella D, Friberg CK, Wellwood I, et al. Continuous EEG monitoring in aneurysmal subarachnoid hemorrhage: a systematic review. Neurocrit Care. 2015;22:450–61.

10 Medical Management of Hemorrhagic Stroke

Jeong-Ho Hong

10.1 Identification of Risk Factors and Outcome in the Acute Stage of Hemorrhagic Stroke

10.1.1 Early Assessment for Risk Factors

Identification of risk factors that can or cannot be modified is a crucial step in acute hemorrhage stroke. Spontaneous intracerebral hemorrhage (ICH) and aneurysmal subarachnoid hemorrhage (SAH) as two common subcategories of hemorrhagic strokes will be mainly discussed in this chapter. Fifty to seventy percent of patients with spontaneous ICH have a history of hypertension, and hypertensive vasculopathy is the most common etiology of spontaneous ICH. Cerebral amyloid angiopathy (CAA) in that amyloid protein deposits within the small- to medium-sized cerebral vessels and leptomeninges is an important cause of primary lobar ICH in the elderly. It is closely related to the presence of cerebral microbleeds (CMBs) reflecting cerebral-hemorrhage-prone status [1]. History of genetic risk and genetic test also helps with initial assessment and treatment. Patients carrying the apolipoprotein E (APOE) ε2 or ε4 alleles appear to be at important risk for CAA-related ICH. Methylenetetrahydrofolate reductase (MTHFR) polymorphism is not uncommon but an important genetic defect of spontaneous ICH. Bleeding diatheses like hematological malignancy and use of antiplatelet agents, anticoagulants like vitamin K antagonist (VKA, e.g., warfarin), and recently introduced non-vitamin K antagonists, so-called new oral anticoagulants (NOAC), increase the risk of ICH. Based on this, a careful history taking and laboratory tests including coagulation profiles should be done.

Rapid neuroimaging, in particular CT of the brain, is an essential tool for diagnosis, management, and follow-up of ICH and SAH patients. It accurately documents the size and location of the hematoma, the presence and extent of mass effect, and the presence of intraventricular hemorrhage (IVH) and hydrocephalus. Cerebral aneurysms and vascular malformations such as arteriovenous malformation, venous angioma, cavernous hemangioma, etc. are the underlying pathological conditions associated with hemorrhagic stroke. Vascular imaging using contrast CT angiography or MR angiography of the intracranial arteries are useful screening tools for this. In particular, the CT angiography can evaluate the size, shape, neck, and count of aneurysm in the SAH patients. It is necessary to confirm the presence of cerebral aneurysm by transfemoral cerebral angiography as gold standard diagnostic tool even if the initial CT angiography is negative [2].

J.-H. Hong
Department of Neurology, Keimyung University
Dongsan Medical Center, Daegu, South Korea

S.-H. Lee (ed.), *Stroke Revisited: Hemorrhagic Stroke*, Stroke Revisited,
https://doi.org/10.1007/978-981-10-1427-7_10

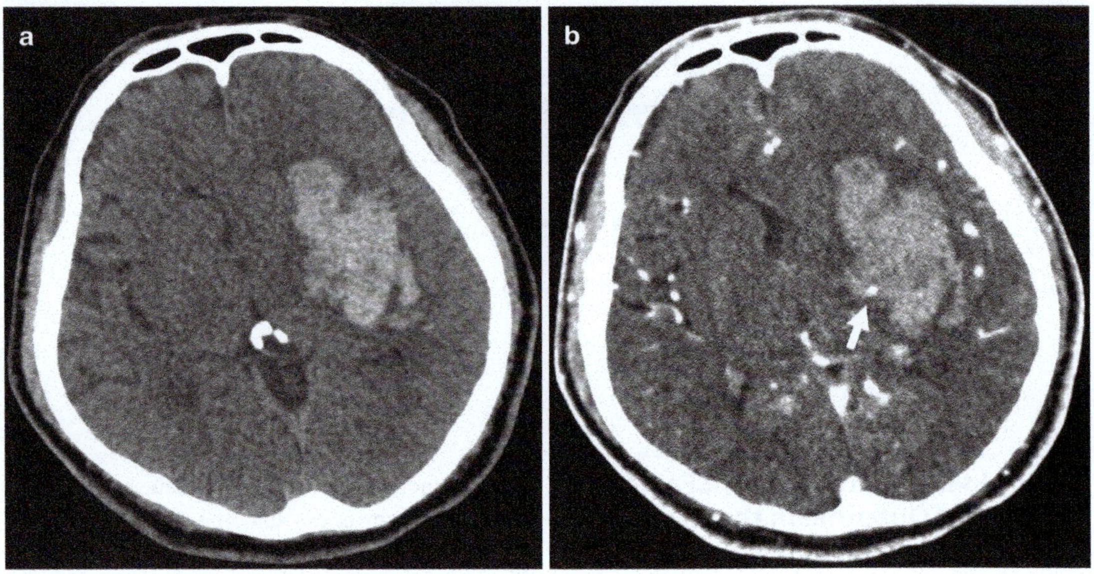

Fig 10.1 Spot sign. Baseline non-contrast computed tomography (CT) (**a**) and CT angiography (**b**). Contrast extravasation (*arrow*), so-called spot sign, seen in the hematoma of a patient with acute intracerebral hemorrhage is shown on only CT angiography

The presence of contrast within the hematoma, called a "spot sign," links closely to ICH expansion, clinical deterioration, and poor outcomes (Fig. 10.1) [3]. Emergency follow-up CT scanning is often required to identify the rapid enlargement of hematoma when there is a change in clinical signs or state of alertness in order to monitor changes in the size of the lesion and ventricular system and to detect shifts. Secondary hematoma expansion occurs about one third of spontaneous ICH within 24 h of onset [4]. Spot sign score calculated by number of the spot sign (≥3 vs. 1–2), maximum axial dimension (≥5 mm vs. 1–4 mm), and maximum attenuation (of Hounsfield units ≥180 vs. 120–179) is one of the strongest factors for significant hematoma expansion in spontaneous ICH (Table 10.1) [5].

10.1.2 Disease Severity and Outcome Prediction

Baseline severity score and initial outcome prediction based on clinical and radiological findings are very important and should be performed because they help physicians to determine the major pathways of treatment. Prognostic model for predicting 30-day mortality among patients with spontaneous ICH is the ICH score allocated points for Glasgow Coma Scale score, ICH volume, presence of intraventricular hemorrhage, age, and infratentorial lesion. It is well validated externally and used widely. Table 10.2 shows detailed ICH score and each mortality [6].

The Fisher grade is the most widely used index of vasospasm risk of SAH. However, some limitations have been raised: lower incidence of

Table 10.1 Spot sign score

Criteria		Pts	SSS	Risk of hematoma expansion (%)
No. of spot signs	1–2	1	0	2%
	≥3	2	1	33%
Maximum axial dimension (mm)	1–4	0	2	50%
	≥5	1	3	94%
Maximum attenuation (HU)	120–179	0		
	≥180	1	4	100%

Reproduced by permission of Stroke [5]
HU Hounsfield units, *Pts* Points, *SSS* Spot sign score

Table 10.2 ICH score

Criteria		Pts	ICH score	Mortality
GCS	3–4	2	0	0%
	5–12	1		
	13–15	0	1	13%
ICH volume	≥30 cm^3	1	2	26%
	<30 cm^3	0		
IVH	Yes	1	3	72%
	No	0	4	97%
Location	Infratentorial	1		
	Supratentorial	0	5	100%
Age	≥80 years	1	6	100%
	<80 years	0		

Reproduced by permission of Stroke [6]
GCS Glasgow Coma Scale, *ICH* intracranial hemorrhage, *IVH* intraventricular hemorrhage, *Pts* Points

Table 10.3 Fisher scale and modified Fisher scale of subarachnoid hemorrhage

		% Classified to grade	% Within grade with symptomatic vasospasm
Fisher scale			
1	Focal thin SAH	8.1	21
2	Diffuse thin SAH	10.9	25
3	Thick SAH present	67.7	37
4	Focal or diffuse thin SAH, with ICH or IVH	13.3	31
Modified Fisher scale			
1	Focal or diffuse thin SAH, no IVH	21.6	24
2	Focal or diffuse thin SAH, with IVH	10.8	33
3	Thick SAH present, no IVH	33.9	33
4	Thick SAH present, with IVH	33.7	40

Reproduced by permission of Neurosurgery [8]

vasospasm in the group 4 than group 3, low correlation between each grade and the incidence of symptomatic vasospasm, and inevitable interpersonal variability in assessing the estimated blood volume. To make up for this, the scale was modified, called the modified Fisher scale (mFS), by Claassen et al. The mFS emphasizes the presence or absence of IVH because IVH increases the risk of symptomatic vasospasm (Table 10.3) [7, 8].

In terms of the severity of SAH, Hunt and Hess grade and the World Federation of Neurological Surgeons (WFNS) grade are the two most commonly used. WFNS grade incorporates the Glasgow Coma Scale for level of consciousness and presence of focal neurological deficits to determine disease severity and to predict outcomes. The presence or absence of a focal neurological deficit defined as either aphasia and/or motor deficit is the criterion for dividing the classifications into grade 2 and 3 (Table 10.4) [9].

Table 10.4 World Federation of Neurosurgical Societies grading scale

Grade	Criteria
I	GCS 15, no focal deficit
II	GCS 13–14, without focal deficit
III	GCS 13–14 with focal neurological deficit
IV	GCS 7–12, with or without deficit
V	GCS <7, with or without deficit

Reproduced by permission of Journal of Neurology, Neurosurgery, and Psychiatry [9]

Hunt and Hess grade was originally intended as an index of surgical risk in patients with intracranial aneurysm [10]. A higher grade predicts a poor clinical outcome and lower likelihood of survival. Although this is also one of the most popular grading systems to categorize the severity of SAH, it has been criticized for poor interobserver reliability and reproducibility and challenging to differentiate between grades 1 and 2. The intensity of headache is subjective and arbitrary: mild headache for grade 1 vs. moderate to severe headache for grade 2 (Table 10.5). While the ICH score, Hunt and Hess grade, and WFNS grade demonstrate the severity of the disease, it does not directly affect treatment modalities.

10.2 General Medical Management in Intracerebral Hemorrhage

Initially, patients with hemorrhagic stroke should be monitored after diagnosis and taken care of in an intensive care unit or dedicated stroke unit with skilled physicians and trained nurses because early neurologic deterioration can often occur within the first 1 or 2 days after onset. Some data showed that the patients admitted to a specialized neuroscience intensive care unit (ICU) showed reduced mortality compared to those admitted to the general ICU. These units should furnish the monitoring of blood pressure (BP), heart rate, electrocardiograph, oxygen saturation, and body temperature. The increased intracranial pressure (ICP), cerebral perfusion pressure (CPP), and continuous intra-arterial BP can be also monitored.

Table 10.5 Hunt and Hess grade

Grade	Criteria	Mortality (%)
I	Asymptomatic or mild headache and slight nuchal rigidity	0–5
II	Severe headache, stiff neck, no neurological deficit except cranial nerve palsy	2–10
III	Drowsy or confused, mild focal neurological deficit	10–15
IV	Stuporous, moderate or severe hemiparesis	60–70
V	Coma, decerebrate posturing	70–100

Reproduced by permission of Journal of Neurosurgery [10]

10.2.1 Reversal of Anticoagulation

First of all, antithrombotics should be discontinued immediately after the onset of hemorrhage in ICH patients, and appropriate agents for reversal of anticoagulant effect should be considered to restrict hematoma expansion and rebleeding (Table 10.6). For patients without antithrombotic-associated ICH, the use of recombinant activated factor VII (rFVIIa) limits hematoma expansion. However, there was an increase in arterial thromboembolic risk with no clear clinical benefit [11]. Hence, the use of rFVIIa is not recommended in noncoagulopathic ICH.

Table 10.6 Guideline for reversal of antithrombotics in intracranial hemorrhage

Antithrombotics	Reversal agent
Vitamin K antagonists	If INR ≥1.4: Vit. K 10 mg IV, plus three- or four-factor PCC IV or fresh frozen plasma 10–15 mL/kg IV if PCC not available
Direct factor Xa inhibitors	Activated charcoal (50 g) within 2 h of ingestion Activated PCC 50 units/kg IV or four-factor PCC 50 units/kg IV Consider andexanet alfa or aripazine (approval pending)
Direct thrombin inhibitors	Activated charcoal (50 g) within 2 h of ingestion Idarucizumab 5 g IV Consider idarucizumab redosing for refractory bleeding after initial administration
Unfractionated heparin	Protamine 1 mg IV for every 100 units of heparin administered in the previous 2–3 h (up to 50 mg in a single dose)
LMWHs (enoxaparin)	Dosed within 8 h: Protamine 1 mg IV per 1 mg enoxaparin (up to 50 mg in a single dose) Dosed within 8–12 h: Protamine 0.5 mg IV per 1 mg enoxaparin (up to 50 mg in a single dose)
Antiplatelet agents	Desmopressin 0.3–0.4 μg/kg IV If neurosurgical intervention: Platelet transfusion

Reproduced by permission of Neurocritical Care [14]
PCC prothrombin complex concentrates, *LMWH* low-molecular-weight heparin, *rFVIIa* recombinant factor VIIa

10.2.1.1 Antiplatelet-Associated Intracerebral Hemorrhage

The effects of antiplatelet drugs on the outcome of ICH are uncertain because some of the research results were conflicting each other. Even the usefulness of platelet transfusions in ICH patients with a history of antiplatelet use still remains unproven. Subgroup analysis of one randomized trial demonstrated platelet transfusion was associated with the decrease rate of postoperative hemorrhage recurrence, disability and mortality, and less postoperative hematoma volume in aspirin-sensitive patients with acute basal ganglia ICH undergoing craniotomy and hematoma evacuation [12]. Most recently, however, the results of PATCH (platelet transfusion in cerebral hemorrhage) trial, which was the first randomized trials to compare the effects of platelet transfusion with standard care in acute antiplatelet medication-related ICH, were reported. PATCH investigators do not recommend platelet transfusion for patients with antiplatelet-associated ICH because of the results on higher rate of serious adverse events and poor clinical outcomes [13]. One clinical trial on the effectiveness of platelet transfusion in patients with ICH is ongoing. Guidelines from neurocritical care society published in 2016 suggest consideration of desmopressin 0.4 μg/kg IV administration for reversal of antiplatelet agents in ICH associate with antiplatelet [14]. Desmopressin, an analog of vasopressin, stimulates the release of von Willebrand factor from endothelial cell and increases the endothelial release of factor VIII and platelet membrane glycoprotein expression, thereby promoting platelet adhesion to the endothelium. However, this recommendation is a low-quality evidence.

10.2.1.2 Anticoagulant-Associated Intracerebral Hemorrhage

With an aging population and an increasing prevalence of atrial fibrillation, VKA and NOAC use has increased. Overall, intraparenchymal hemorrhage occurs in 0.3–1.1% of patients on vitamin K antagonist therapy. Patients with VKA-associated ICH are more likely to die than other ICH patients because of more hemorrhage expansion. Immediate discontinuation of VKA and urgent reversal should be warranted in ICH patients with an elevated international normalized ratio (INR) due to administration of VKA. Although agents for reversal of VKA including vitamin K, fresh frozen plasma (FFP), prothrombin complex concentrates (PCC), and rFVIIa can reduce the INR, their efficacy, safety, and timeliness differ. Intravenous administration of vitamin K 5–10 mg should be initiated in the first hour of symptom onset. Intravenous administration of vitamin K is more effective to reverse INR level than oral and subcutaneous one. Anaphylactic shock is one of the important adverse effects with intravenous administration, and the slow infusion rate can reduce the risk. However, there is no high-quality evidence on efficacy of vitamin K monotherapy. Onset of action begins by 2 h and maximal effect is shown in the first 24 h after given. The INR reduction <1.4 may take up to 24 h. On the other hand, most hematoma expansion occurs in the first hour after onset. For these reasons, vitamin K monotherapy is insufficient for preventing hematoma growth in the acute phase of ICH, and other rapid reversal agents are coadministrated with vitamin K intravenously.

Theoretically, FFP can reverse the effects of VKA because FFP includes all of the coagulation factors. Several studies reported the utility of FFP to normalize the INR after VKA-related ICH. However, the evidence supporting its use in VKA-related ICH is originated by small cohort studies. FFP monotherapy is also problematic because the degree of normalization relies on the initial INR and the dose of FFP administered. Volume overload may cause pulmonary edema and heart failure. Additionally, FFP leads to a durable reversal of anticoagulant activity as vitamin K. One clinical trial showed that no patient had an INR <1.4 within 1 h of initiation of FFP administration.

PCCs are another option to reverse to normalize the level of the INR after ICH caused by VKA. All PCCs contain variable coagulation factors such as factors II, IX, and X, and the inclusion of factor VII distinguished three-factor PCCs from four-factor PCCs. Many studies observed the strength of PCC: fast preparation because of no need for cross matching, rapid INR reversal, and small volume. The results of some randomized clinical trials on effectiveness of PCC compared to FFP in VKA-related ICH demonstrated faster INR reversal, less hematoma expansion, less complication leading from volume overload, and better functional outcome. Thromboembolic events were similar between PPC and FFP groups. In one randomized trial comparing FFP monotherapy and combination of PCC and FFP, FFP alone developed higher volume overload-related complications. A multicenter retrospective study reported combination of PCC and FFP may be associated with lower mortality compared to FFP monotherapy or even PCC monotherapy. While rFVIIa leads to rapid INR reversal similar to that of PCC, it has quite high rate of thromboembolic complications. Therefore, the use of rFVIIa alone is not recommended in VKA-associated ICH.

In summary of treatment for VKA-related ICH, the first step is to quit the antithrombotics. The second step is the administration of intravenous vitamin K plus PCC immediately. Rapid INR normalization for PCCs and reversal durability for vitamin K complement each other. If PCCs are not available or contraindicated, FFP might be considered as alternatives.

NOACs are increasingly used as alternatives to VKA therapy. While there is less clinical experience with reversal of NOAC-related ICH, a number of measures have been suggested to guide treatment in the setting of hemorrhagic complications. In the literature reviews, the incidence of ICH caused to VKA is less then NOAC and outcome of NOAC-associated ICH appears favorable compared to VKA, but bleeding complications always can be life-threatening. For treatment of NOAC-related ICH, discontinuation is the first step too, because of short elimination half-lives. Recently, a specific antidote (idarucizumab) for direct thrombin inhibitor (dabigatran) is available but not for direct factor Xa inhibitors (rivaroxaban, apixaban, edoxaban, and betrixaban). Oral active charcoal can be considerable if the last NOAC dose was taken in the previous few hours. Hemodialysis is recommended as an option for dabigatran. There is no recommendation because of the lacking data regarding other specific reversal agents for NOACs.

10.2.2 General Medical Care

10.2.2.1 Fever and Temperature Control

Fever after ICH is not uncommon, especially in patients with IVH. Fever is correlated with hematoma growth and neurologically worsening, and the duration of fever is related to clinical outcome in ICH patients. These results provide an adequate rationale for treatment of fever in ICH patients. However, therapeutic normothermia has not been clearly demonstrated as clinical benefits. With respect to hypothermia in ICH patients, two preliminary data demonstrated that therapeutic hypothermia reduced perihemorrhagic edema after large supratentorial ICH [15, 16]. Therapeutic hypothermia has not been sufficiently studied in ICH patients and has yet to be given high level of evidence. Two clinical trials on the therapeutic hypothermia in ICH patients are ongoing: cooling in intracerebral hemorrhage (CINCH) and targeted temperature management after intracerebral hemorrhage (TTM-ICH). Considering these data, the control of fever is reasonable, and therapeutic hypothermia should be considered investigational to prevent secondary brain injury for ICH patients.

10.2.2.2 Seizure

The frequency of seizures depends on the duration of monitoring and presence of cortical involvement. Some studies demonstrated that early symptomatic seizures within 7 days of ICH onset account for 10–15%, increasing to 31% when subclinical seizures using continuous electroencephalographic monitoring are considered [17]. Although the association between electrographic seizures and clinical outcome remains unclear, both clinical seizure and electrographic seizures in patients with decreased consciousness should be treated with antiepileptic drug to prevent seizure recurrence. In terms of prophylactic treatment, guidelines from the American Heart Association/American Stroke Association (AHA/ASA) and European Stroke Organization (ESO) recommend against routinely administration for seizure prophylaxis in acute ICH because it can increase the rate of death and disability with no difference regarding the overall incidence of seizures.

10.2.2.3 Glucose Management

Many data demonstrate hyperglycemia and hypoglycemia after ICH is related with poor outcomes, independent of the presence of diabetes mellitus. However, the optimal management of hyperglycemia in ICH and the exact target level of glucose remains unclear because of limited information regarding ICH-specific issues related to glucose treatment. One randomized trial regarding intensive (81–108 mg/dL) versus conventional glucose control (<180 mg/dL) in critically ill patients, even not ICH patients, reported intensive group increased the risk of mortality at 3 months with significant high rate of severe hypoglycemia compared to conventional group [18]. This is in concordance with result of other study recruited patients with traumatic brain injury [19]. Thus, both hyperglycemia and hypoglycemia should be avoided, and close monitoring of glucose levels is necessary.

10.2.2.4 Prophylaxis and Treatment of Venous Thromboembolism

Patients with ICH are at high risk for venous thromboembolism: deep venous thrombosis (DVT) and pulmonary thrombosis. In particular, women and blacks may be at greater risk. The CLOTS (Clots in Legs Or sTockings after Stroke) trials 1, 2, and 3, regarding assessing the effectiveness among different treatments (elastic stocking alone vs. none, thigh-high graduated compression stockings vs. calf-high stockings, and intermittent pneumatic compression (IPC) vs. none) indicated that early IPC in immobile patients with ICH reduced the occurrence of proximal DVT, while graduated compression stockings were ineffective [20–23]. Net benefit and risk of anticoagulants for thromboprophylaxis remains unclear. A meta-analysis comparing anticoagulants (low-molecular-weight heparin, low-dose subcutaneous unfractionated heparin or heparinoids) with treatments other than anticoagulants (elastic stockings, IPC, or placebo) indicated early anticoagulation is related with a significant reduction in pulmonary embolism, nonsignificant reduction in death and DVT, and nonsignificant increase in hematoma expansion [24]. Based on these results, IPC should be applied for prevention of thromboprophylaxis in patients with acute ICH. The caution should be given to intervene pharmacological drugs for venous thromboembolism. However, guidelines from AHA/ASA have recommended that after documentation of cessation of bleeding, low-molecular-weight heparin or low-dose subcutaneous unfractionated heparin may be considered for prevention of venous thromboembolism in immobile patients after 1–4 days from onset.

In terms of optimal treatment for acute ICH patients presenting with venous thromboembolism, there are insufficient high-quality data. One study estimated the risk of fatal pulmonary embolism in acute ICH patients to be about 25% for those who were untreated for DVT or nonfatal pulmonary embolism, which risk is too high to deny treatment for VTE to patients with an acute ICH. On the other hand, VTE are most likely to occur after the period of highest risk of hematoma enlargement, and the risks of worsening of an ICH with anticoagulation therapy during this period are fully unknown. Based on the estimates studied about these concerns, which have not been confirmed by clinical studies, the risk of recurrent ICH during anticoagulation appears to be substantially less than that of a fatal pulmonary embolism in an acute/subacute ICH patients presenting with VTE. Withholding anticoagulation with serial monitoring to detect extension of the thrombosis proximally is reasonable for ICH patients who have isolated distal DVT located below the knee. Inferior vena cava (IVC) filters are not routinely inserted in ICH patients with symptomatic DVT or pulmonary embolism although guidelines from AHA/ASA suggest that IVC filter placement is probably indicated in ICH patients with symptomatic DVT or pulmonary embolism in this setting. Physicians should be cautioned with regard to the high rate of long-term complications as placing the IVC filter. The efficacy of IVC filter placement in patients with symptomatic DVT is still unknown. Consequently, treatment with anticoagulants for symptomatic

DVT and pulmonary embolism is considered in selected ICH patients with favorable benefit-to-risk, depending on time from ICH onset, hematoma stability, site and size of hemorrhage, cause of ICH, and overall patient condition. However, IVC filter placement can be considered as anticoagulation therapy is contraindicated.

10.3 Blood Pressure Management in Intracerebral Hemorrhage

10.3.1 The Key Point to Debate About BP Management During the Acute Stage of Intracerebral Hemorrhage

BP is often elevated in patients with acute ICH. BP monitoring and treatment is a critical issue. The target goal of BP in the acute stage has continued to stir up controversy. Despite possible beneficial effect on decreased risk of rebleeding and hematoma expansion, the reduction of BP in the acute phage of ICH might be a double-edged sword because of the potential risk of exacerbating tissue ischemia at the hypoperfused penumbra zone in the perihematomal area, leading to neurologic worsening. However, studies addressing the effect of BP lowering on regional cerebral blood flow (CBF) and ischemic insults have also found conflicting results. Some studies showed that cerebral ischemia on diffusion-weighted imaging occurred in one third of patients with ICH, which was related with early reduction in mean arterial pressure [25, 26]. On the other hand, the Intracerebral Hemorrhage Acutely Decreasing Arterial Pressure Trial (ICH ADAPT) investigators demonstrated that rapid BP lowering after acute ICH did not reduce relative CBF in the perihematomal region [27].

Many patients with ICH have a chronic hypertension, and their brain autoregulation is shifted to the right. That means hypertensive ICH patients can be at risk of hypoperfusion for tolerable levels of MAP in normotensive ICH patients. Based on this, previous guidelines from the European Stroke Initiative (2006) suggested individual BP target according to history of chronic hypertension: target BP of 170/100 mmHg or MAP of 125 mmHg for ICH patients with prior hypertension and target BP of 150/90 mmHg or MAP of 110 mmHg for ICH patients without known hypertension. Additionally, they did not recommend the routine BP lowering and also suggested starting time to lower BP individually. Systolic BP of 180 mmHg and diastolic BP of 105 mmHg for hypertensive ICH patients and 160/95 mmHg for non-hypertensive ICH patients were recommended as an upper limit.

The other concern we should be considered is CPP. Based on the classic formula as CPP = MAP – ICP, raising MAP raises CPP and raising ICP lowers CPP. In this sense, every increased ICP can cause a change in brain tissue perfusion in hemorrhagic stroke. Rising ICP and declining CPP are associated with mortality. Recent guidelines from AHA/ASA recommend that a CPP of 50–70 mmHg may be reasonable to maintain depending on the status of cerebral autoregulation. However, this recommendation is based upon traumatic brain injury because of limited data regarding ICP and CPP in ICH.

10.3.2 Safety of Intensive BP Reduction in the Early Phase of Intracerebral Hemorrhage

These recommendations were before the results of the ongoing trials were published. One systematic review including 32 studies and 10,892 patients showed the positive correlation between high BP and the rate of increased disability and mortality [28] and formed the basis for 2 pilot trials: the Intensive Blood Pressure Reduction in Acute Cerebral Hemorrhage (INTERACT)-1 trial in 2008 and the Antihypertensive Treatment of Acute Cerebral Hemorrhage (ATACH)-1 trial in 2010. INTERACT-1 trials randomly assigned 404 ICH patients within 6 h of onset to either intensive BP lowering (target systolic BP

<140 mmHg within 1 h) or the earlier AHA/ASA guideline-based management (target systolic BP <180 mmHg) to investigate proportional change in the hematoma volume at 24 h in 2 different groups. The results of INTERACT-1 trial found early reduction of systolic BP to less than 140 mmHg to be safe [29].

The ATACH-1 trial was conducted to determine the safety and feasibility of reducing BP in the acute phase of ICH [30]. The patients with ICH within 6 h of symptom onset, systolic BP ≥170 mmHg, and hematoma volume <60 cc were assigned to three tiers, 170–200 mmHg, 140–170 mmHg, and 110–140 mmHg, according to the systolic BP-lowering goals. The investigators found no significant relationship between systolic BP and any of the outcomes (hematoma expansion, perihematomal edema, and 3-month functional outcome). These two pilot trials failed to show efficacy of rapidly intensive BP reduction. However, results of two pilot trials provided an important proof of concept for early intensive BP lowering in patients with acute ICH.

10.3.3 Efficacy of Intensive BP Reduction in the Early Phase of Intracerebral Hemorrhage

Following the promising data supporting safety from two pilot trials, two landmark clinical trials were performed to evaluate the efficacy of intensive BP reduction in patients with acute ICH. In 2013, the results of the INTERACT-2 trials enrolling 2839 patients were published [31]. Subjects with a systolic BP between 150 and 220 mmHg within 6 h of the ICH onset were randomly assigned to either intensive treatment to lower BP to a target systolic BP of <140 mmHg within 1 h or guideline-based treatment of systolic BP <180 mmHg. Intensive BP lowering demonstrated a trend ($P = 0.06$) to association with primary outcome defined as modified Rankin scale score of 3–6, but the relationship did no achieve statistical significance. However, a predefined ordinal analysis of a modified Rankin score as secondary outcomes showed a 13% improvement in the modified Rankin score with intensive treatment group ($P = 0.04$). Nonfatal serious adverse events and mortality were similar in the two treatment groups. The difference in hematoma growth between groups was also not significant.

Recently, the results of another randomized clinical study, the ATACH-2 trial, were reported [32]. The study compared treating the systolic BP <140 mmHg versus <180 mmHg in 1000 patients with ICH within 4.5 h of onset, systolic BP ≥180 mmHg, and hematoma volume <60 cc. Single agent as intravenous nicardipine was used in this trial, while multiple agents depending on physician's discretion were administrated in the INTERACT-2 trial. The study results demonstrated no difference in the rate of death or disability as a score of 4–6 on the modified Rankin scale at 3 months between the two groups. In the intensive BP reduction group, there was a trend, though not significant, toward a lower rate of hematoma growth (19% versus 24%, $P = 0.09$).

Current guidelines indicated that rapidly lowering of systolic BP to 140 mmHg is safe in ICH patients presenting with systolic BP of 150–200 mmHg and can be effective for improving functional outcomes.

10.4 General Medical Management in Aneurysmal Subarachnoid Hemorrhage

Good outcome in aneurysmal SAH is closely related with treatment volume and availability of endovascular treatment and neurointensive care services. Low-volume centers should consider early transfer to high-volume centers. Patients with aneurysmal SAH should be admitted to an intensive care unit for hemodynamic and neurologic monitoring. Neurologic deteriorations occurred in about one third of patients within the first day. Life-threatening medical complication is 40%. Especially, pulmonary edema and cardiac arrhythmias complicate 23% and 35%, respectively. Nearly half of pulmonary complications occurred on days 3–4, and the peak occurrence rate of cardiac arrhythmias occurred on days 2–3 [33]. Hence, chest X-ray, troponin levels, and ECG should be checked regularly. Cardiopulmonary complications and management will be discussed later in this chapter. Absolute bed rest, sufficient analgesics to relieve pain, and avoidance of stimulus maneuvers are also recommended.

The initial care of aneurysmal SAH should include prevention and management of rebleeding, increased ICP, vasospasm, and hydrocephalus. Rebleeding after aneurysmal SAH is highly associated with increased mortality and poor functional outcome. The risk of rebleeding is 4–14% within the first 24 h, and of these, more than one third of rebleeding occurs within the first 3 h of symptom onset [34]. Although there are few studies, antithrombotics should be discontinued after SAH, and appropriate reversal agents should be considered until the aneurysm is definitively repaired by interventions. The early surgical clipping or endovascular coiling for the ruptured aneurysm should be performed to prevent the rebleeding after aneurysmal SAH. In addition to the late procedure, one of the risk factors associated with early rebleeding is systolic BP >160 mmHg [35]. The revised guidelines from the AHA/ASA indicated that the goal of systolic BP should be less than 160 mmHg until the surgical or endovascular procedure is performed. Figure 10.2 shows the summary of management for subarachnoid hemorrhage.

10.4.1 Management and Monitoring of Cerebral Vasospasm

Cerebral vasospasm and its associated delayed cerebral ischemia (DCI) are not uncommon in aneurysmal SAH. It most frequently occurs between post-bleeding day 4 and day 14 and often results in significant morbidity and mortality. Patients should be closely monitored using transcranial Doppler (TCD) and continuous electroencephalography (cEEG) during these periods.

TCD is widely used for diagnosis and monitoring of cerebral vasospasm after SAH. Lindegaard ratio (LR) is defined as mean flow velocity (MFV) in the middle cerebral artery

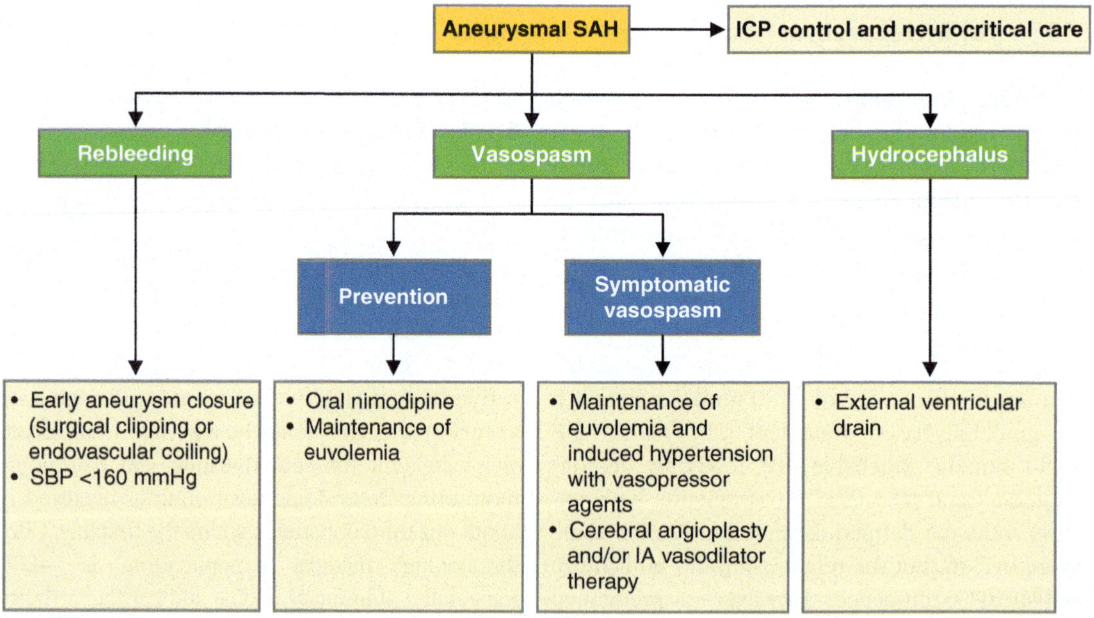

Fig 10.2 Summary of management for subarachnoid hemorrhage. *SAH* subarachnoid hemorrhage, *ICP* intracranial pressure, *SBP* systolic blood pressure, *IA* intra-arterial

(MCA)/MFV in the extracranial internal carotid artery (ICA). High MFV in the MCA (>120 cm/s) may be due to hyperemia or vasospasm. At this time, the LR helps differentiation between hyperemia and vasospasm. As MFV in the MCA rises up suddenly, the LR less than 3.0 means hyperemia and the value higher than 3.0 may indicate hyperemia, and when the value is higher than 6.0, vasospasm is almost always present. However, the criticisms regarding the low correlation between high MVF and high LR and exact cutoff points remain still. Although daily TCD testing might help to detect vasospasm with a trend, the role of TCD as a real-time detection tool has been criticized for its poor temporal resolution. Other criticisms are that TCD can be very limited in patients with poor acoustic windows, ranging to 10–20%, and is also not useful to detect vasospasm in more distal branches.

One of the important goals in the management of SAH is to predict and forestall secondary brain injury timely. cEEG severs this purpose well. Alpha/delta ratio (ADR) is the strongest indicator associated with DCI, and clinical cutoffs were defined as six consecutive clips with less than 10% decrease in ADR from baseline and any single clip with less than 50% (Fig. 10.3) [36]. Brain symmetry index using specific processing software is the other useful index. cEEG is also helpful in detecting vasospasm and nonconvulsive seizures in high-grade SAH patients with limited the neurologic examination due to unconsciousness. Subclinical seizure is frequently seen in patients with SAH. Perfusion image of brain

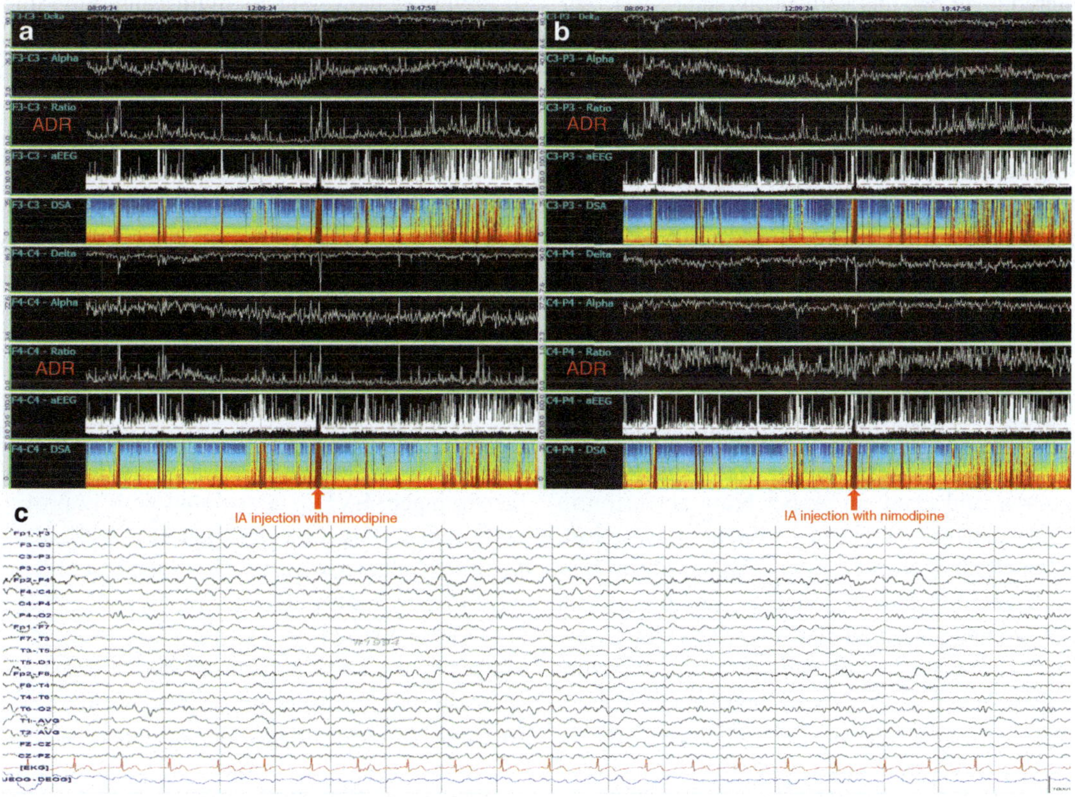

Fig. 10.3 Continuous electroencephalogram (EEG). Continuous EEG data from two bipolar channels in the bilateral fronto-central (F3-C3, F4-C4) and centro-parietal (C3-P3, C4-P4) regions showing progressive decrement of the alpha-delta ratio after 10 a.m. on the left hemisphere with more prominence on the centro-parietal than fronto-central region, and an increase of alpha-delta ratio after intra-arterial injection with nimodipine (**a** and **b**). Raw EEG data just before angioplasty, showing the rise in asymmetry with delta slowing on the left hemisphere (**c**). *ADR* alpha-to-delta ratio, *DSA* density spectral array, *EEG* electroencephalogram, *aEEG* amplitude EEG. Reproduced from Journal of Korean Neurosurgical Society [36]

can be one of the other options to identify regions of potential brain ischemia.

Unfortunately, no effective preventive therapy for vasospasm has been developed to date. The calcium channel blocker, nimodipine, has been originally designed for prevention of vasospasm because of the vasodilatory effects on cerebral vessels. However, nimodipine has no convincing evidence regarding prevention of vasospasm. On the other hand, meta-analysis on efficacy of prophylactic nimodipine after SAH showed neurological outcomes were improved and mortality was slightly, though not significantly, reduced in the nimodipine group [37]. Nimodipine was given orally between the fourth and twenty-first days after bleeding in most of clinical trials. Current guidelines recommend oral nimodipine (60 mg every 4 h for 3 weeks) should be administered to all patients with aneurysmal SAH. The effectiveness of nimodipine given intravenously remains uncertain. Nimodipine is not recommended in traumatic SAH because of one systematic review showing nimodipine did not affect long-term clinical outcome [38]. Recent clinical trials regarding the utility of statin (regardless of dose regimens), magnesium sulfate, and clazosentan (an endothelin receptor antagonist) failed to show the effectiveness on DCI or functional outcome after aneurysmal SAH.

Traditionally, hemodynamic augmentation has consisted of hemodilution, hypervolemia, and hypertensive therapy, called the "triple-H." In decades, triple-H therapy has been used to improve and maintain proper brain perfusion in SAH patients with or without vasospasm, although there have been no evidences from randomized clinical trials. Triple-H therapy is associated with increased risk of rebleeding at the aneurysm site if it has not been closed. Achieving hypervolemia is associated undesirable effects including fluid overload and pulmonary edema, and hypovolemia is also should be avoided because of the risk of ischemic complications. Therefore, any prophylactic hemodynamic augmentation appears unuseful for the vasospasm, and euvolemic normotensive normal cardiac performance is recommended with normal saline, which should be checked by documentation of fluid input and output. Central venous pressure (CVP) is a poor surrogate for volume status. Other useful tools for hemodynamic monitoring will be explained in more detail later in this chapter. Synthetic colloids and routine blood transfusion may be associated with poor clinical outcomes.

Triple-H therapy has not been found effective in even symptomatic or laboratory vasospasm. Accumulating literature on treating symptomatic vasospasm has shifted the focus from this triple-H therapy to the maintenance of euvolemia and induced hypertension with vasopressor agents. Intra-arterial (IA) injection of nimodipine, nicardipine, and verapamil may lead to irreversible ischemic injury (Fig. 10.4). IA balloon angioplasty is also useful in treating symptomatic vasospasm. IA infusion of vasodilation therapy is relatively safe, but the positive effect may not last long, whereas IA balloon angioplasty has the risk of rupture of the vessel but higher durability than IA infusion. For refractory symptomatic vasospasm, both intra-aortic balloon counterpulsation therapy and partial aortic occlusion are considerable to improve CBF and reduce permanent neurologic damages.

10.4.2 Management of Hydrocephalus

Aneurysmal SAH-associated acute symptomatic hydrocephalus occurs in 15–87% and leads to poor neurological condition. It can be managed by external ventricular drainage (EVD) or lumbar drainage. EVD is associated with improved neurological outcome. If patients with acute hydrocephalus associated with aneurysmal SAH have concomitant IVH and increased ICP, EVD should be applied as an important early step. However, it should be cautioned that EVD can increase risk for rebleeding and ventriculitis. Lumbar drainage might be safe and has no increase in the risk of rebleeding in aneurysmal SAH without IVH. Preliminary data showed the decreased incidence of vasospasm after lumbar drainage in nontraumatic SAH. However, the effectiveness of lumbar drainage has been derived from small retrospective studies, and the theoretical risk of downward herniation after lumbar drainage should be considered with caution in patients with suspicious severe intracra-

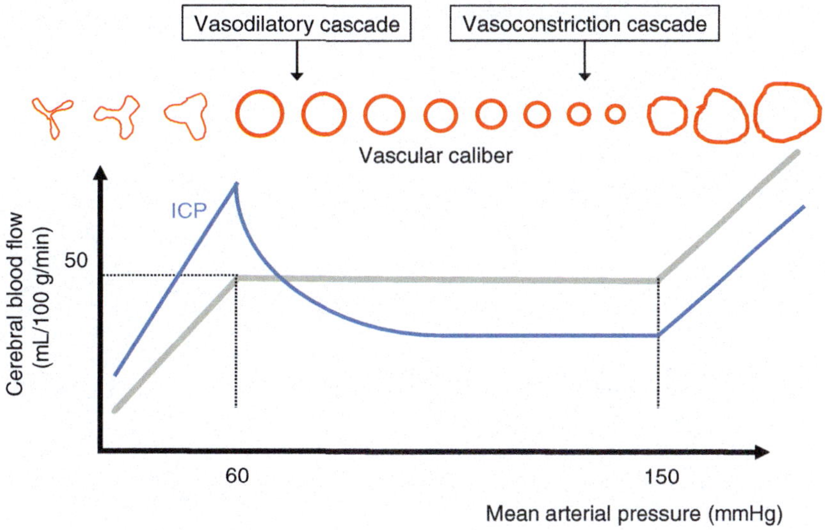

Fig 10.5 Cerebral autoregulation. Reproduced by permission of Critical Care Clinics [39]

cerebral herniation, cerebral edema, and reduced CPP as secondary brain injury. Traditionally, secondary brain injury is partially reversible and preventable if identified early and treated appropriately. ICP monitoring is one of the best ways for early detection of secondary brain injury and can provide understanding of cerebral hemodynamics as well as direct pressure. Precise monitoring of the ICP is performed by inserting a catheter into four different anatomical sites: epidural, subarachnoid, intraparenchymal, and intraventricular. External ventricular drain (EVD) allows both ICP monitoring and therapeutic drainage of CSF, which is considered the gold standard for ICP measurement. The ICP zero point is defined as the center of the head or at the level of the foramen of Monro, which is anatomically close to the tragus of the outer ear.

The ICP waveform is important because its morphology provides clues to the pressure-volume relationship within the intracranial vault [41]. The shape of the ICP waveform has three distinct upstrokes, typical feature of vascular origin: the first peak (percussion wave, P1) representing arterial pulsation, the second peak (tidal wave, P2) representing intracranial compliance, and last peak (dicrotic wave, P3) representing aortic valve closure. When ICP is normal and a compensated pressure-volume relationship exists within the cranium, P1 should have the highest upstroke, P2 in-between upstroke, and P3 the lowest upstroke. If P2 is higher than P1, it indicates intracranial hypertension (Fig. 10.6).

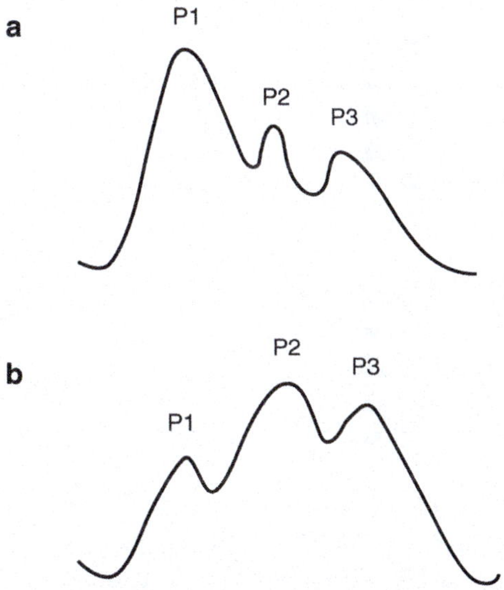

Fig. 10.6 Intracranial pressure waveforms in conditions of normal (**a**) and poor (**b**) intracranial compliance. Adapted from Journal of Neurocritical Care [41]

Lundberg suggested three different types of ICP variations: A, B, and C waves (Fig. 10.7). Lundberg A waves, known as "plateau waves," are clinically very important and pathological waves because they indicate reduced intracranial compliance. They are steep increases in ICP to 50 mmHg or more and last 5–20 min and then return precipitously to below the original level or slightly elevated baseline. Lundberg B wave was defined as repetitive changes in ICP due to CBF fluctuations that lead to changes in CBV and ICP. They rise from a variable baseline to a level

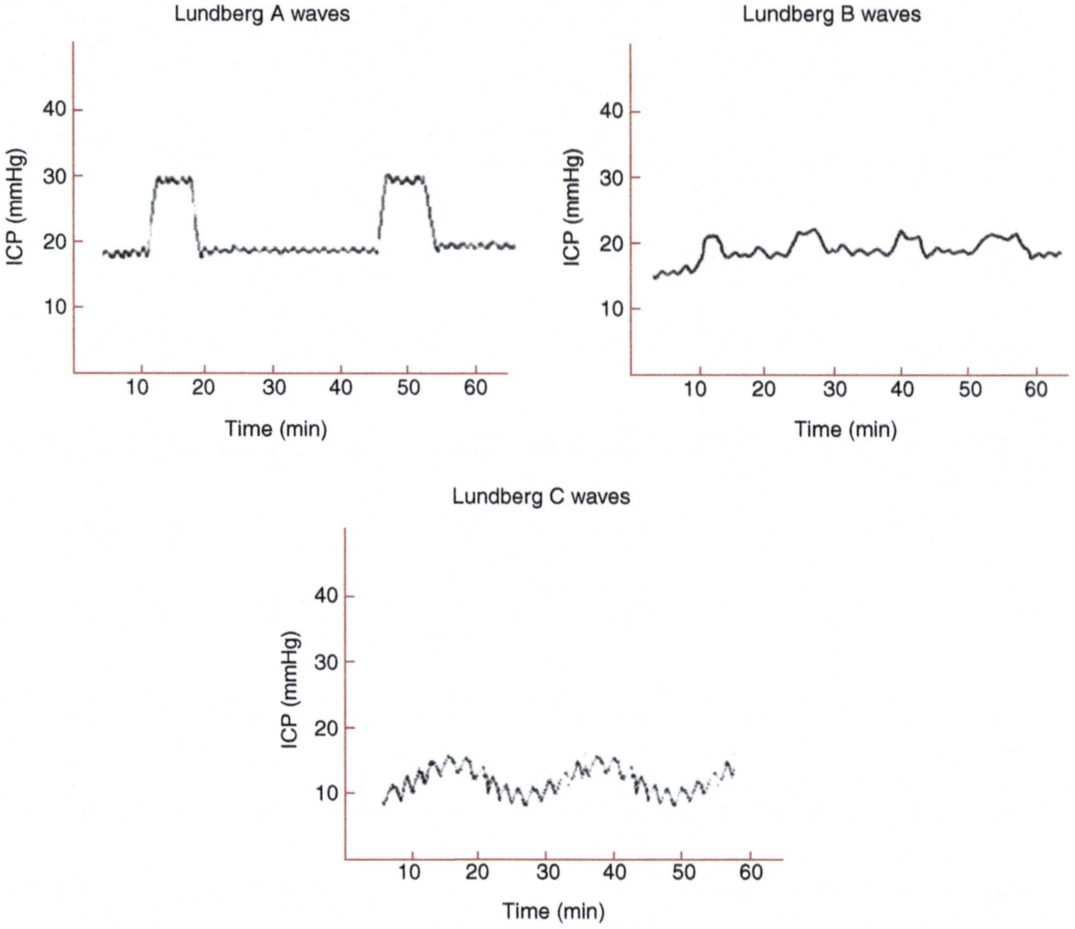

Fig. 10.7 Pathologic intracranial pressure waves. (**a**) Lundberg A (plateau) waves. (**b**) Lundberg B waves. (**c**) Lundberg C waves. Adapted from Journal of Neurocritical Care [41]

20–30 mmHg higher and then fall abruptly. They occur at frequencies of 0.5–2 waves/min and last over 0.5–3 min. Lundberg C waves occur at a rate of 4–8 waves/min and are probably caused by interaction between the cardiac and respiration cycles. Therefore, they are little pathological significance. The ICP waveform provides insight into intracranial compliance and is important to recognize [42].

10.5.1.2 Management of Intracranial Pressure

If cerebral herniation or ICP crisis is suspected, immediate brain imaging and treatment must be initiated. Surgical decompression is the most effective way to reduce ICP. Intraventricular hemorrhage with/without acute hydrocephalus, high-grade subarachnoid hemorrhage, and any symptoms of increased ICP or herniation are good indications for placing EVD because of monitoring and managing ICP at the same time. If surgical treatment is not an option, the following medical steps can be considered as shown in Fig. 10.8.

Sedatives and analgesics can be used to relieve patients from agitation and pain, but they can also interfere with assessment of consciousness. Although a light level of sedation is associated with improved clinical outcomes, a deep level of sedation may be required in severely increased ICP. Systemic and cerebral physiologic effects of sedatives and analgesics used commonly in patients with hemorrhagic stroke are provided in Table 10.7. Short-acting drugs are usually recommended.

Osmotherapy with either mannitol or hypertonic saline has a role to help to remove water

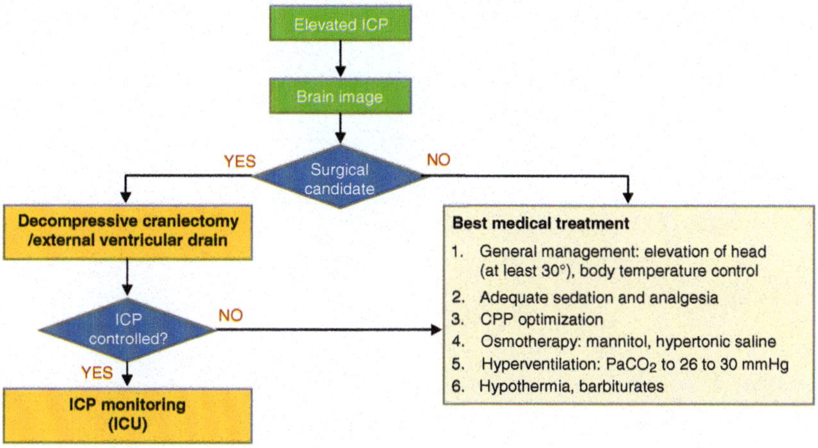

Fig. 10.8 Algorithm for management of elevated intracranial pressure. *ICP* intracranial pressure, *ICU* intensive care unit, *CPP* cerebral perfusion pressure

Table 10.7 Systemic and cerebral physiologic effects of sedatives and analgesics

	Rapid onset (min)	Fast recovery	Sedative effect	Analgesic effect	ICP	MAP	Seizure	Unique effects
Fentanyl	+++ (1–2)	++	+	+++	↓/—	↓	—	Accumulative effects with repeated or prolonged administration
Remifentanil	+++ (1–2)	+++	+	+++	↓/—	↓↓	—	Prompt reversal upon discontinuation: Possible frequent neurologic examination No accumulation in renal or hepatic insufficiency Hypotension
Morphine	++ (10)	++	+	+++	↑	↓	—	Nausea, respiratory depression, coughing response↓ Accumulate in hepatic or renal dysfunction and prolong effects (50%↓in renal failure)
Propofol	+++ (<1~2)	+++	+++	–	↓↓	↓↓	↓	Shivering↓, $CMRO_2$↓, respiratory depression Rare but potentially fatal propofol infusion syndrome Infection risk↑, triglyceride↑ Hypotension, bradycardia, injection site pain Unaltered metabolism in hepatic or renal insufficiency
Ketamin	+++ (0.5)	+++	+++	++	↑/—	↑/—	↓	Bronchodilatation No respiration depression Sympathetic stimulation Hallucinations, delirium upon withdrawal, hypersalivation

(continued)

Table 10.7 (continued)

	Rapid onset (min)	Fast recovery	Sedative effect	Analgesic effect	ICP	MAP	Seizure	Unique effects
Midazolam	+++ (2–5)	++	+++	–	↓/—	↓	↓	Accumulate and cause prolonged sedation if delivered long-term Prolonged half-life in hepatic or renal impairment Delirium↑
Lorazepam	+ (5–20)	+	++	–	↓/—	↓	↓	Delirium↑ Safety in mild to moderate hepatic and renal insufficiency High dosing causing metabolic acidosis
Thiopental	++	++	+++	–	↓	↓↓	↓	$CMRO_2$↓, respiration depression, hypotension, cardiac depression, ileus Accumulative effects with repeated or prolonged administration
DEX	++ (15)	++	++	++	↓/—	↓	—	Sympatholysis, cooperative sedation No respiration depression, delirium↓, shivering↓, GFR↑, cardioprotection Bradycardia, hypotension, hypertension upon abrupt discontinuation

$CMRO_2$ cerebral metabolic rate of oxygen, *GFR* glomerular filtration rate, *DEX* Dexmedetomidine

from brain tissue across the blood-brain barrier by creating an osmotic gradient that draws water from the interstitium into the vascular space. Mannitol is not metabolized and excreted unchanged in the urine after infusion. Therefore, it acts as a potent osmotic diuretic, and the effects of ICP reduction are usually seen within 15 min, peak 15–120 min, and last from 1 to 5 h. There is a significant dose-response relationship when using mannitol, so rapid bolus IV infusion at a usual dose of 0.5–1 g/kg is effective in reducing ICP. Doses less than 0.5 g/kg appear to be less efficacious. The important concern regarding mannitol use is acute kidney injury. Using serum osmolarity of 320 mOsm/kg as the threshold to stop mannitol to prevent this complication is likely relative, and serum osmolarity may be tolerated up to 340 mOsm/kg [43]. Instead of checking serum osmolarity, frequent monitoring of osmolar gap, which is the difference between the calculated and the measured osmolality, is recommended. This complication is rare, if the osmolar gap is less than 55 [44].

Hypertonic saline has a similar osmotic effect as mannitol but is a less potent diuretic, which can increase BP, cardiac output, and CBF by expanding the intravascular volume [45]. Hypertonic saline is currently the preferred agent of a majority of neurointensivists. Some meta-analysis showed that hypertonic saline is more effective than mannitol for the management of ICP [46]. Hypertonic saline comes in several different concentrations: 3, 7.5, 11.7, and 23.4%. Use of a hypertonic solution can cause complications such as hypokalemia, hypernatremia, cardiac failure, pulmonary edema, and kidney damage. When hyponatremia exists as baseline, central pontine myelinolysis may occur because of rapid increased sodium level. When administering more than 7.5% concentration, it is preferably injected through a central vein than the peripheral vein to minimize phlebitis. Although

Table 10.8 Comparison of mannitol and hypertonic saline

	Mannitol	Hypertonic saline
Dose	1. 0.5–1.5 g/kg/dose, repeatedly every 4–8h	1. 2%, 3% hypertonic saline: 1–2 mL/kg/h, 250 mL bolus over 30 min if more aggressive therapy is desired 2. 23.4% 30 mL hypertonic saline bolus infusion (11.7% 60 mL) over 10 min
Monitoring	2. Follow osmolar gap (<55) 3. Achieve hypernatremia s systemic hypovolemia 4. BUN/Cr	3. Prespecified Na ranges (e.g., 150–160) 4. Avoid exceeding 160 mEq/L
Advantage	1. Rapid effect in reducing ICP even before the onset of osmotic diuresis 2. No need for central venous access	1. 23.4% 30 mL bolus (11.7% 60 mL) has an immediate effect in ICP reduction 2. Hypertonic saline permeability coefficient 1 vs. 0.9 for mannitol 3. Volume expander 4. Positive inotropic 5. Immunomodulatory results
Disadvantage	1. Could lead to reduction of intravascular volume and compromise of MAP/CPP 2. Impaired clearance can lead to nephrotoxicity 3. Accumulation into injured brain via disrupted BBB and rebound edema	1. Hyperchloremic metabolic acidosis 2. Accumulation into injured brain via disrupted BBB and rebound edema 3. Hyperoncotic hemolysis 4. Requires central venous access 5. Bolus administration (esp. 23.4%) can lead to transient hypotension

Reproduced by permission of Neurocritical Care [47]
BUN blood urea nitrogen, *Cr* creatinine, *MAP* mean arterial pressure, *CPP* cerebral perfusion pressure, *BBB* blood-brain barrier, *ICP* intracranial pressure

serum sodium concentration below 160 mEq/L is recommended, concentration as high as 180 mEq/L has been tolerated without complications. Table 10.8 shows the comparison of mannitol and hypertonic saline [47].

Use of a ventilator to lower $PaCO_2$ to 26–30 mmHg arbitrarily causes hyperventilation, inducing respiratory alkalosis and cerebrovascular constriction, eventually reducing ICP. However, the effectiveness of hyperventilation treatment is very short (11–20 h) due to a rapid adaptation to the new $PaCO_2$ which causes a low pH in the CSF, and the vasoconstriction induced by prolonged hyperventilation can cause ischemia [48]. Therefore, therapeutic hyperventilation should be considered as an urgent but temporary intervention (bridge therapy) when ICP is elevated.

Therapeutic hypothermia which maintains body temperature at 32–35 °C in order to reduce cerebral metabolism can also be attempted. Cooling results in 6–10% decrease in cerebral metabolism for every 1 °C reduction. In addition to reducing ICP, several studies showed therapeutic hypothermia attenuated perihematomal edema growth in patients with intracerebral hemorrhage [49]. During hypothermia, it is important to prevent the patient from shivering, as this can increase ICP. Buspirone, dexmedetomidine, meperidine, magnesium sulfate, or propofol can be used to control the shivering. If not abolished, neuromuscular blockade may be used. Antishivering protocol is showed in Table 10.9 [50].

Barbiturate coma therapy is also a useful method to control increased ICP patients. Barbiturate coma therapy (10–30 mg/kg as an initial dose and 1–3 mg/kg per hour for maintenance) decreases brain metabolism and CBF. It can be complicated by hypotension and cardiac output due to suppressing the heart, possibly requiring vasopressor support. Thus, using the continuous electroencephalogram (EEG) monitoring allows pharmacologic adjustment to maintain enough suppression of the EEG background (burst suppression) while minimizing adverse effects.

Preventing conditions that can elevate ICP is also important. Turning the head and neck to one side and tightly wrapping the neck in order to

Table 10.9 The Columbia anti-shivering protocol

Step		Intervention	Dose
0	Baseline	Acetaminophen	650–1000 mg Q 4–6 h
		Buspirone	30 mg Q 8 h
		Magnesium sulfate	0.5–1 mg/h IV goal (3–4 mg/dL)
		Skin counterwarming	43 °C/MAX temp
1	Mild sedation	Dexmedetomidine	0.2–1.5 μg/kg/h
		or Opioid	Fentanyl starting dose 25 μg/h Meperidine 50–100 mg IM or IV
2	Moderate sedation	Dexmedetomidine and opioid	Doses as above
3	Deep sedation	Propofol	50–75 μg/kg/min
4	Neuromuscular blockade	Vecuronium	0.1 mg/kg IV

Reproduced by permission of Neurocritical Care [50]

maintain intubation can increase ICP by interfering with the return of blood in the jugular vein. Putting the head in a neutral position and elevating 30–40° can improve cerebral venous and CSF flow, eventually lowering ICP. An increase in body temperature leads to an increase in metabolism, cerebral blood CBF, and swelling of the brain. Antipyretic drugs should be used, and passive temperature management, such as cold blankets, can be used if needed. These general managements apply to all patients with elevated ICP.

10.5.2 Hemodynamic Monitoring

If hypotension is observed in patients with hemorrhagic stroke, rapid identification of the cause—whether it is due to low circulating blood volume or heart failure—is required. If the problem is due to low circulating blood volume, first, sufficient fluid infusion should be provided, and then a vasopressor or inotropics should be used. If the low BP is due to heart disease and the circulating blood volume is normal, excessive infusion can increase the burden on the heart, reduce cardiac output, cause pulmonary edema, and degenerate gaseous exchange, eventually worsening the patient's condition. Therefore, it is crucial to monitor the circulating blood volume.

10.5.2.1 Central Venous Pressure

CVP allows estimation of preload on the left ventricle (left ventricular end-diastolic pressure). An estimate of the central venous pressure can help determine a patient's volume status; however, the CVP can be affected by a patient's cardiopulmonary disease. Many studies thus far have indicated that the accuracy of CVP is only about 50% and the CVP does not adequately predict whether or not an intravenous fluid challenge will increase stroke volume. Therefore, this should not be used independently, but along with other indicators, when assessing the cardiovascular reaction after providing an infusion. However, low CVP is a relatively good indicator of hemodynamic response to a fluid challenge.

10.5.2.2 Stroke Volume Variation and Pulse Pressure Variation

In patients with mechanical ventilation and no spontaneous breathing activity, stroke volume variation (SVV) and pulse pressure variation (PPV) can be used as a dynamic index to predict fluid responsiveness [51]. Positive pressure ventilation reduces right ventricular preload due to compression of the superior and inferior vena cava (IVC). The cyclic variations of venous return induced by mechanical ventilation lead to the cyclic variation of stroke volume. PPV is caused by inspiration and expiration over a single respiratory. If patients have low circulating blood volume, these variations increase. SVV more than 10% or PPV greater than 13% are good predictor of fluid responsiveness. SVV and PPV are known to be better indicators than CVP when assessing fluid responsiveness. However, in cases of increased pulmonary arterial pressure, spontaneous breathing, and atrial fibrillation, these indexes are less effective.

10.5.2.3 Inferior Vena Cava Diameter

The IVC diameter is easy to measure and reflects the right chambers' preload. Using ultrasound, changes in the internal diameter of the IVC can be monitored according to changes in breathing. The transducer position is just below the xiphoid process 1–2 cm to the right of the midline, and IVC is detected usually about 1 cm below the pulmonary vein. The normal diameter of the IVC is between 1.5 and 2.5 cm. If the diameter is reduced to below 1 cm and complete collapse occurs as breathing changes, this is a good indication of a low circulating blood volume [52]. This simple test is useful in the neuro ICU, where rapid hemodynamic assessment is required, or in emergency patients who are unable to undergo invasive intervention. However, there are other factors aside from circulating blood volume—such as intrathoracic pressure and the function of the right heart—that affect the internal diameter. Therefore, careful examination of the patient and other hemodynamic index should be considered together.

10.5.2.4 Passive Leg Raising Test

When both legs are raised to 45–60° from the supine position, venous blood from the deep veins of the legs moves to the central vascular system through the inferior vena cava. This posture provides temporarily increased circulating blood volume by around 300 mL, causing increased cardiac output. This is the simplest method to see if the patients in ICU require fluid resuscitation. The maneuver might be reinforced in a clinical setting by moving the patient's bed from a semi-Fowler position to a supine position with the legs raised. Repeated assessment is available, and the simultaneous monitoring of BP or pulse rate is mandatory.

10.6 Management of General Medical Complications in Hemorrhagic Stroke

Patients with hemorrhagic stroke are exposed to systemic complications, due to not only the primary disease but also the ICU environment (prone to infections). Approximately 50% of deaths after 7 days of stroke onset are due to medical complications. Most of problems are cardiopulmonary complications. The most common medical problem is pneumonia (5.6%) followed by aspiration (2.6%) and respiratory failure/distress (2%) [53]. Many patients present with decreased consciousness and are required supporting intubation with/without mechanical ventilation. Dysphasia is very common and a major risk factor for developing aspiration pneumonia. Therefore, initial screening for dysphasia should be carried out before the beginning of oral intake to reduce the risk of pneumonia. The second common complications are cardiac problems as follows: acute myocardial infarction, heart failure, arrhythmias, and cardiac arrest. Concurrent stroke and acute myocardial infarction are not uncommon. Sudden cardiovascular or pulmonary events after a brain hemorrhagic insult sometimes can occur without pre-existing cardiopulmonary pathology: stress-induced cardiomyopathy and neurogenic pulmonary edema. The following are common and serious secondary systemic complications due to hemorrhagic stroke.

10.6.1 Ventilator-Associated Pneumonia

Ventilator-associated pneumonia (VAP) is an infection occurring within 48 h post-mechanical ventilation. Since many patients with hemorrhagic stroke use ventilators, VAP is an important complication when managing these patients. More than 85% of pneumonia seen in the ICU is VAP. The occurrence rate is 2–3% per day of mechanical ventilation, and this applies to 8–38% of all patients who receive mechanical ventilation. The frequency increases with prolongation of the mechanical ventilation, but recent studies indicate that the frequency increases for 5 days after the commencement of ventilation and decreases afterward. Therefore, monitoring the early stages of mechanical ventilation is essential.

VAP is divided into early VAP (occurring before day 4 of mechanical ventilation) and late

VAP (occurring after day 5). Early VAP is a type of community-acquired infection and is often caused by *Streptococcus pneumoniae*, *Haemophilus influenzae*, *Staphylococcus aureus*, and antibiotic-resistant intestinal gram-negative bacilli. Late VAP is considered a hospital-acquired infection and is often caused by *Pseudomonas aeruginosa*, resistant *Klebsiella pneumoniae*, *Acinetobacter baumannii*, and methicillin-resistant *Staphylococcus aureus*. Late VAP has a high mortality rate, and early VAP does not always have a good prognosis, as the infection can be a hospital-acquired infection from a previous center. Causes include direct inhalation from the oropharynx, inhalation from the oropharynx following gastric reflux, direct infection from the pleura, infection from urinary catheters, and hematogenous spread. The most important route of infection is direct inhalation from the oropharynx. Intubation hinders the normal defense mechanisms of the bronchial tubes, by suppressing the cough reflex, damaging the mucosal epithelium, and suppressing ciliary movement. Most importantly, intubation can act as a direct route of infection.

The procedure for diagnosis and treatment is identical to other hospital-acquired pneumonias. Since VAP is often caused by multidrug-resistant bacteria, treatment is difficult and mortality is high. Therefore, prevention is as important as diagnosis and treatment. Preventative measures include providing education to medical staff, washing hands, isolating patients infected with multidrug-resistant bacteria, and operating a program to monitor infections in the ICU. The best method is to avoid intubation where possible and consider other noninvasive ventilation methods. Intubation tubing is also better if it is silver-coated. The pressure of the cuff should be maintained no lower than 20 cm H_2O. Head-of-bed elevation of 30–45° in mechanically ventilated patients with hemorrhagic stroke decreased the risk of developing VAP. Oral hygiene should be maintained by providing frequent disinfection and suction. Antacids should be avoided as much as possible, and changing of the tubing or the ventilator circuit should also be minimized. The nutrition tube undoubtedly causes aspiration pneumonia, but considering the risks of malnutrition or parenteral nutrition, it is best to start using nutrition tubes for a better prognosis.

10.6.2 Neurogenic Pulmonary Edema

Neurogenic pulmonary edema refers to pulmonary edema that occurs within a short period after central nerve system (CNS) damage. Neurogenic pulmonary edema frequently occurs even without underlying diseases of the lungs or heart. More than 70% of cases occur after cerebral hemorrhage [54]. Causes include a rapid ICP increase, pulmonary vasoconstriction due to an adrenergic response after damage to the solitary tract nucleus, and increased permeability of lung capillaries due to increased pressure. The inflammatory response due to increased permeability also worsens the pulmonary edema.

There is no special diagnostic tool, but changes in chest imaging or difficulties in breathing in the early stages of acute brain damage can indicate pulmonary edema. It is difficult to differentiate from aspiration pneumonia or ventilator-associated pneumonia. However, neurogenic pulmonary edema typically occurs within hours of the brain damage, and aspiration pneumonia occurs 24–48 h after damage. Moreover, neurogenic pulmonary edema occurs bilaterally in the lungs, while aspiration pneumonia is typically localized to one lung. The treatment procedure includes appropriate mechanical ventilation to prevent damage to the heart and lungs. If the causative brain condition improves, neurogenic pulmonary edema is also improved.

10.6.3 Pulmonary Embolism

Pulmonary embolism is not a rare complication and has a high mortality rate. Pulmonary embolism can be acute or chronic, and patients with hemorrhagic stroke often exhibit acute pulmonary embolism. Acute pulmonary embolism is clinically divided into massive and sub-massive pulmonary embolism. Massive pulmonary embolism occurs when systolic pressure drops below 90 mmHg or 40 mmHg from the standard for longer than 15 min. If symptoms such as acute myocardial infarction, tension pneumothorax, cardiac tamponade, or newly developed arrhythmias are not accompanied yet central venous pressure is increasing and BP is decreasing, massive pulmonary embolism should be questioned. There is a high frequency of left ventricular collapse or death. As death can occur any time from 1 to 2 h until 72 h from the start of symptoms, these patients should be monitored with caution. The mortality rate is 30% when untreated but is lowered to 8% with aggressive treatment.

In more than 40% of cases, there is an association with DVT. Symptoms are similar to other pulmonary diseases and are not helpful for diagnosis, but common symptoms include difficulty in breathing, exhaustion, pleural pain, cough, edema in the legs, and pain in the legs. A more specific symptom is that the difficulty in breathing occurs within a few minutes. Diagnosis is performed using D-dimer, spiral CT, V/Q scan, and pulmonary angiography. The D-dimer test has a low sensitivity but high specificity. Therefore, in patients with a low or moderate suspicion of pulmonary embolism, D-dimer level below 500 ng/mL is enough to exclude the possibility of pulmonary embolism. Since massive pulmonary embolism has a high mortality rate, an emergency ECG to check for pulmonary hypertension or overload on the right ventricle should be performed. If the ECG results suggest these conditions, emergency thrombolysis should be performed. When the patient is stable, a spiral CT should be performed to identify other causes of shock.

Hemodynamic stability is the first thing to consider when treating massive pulmonary embolism. BP should be elevated using a heart stimulant such as dopamine or dobutamine. Although the oxygen supply is effective, massive infusion therapy is still questionable. If any contraindications such as acute ICH and untreated aneurysmal SAH are present in patients with hemodynamically unstable pulmonary embolism, embolectomy is recommended, not thrombolytics. For the treatment of sub-massive pulmonary embolism or maintenance treatment for massive pulmonary embolism, low-molecular-weight heparin is used. This is later exchanged for warfarin, but if the INR reaches 2–3, then low-molecular-weight heparin is stopped. Non-vitamin K antagonist oral anticoagulants have also been recently used. These oral anticoagulants are given for 3 months if a correctable risk factor is present and 6 months or longer if there is no special risk factor.

10.6.4 Stress-Induced Cardiomyopathy

Stress-induced cardiomyopathy is an acute and transient dysfunction of the apical left ventricle after emotional or physical stress. The shape of the lesion is similar to a jar used to catch octopus in Japan and is also known as takotsubo cardiomyopathy [55]. Although there is little known regarding its etiology, it is thought to be due to temporary twitching of the coronary artery due to excessive secretion of catecholamines. Clinically, it can mimic acute coronary syndrome. Although increased levels of troponin and creatine kinase-MB (CK-MB) are observed in stress-induced cardiomyopathy, the level of increase is smaller than that of ST segment elevation myocardial infarction. Cardiac function is the presence of severely reduced ejection fraction with large regions of akinesia. There are ST segment elevation in 40–80% and T-wave inversion in about 65%. However, coronary angiography shows no stenosis in stress-induced cardiomyopathy. Moreover, it is reversible. About 50% of the patients can develop acute heart failure, and the treatment follows that regularly used for acute heart failure. If patients are hemodynamically stable with congestion, diuretic drugs can be administrated. In addition, angiotensin-converting enzyme inhibitors, angiotensin receptor blockers, and beta-blockers can be given until left ventricular function recovers. If hemodynamically unstable, positive inotropic agents are used to promote myocardial contractility. The patient improves in a few weeks, and the mortality rate is only about 1–2% but had been reported to reach 16% in severely affected patients.

10.6.5 Paroxysmal Sympathetic Hyperactivity

Paroxysmal sympathetic hyperactivity can occur in patients with severe hemorrhagic stroke. Early diagnosis and treatment is essential because of prolonged length of ICU stay and poor prognosis. It is often caused by paroxysmal hyperactivity of the sympathetic system, and common symptoms include tachycardia (more than 120 beats/min), hyperventilation (more than 30 breaths/min), fever (greater than 38.5 °C), increased BP (systolic pressure greater than 160 mmHg), dilated pupils, perspiration, and more. Abruptly stopping sedatives can induce similar symptoms, and this condition should be differentiated from symptoms caused by sepsis, neuroleptic malignant syndrome, or malignant hyperthermia. Although the pathophysiology is unknown, disconnection between autonomic center of the diencephalon cortex, subcortex, and brainstem is thought to cause this condition. Morphine is commonly used as a treatment, and to control elevated BP, a presynaptic alpha-2 receptor agonist, such as dexmedetomidine or clonidine, and propranolol (beta-receptor blockers) are used in addition. In cases of increased muscle tone, baclofen (GABA-B receptor agonists) can also be useful [56].

References

1. Kim BJ, Lee SH. Cerebral microbleeds: their associated factors, radiologic findings, and clinical implications. J Stroke. 2013;15:153–63.
2. Connolly ES Jr, Rabinstein AA, Carhuapoma JR, et al. Guidelines for the management of aneurysmal subarachnoid hemorrhage: a guideline for healthcare professionals from the American Heart Association/American Stroke Association. Stroke. 2012;43:1711–37.
3. Becker KJ, Baxter AB, Bybee HM, et al. Extravasation of radiographic contrast is an independent predictor of death in primary intracerebral hemorrhage. Stroke. 1999;30:2025–32.
4. Brott T, Broderick J, Kothari R, et al. Early hemorrhage growth in patients with intracerebral hemorrhage. Stroke. 1997;28:1–5.
5. Delgado Almandoz JE, Yoo AJ, Stone MJ, et al. Systematic characterization of the computed tomography angiography spot sign in primary intracerebral hemorrhage identifies patients at highest risk for hematoma expansion: the spot sign score. Stroke. 2009;40:2994–3000.
6. Hemphill JC III, Bonovich DC, Besmertis L, et al. The ICH score: a simple, reliable grading scale for intracerebral hemorrhage. Stroke. 2001;32:891–7.
7. Claassen J, Bernardini GL, Kreiter K, et al. Effect of cisternal and ventricular blood on risk of delayed cerebral ischemia after subarachnoid hemorrhage: the Fisher scale revisited. Stroke. 2001;32:2012–20.
8. Frontera JA, Claassen J, Schmidt JM, et al. Prediction of symptomatic vasospasm after subarachnoid hemorrhage: the modified fisher scale. Neurosurgery. 2006;59:21–7.
9. Teasdale GM, Drake CG, Hunt W, et al. A universal subarachnoid hemorrhage scale: report of a committee of the World Federation of Neurosurgical Societies. J Neurol Neurosurg Psychiatry. 1988;51:1457.
10. Hunt WE, Hess RM. Surgical risk as related to time of intervention in the repair of intracranial aneurysms. J Neurosurg. 1968;28:14–20.
11. Mayer SA, Brun NC, Begtrup K, et al. Efficacy and safety of recombinant activated factor VII for acute intracerebral hemorrhage. N Engl J Med. 2008;358:2127–37.
12. Li X, Sun Z, Zhao W, et al. Effect of acetylsalicylic acid usage and platelet transfusion on postoperative hemorrhage and activities of daily living in patients with acute intracerebral hemorrhage. J Neurosurg. 2013;118:94–103.
13. Baharoglu MI, Cordonnier C, Al-Shahi Salman R, et al. Platelet transfusion versus standard care after acute stroke due to spontaneous cerebral haemorrhage associated with antiplatelet therapy (PATCH): a randomised, open-label, phase 3 trial. Lancet. 2016;387:2605–13.
14. Frontera JA, Lewin JJ III, Rabinstein AA, et al. Guideline for reversal of antithrombotics in intracranial hemorrhage: a statement for healthcare professionals from the Neurocritical Care Society and Society of Critical Care Medicine. Neurocrit Care. 2016;24:6–46.
15. Kollmar R, Staykov D, Dorfler A, et al. Hypothermia reduces perihemorrhagic edema after intracerebral hemorrhage. Stroke. 2010;41:1684–9.
16. Staykov D, Wagner I, Volbers B, et al. Mild prolonged hypothermia for large intracerebral hemorrhage. Neurocrit Care. 2013;18:178–83.
17. Claassen J, Jette N, Chum F, et al. Electrographic seizures and periodic discharges after intracerebral hemorrhage. Neurology. 2007;69:1356–65.
18. Investigators N-SS, Finfer S, Chittock DR, et al. Intensive versus conventional glucose control in critically ill patients. N Engl J Med. 2009;360:1283–97.
19. Australian N-SSIFT, New Zealand Intensive Care Society Clinical Trials Group, The Canadian Critical Care Trials Group, et al. Intensive versus conventional glucose control in critically ill patients with traumatic brain injury: long-term follow-up of a subgroup of

patients from the NICE-SUGAR study. Intensive Care Med. 2015;41:1037–47.
20. Collaboration CT. Thigh-length versus below-knee stockings for deep venous thrombosis prophylaxis after stroke: a randomized trial. Ann Intern Med. 2010;153:553–62.
21. Collaboration CT, Dennis M, Sandercock P, et al. The effect of graduated compression stockings on long-term outcomes after stroke: the CLOTS trials 1 and 2. Stroke. 2013;44:1075–9.
22. Collaboration CT, Dennis M, Sandercock PA, et al. Effectiveness of thigh-length graduated compression stockings to reduce the risk of deep vein thrombosis after stroke (CLOTS trial 1): a multicentre, randomised controlled trial. Lancet. 2009;373:1958–65.
23. Collaboration CT, Dennis M, Sandercock P, et al. Effectiveness of intermittent pneumatic compression in reduction of risk of deep vein thrombosis in patients who have had a stroke (CLOTS 3): a multicentre randomised controlled trial. Lancet. 2013;382:516–24.
24. Paciaroni M, Agnelli G, Venti M, et al. Efficacy and safety of anticoagulants in the prevention of venous thromboembolism in patients with acute cerebral hemorrhage: a meta-analysis of controlled studies. J Thromb Haemost. 2011;9:893–8.
25. Menon RS, Burgess RE, Wing JJ, et al. Predictors of highly prevalent brain ischemia in intracerebral hemorrhage. Ann Neurol. 2012;71:199–205.
26. Garg RK, Liebling SM, Maas MB, et al. Blood pressure reduction, decreased diffusion on MRI, and outcomes after intracerebral hemorrhage. Stroke. 2012;43:67–71.
27. Butcher KS, Jeerakathil T, Hill M, et al. The intracerebral hemorrhage acutely decreasing arterial pressure trial. Stroke. 2013;44:620–6.
28. Willmot M, Leonardi-Bee J, Bath PM. High blood pressure in acute stroke and subsequent outcome: a systematic review. Hypertension. 2004;43:18–24.
29. Anderson CS, Huang Y, Wang JG, et al. Intensive blood pressure reduction in acute cerebral haemorrhage trial (INTERACT): a randomised pilot trial. Lancet Neurol. 2008;7:391–9.
30. Qureshi AI, Palesch YY, Martin R, et al. Effect of systolic blood pressure reduction on hematoma expansion, perihematomal edema, and 3-month outcome among patients with intracerebral hemorrhage: results from the antihypertensive treatment of acute cerebral hemorrhage study. Arch Neurol. 2010;67:570–6.
31. Anderson CS, Heeley E, Huang Y, et al. Rapid blood-pressure lowering in patients with acute intracerebral hemorrhage. N Engl J Med. 2013;368:2355–65.
32. Qureshi AI, Palesch YY, Barsan WG, et al. Intensive blood-pressure lowering in patients with acute cerebral hemorrhage. N Engl J Med. 2016;375:1033–43.
33. Solenski NJ, Haley EC Jr, Kassell NF, et al. Medical complications of aneurysmal subarachnoid hemorrhage: a report of the multicenter, cooperative aneurysm study. Participants of the Multicenter Cooperative Aneurysm Study. Crit Care Med. 1995;23:1007–17.
34. Tanno Y, Homma M, Oinuma M, et al. Rebleeding from ruptured intracranial aneurysms in North Eastern Province of Japan. A cooperative study. J Neurol Sci. 2007;258:11–6.
35. Ohkuma H, Tsurutani H, Suzuki S. Incidence and significance of early aneurysmal rebleeding before neurosurgical or neurological management. Stroke. 2001;32:1176–80.
36. Hong JH, Bang JS, Chung JH, et al. Protocol based real-time continuous electroencephalography for detecting vasospasm in subarachnoid hemorrhage. J Korean Neurosurg Soc. 2016;59:154–7.
37. Barker FG II, Ogilvy CS. Efficacy of prophylactic nimodipine for delayed ischemic deficit after subarachnoid hemorrhage: a metaanalysis. J Neurosurg. 1996;84:405–14.
38. Vergouwen MD, Vermeulen M, Roos YB. Effect of nimodipine on outcome in patients with traumatic subarachnoid haemorrhage: a systematic review. Lancet Neurol. 2006;5:1029–32.
39. Wartenberg KE, Schmidt JM, Mayer SA. Multimodality monitoring in neurocritical care. Crit Care Clin. 2007;23:507–38.
40. Rose JC, Mayer SA. Optimizing blood pressure in neurological emergencies. Neurocrit Care. 2004;1:287–99.
41. Hirzallah MI, Choi HA. The monitoring of brain edema and intracranial hypertension. J Neurocrit Care. 2016;9:92–104.
42. Lundberg N. Continuous recording and control of ventricular fluid pressure in neurosurgical practice. Acta Psychiatr Scand Suppl. 1960;36:1–193.
43. Diringer MN, Zazulia AR. Osmotic therapy: fact and fiction. Neurocrit Care. 2004;1:219–33.
44. Garcia-Morales EJ, Cariappa R, Parvin CA, et al. Osmole gap in neurologic-neurosurgical intensive care unit: its normal value, calculation, and relationship with mannitol serum concentrations. Crit Care Med. 2004;32:986–91.
45. Suarez JI, Qureshi AI, Bhardwaj A, et al. Treatment of refractory intracranial hypertension with 23.4% saline. Crit Care Med. 1998;26:1118–22.
46. Kamel H, Navi BB, Nakagawa K, et al. Hypertonic saline versus mannitol for the treatment of elevated intracranial pressure: a meta-analysis of randomized clinical trials. Crit Care Med. 2011;39:554–9.
47. Hays AN, Lazaridis C, Neyens R, et al. Osmotherapy: use among neurointensivists. Neurocrit Care. 2011;14:222–8.
48. Muizelaar JP, Marmarou A, Ward JD, et al. Adverse effects of prolonged hyperventilation in patients with severe head injury: a randomized clinical trial. J Neurosurg. 1991;75:731–9.
49. Fischer M, Schiefecker A, Lackner P, et al. Targeted temperature management in spontaneous intrace-

rebral hemorrhage: a systematic review. Curr Drug Targets. 2016;18(12):1430–40.
50. Choi HA, Ko SB, Presciutti M, et al. Prevention of shivering during therapeutic temperature modulation: the Columbia anti-shivering protocol. Neurocrit Care. 2011;14:389–94.
51. Berkenstadt H, Margalit N, Hadani M, et al. Stroke volume variation as a predictor of fluid responsiveness in patients undergoing brain surgery. Anesth Analg. 2001;92:984–9.
52. Charron C, Caille V, Jardin F, et al. Echocardiographic measurement of fluid responsiveness. Curr Opin Crit Care. 2006;12:249–54.
53. Lyden PD, Shuaib A, Lees KR, et al. Safety and tolerability of NXY-059 for acute intracerebral hemorrhage: the CHANT trial. Stroke. 2007;38:2262–9.
54. Baumann A, Audibert G, Mcdonnell J, et al. Neurogenic pulmonary edema. Acta Anaesthesiol Scand. 2007;51:447–55.
55. Lee VH, Connolly HM, Fulgham JR, et al. Tako-tsubo cardiomyopathy in aneurysmal subarachnoid hemorrhage: an underappreciated ventricular dysfunction. J Neurosurg. 2006;105:264–70.
56. Choi HA, Jeon SB, Samuel S, et al. Paroxysmal sympathetic hyperactivity after acute brain injury. Curr Neurol Neurosci Rep. 2013;13:370.

11 Principles and Techniques of Surgical Management of ICH

Josephine U. Pucci, Shyle H. Mehta, Brandon R. Christophe, and Edward S. Connolly Jr

Spontaneous or nontraumatic ICH is a focal collection of blood within the brain parenchyma. ICH is the second most common form of stroke, accounting for 10–30% of all cases [1–3]. With about a 40% mortality rate at 1 month [1] and a 40% disability rate at 1 year [4], ICH is one of the leading causes of stroke-related mortality and morbidity. Many acute complications are associated with worsening patient outcomes following ICH, including hematoma expansion and perihematomal edema (PHE) [5]. The etiology by which these complications lead to worse outcomes is likely explained by blood expansion leading to mass effect and/or increased intracerebral pressure (ICP) and secondary neuronal injury triggered by hemotoxicity. Management options include both medical and surgical intervention. Goals of surgical procedures include minimizing the pathophysiological impact of the hematoma on the surrounding tissue, decreasing edema from blood product breakdown in order to facilitate survival of penumbra of functionally impaired but potentially viable surrounding tissue [5], reducing ICP, and/or preventing herniation.

Indications for surgery in patients with ICH are greatly dependent on the site and size of hemorrhage, age of patient, level of consciousness, and time elapsed since ICH ictus. Yet, research in ICH approach, management, surgical indications, and technical management insufficiently addresses some of the most common complications. In 2015, the American Heart Association/American Stroke Association (AHA/ASA) provided comprehensive recommendations for the diagnosis and treatment of spontaneous ICH [6]. Overall, the treatment of hemorrhages large in volume, enlarging, or atypically located in younger patients was recommended with aggressive treatment, such as surgical hematoma evacuation. This is in addition to conservative measures, such as management addressing blood pressure, glucose levels, temperature, hemostasis, coagulopathy, and deep vein thrombosis [5, 6]. Although much research discusses conventional craniotomies, its effectiveness in ICH patients remains controversial. Ongoing trials explore other surgical options to address ICP and mass effect following ICH, such as minimally invasive surgery (MIS) techniques and decompressive craniectomy (DC).

J. U. Pucci · S. H. Mehta · B. R. Christophe
Columbia University Medical Center, Columbia University, New York, NY, USA
e-mail: jup2102@cumc.columbia.edu; brc2119@cumc.columbia.edu

E. S. Connolly Jr (✉)
Department of Neurological Surgery, Columbia University, New York, NY, USA
e-mail: esc5@cumc.columbia.edu

S.-H. Lee (ed.), *Stroke Revisited: Hemorrhagic Stroke*, Stroke Revisited,
https://doi.org/10.1007/978-981-10-1427-7_11

11.1 Craniotomy

Following primary ICH, a standard craniotomy can evacuate hemorrhage (Fig. 11.1a). Although randomized trials have not clearly indicated the effectiveness of craniotomy clot removal on patient outcome [6], numerous clot removals are performed annually. In 2015, the AHA/ASA recommended a standard craniotomy hematoma evacuation in patients with clots greater than 30 mL within 1 cm of the cortical surface; due to the lobar location, clots can be assessed with minimal damage to brain tissue [5]. These AHA/ASA recommendations mainly drew upon a series of randomized trials, most notably STICH I and STICH II.

In 2008, a meta-analysis reviewed ten randomized trials including 2059 patients [7]. According to the results of this meta-analysis, craniotomy was linked to a reduced risk of death and dependency (OR 0.71), but this benefit was not robust. The largest of the ten randomized trials was the STICH trial; patients assigned to early hematoma evacuation (defined as a median time to surgery of 30 hours after onset of hemorrhage) were marginally likelier to have better outcome at 6 months than those who received initial conservative treatment, but this benefit was not significant [8]. In addition, patients with hematoma within 1 cm of the cortical surface who received a craniotomy were more likely to benefit, though this effect was not significant either. A major limitation to the study was high crossover rate: 26% of patients received surgical evacuation even though they were initially assigned to the group that received conservative medical management. This could compromise the study's ability to demonstrate benefit from surgery [9].

The STICH II trial found that the rates of adverse outcomes at 6 months were similar between patients who underwent early hematoma evacuation (defined as within 48 hours of hemorrhage onset) and patients who received conservative medical management (59% vs. 62%) [10]. This study has limitations, however, including the state of treated patients (conscious and without intraventricular extension) and the high crossover rate (21% of patients received surgical evacuation even though they were initially assigned to the group that received conservative medical management).

When the data from the STICH II trial were combined with those from 14 other randomized

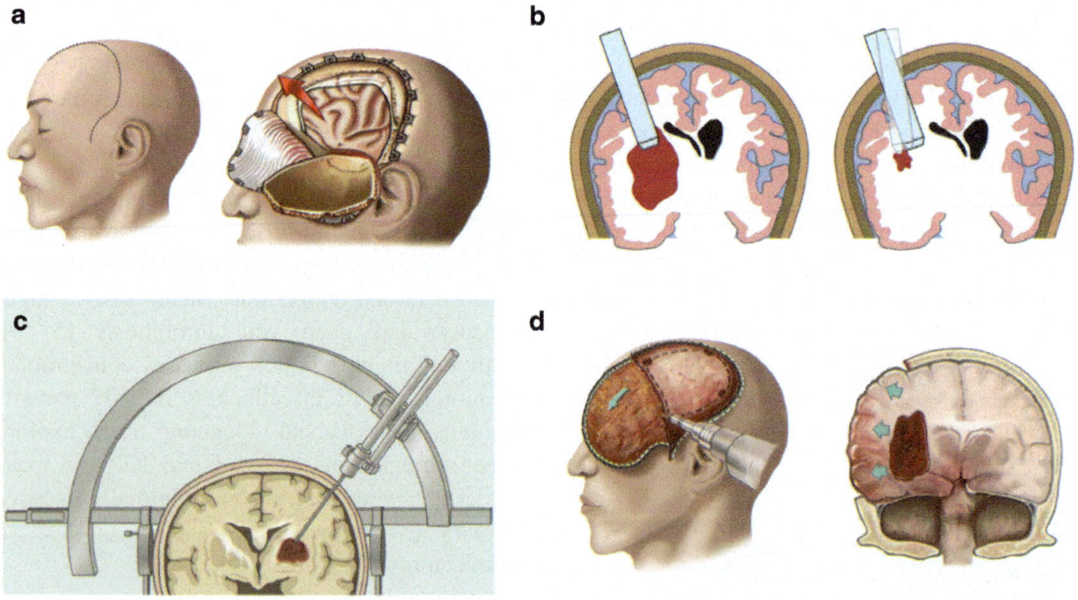

Fig. 11.1 Illustrations of surgical techniques of intracerebral hemorrhage (ICH). (**a**) Craniotomy. (**b**) Endoscopic evacuation. (**c**) Stereotactic aspiration. (**d**) Decompressive craniectomy

trials, a survival benefit for surgical hematoma evacuation was observed for certain patient subgroups: patients with (1) poorer prognosis on presentation of hemorrhage, (2) patients whose condition deteriorated following presentation, and (3) patients with superficial ICH and without intraventricular extension [10] (Fig. 11.2). Since certain subgroups were excluded from trial

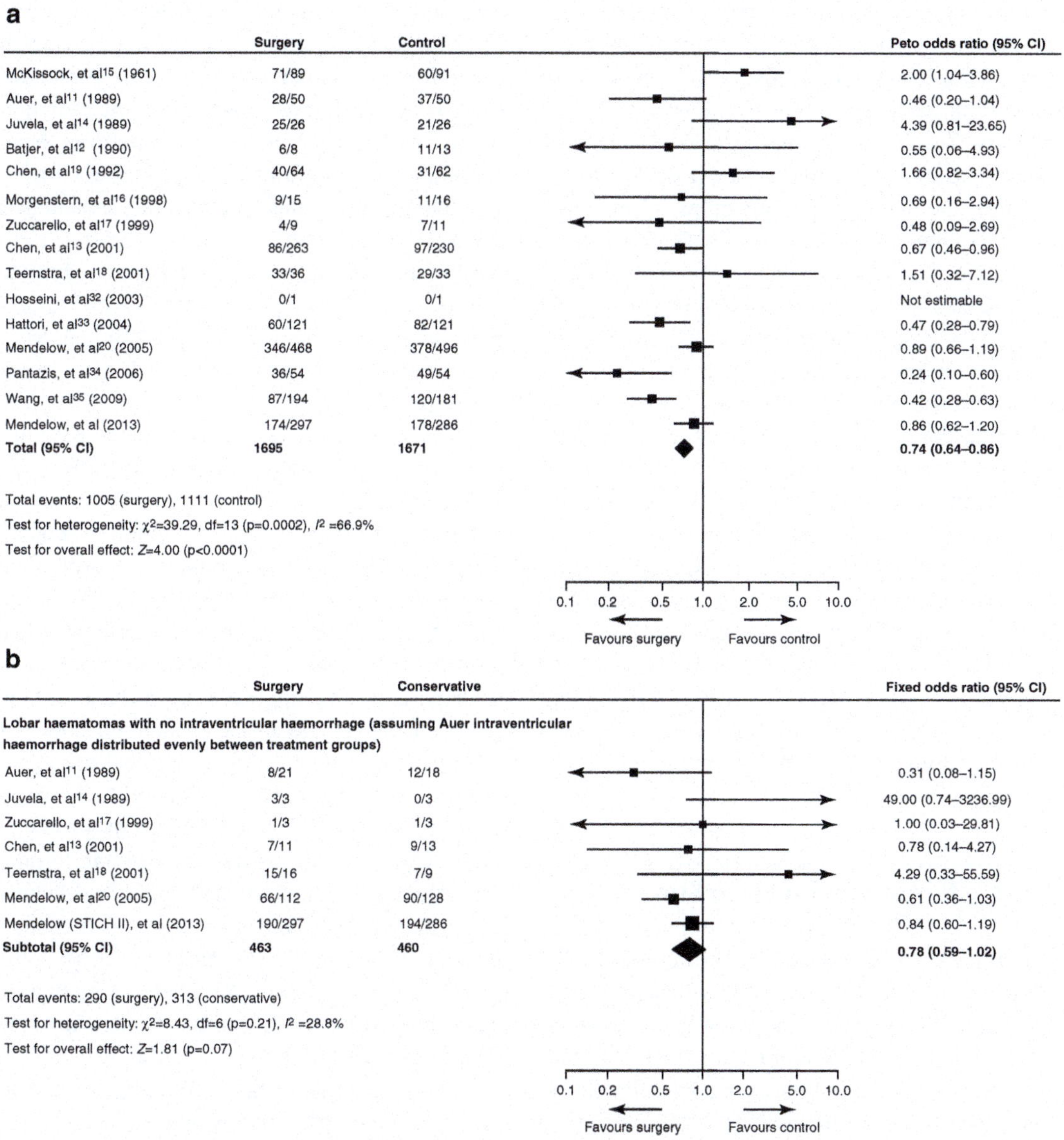

Fig. 11.2 (**a**) Meta-analysis of surgery trials in patients with intracerebral hemorrhage (ICH). Incorporation of the results from "Early surgery versus initial conservative treatment in patients with spontaneous supratentorial lobar intracerebral haematomas (STICH II)" trial (583 patients) with the previous meta-analysis of 14 trials of surgery shows a significant advantage for surgery with an odds ratio of 0.74 (95% CI 0.64–0.86; $p < 0.0001$). There is significant heterogeneity (p = 0.0002) because the studies included different patient groups and different types of surgery. (**b**) Meta-analysis of patient cases of lobar hematomas with no intraventricular hemorrhage (IVH). There is no evidence of heterogeneity (p = 0.21), and there is not a significant benefit from surgery (n = 923; 0.78, 0.59–1.02; p = 0.07). The results of the meta-analyses suggest that there is a role for surgery in patients with intracerebral hemorrhage, but that there is still some uncertainty about which patients benefit most. Adapted by permission of Lancet [10]

evidence, more studies are necessary to conclusively decide which patient subgroups should receive surgical hematoma evacuation.

Although surgical procedures may be controversial in some cases, patients with cerebellar hemorrhages larger than 3 cm (in diameter), with brainstem compression, and hydrocephalus caused by ventricular obstruction should all receive surgical removal of the hemorrhage [11]. It is also recommended that external drainage be done with decompression of the posterior fossa, as drainage without this decompression could possibly lead to cerebellar mass herniation. Typically, hemorrhages that involve the brainstem are associated with a dismal prognosis that surgery is unlikely to influence. Because of the narrow confines of this space, hemorrhage can cause obstructive hydrocephalus or local mass effect on the brainstem, both of which are devastating to patients [6].

Although craniotomies can result in lengthy operations, high blood loss, and additional tissue insult, they may still benefit specific patient subsets, including those with supratentorial and posterior fossa hemorrhages. Currently, no other patient group is recommended for surgery, and no surgical method other than standard craniotomy is supported, although ongoing clinical trials are likely to change this recommendation.

11.2 Minimally Invasive Surgery

Given the advances made in MIS in other fields, it is possible that a similar approach may be safer and more effective than craniotomy clot evacuations. MIS could evacuate hemorrhages in locations in which craniotomies cannot reach without extensive tissue insult. STICH failed to significantly justify the use of surgery in deeply seated hemorrhages, but MIS may be particularly beneficial in these cases. The effectiveness of minimally invasive clot evacuation utilizing either endoscopic or stereotactic aspiration with or without thrombolytic usage is still considered investigational [6, 11].

11.2.1 Endoscopy

Endoscopic evacuation of ICH aims to remove clots and minimize secondary injury due to parenchymal manipulation. Intracranial access is gained through a small burr hole, and hematoma is generally evacuated through a sheath under direct visualization (Fig. 11.1b). An endoscope is introduced to view the volume of irrigation to ensure that no blood is coming from vessels, as this might need coagulation. Current parameters for which endoscopic evacuation could be considered are supratentorial clots greater than 30 mL, with a technical goal to reduce the clot burden to less than 15 mL [5]. As more data becomes available, the clinical criterion for endoscopic evacuation of ICH is likely to evolve [5].

Most recently, ICES, a multicenter randomized, controlled trial, concluded that early computerized tomographic image-guided endoscopic surgery is a safe and effective method to remove acute ICH and could also enhance neurological recovery compared to medically treated patients. In ICES, one of the three preapproved approaches was selected: anterior frontal lobe approach, posterior parietal lobe approach, or surface cortical approach. An image probe positioned over the candidate entry point guided the ideal trajectory selected. Each approach was devised to be parallel and in the middle of the long axis of the hematoma. It was imperative that the Sylvian fissure, internal capsule, white matter tracts, and ventricles were avoided. The endoscope was manually inserted into the cortex upon releasing the hydraulic break. The endoscope sheath was placed approximately two thirds of the way to the hematoma's distal margin parallel to its long axis. Using irrigation and aspiration, the hematoma was removed. Upon achieving hemostasis, the endoscope sheath was retracted so that it was one third of the way into the hematoma cavity. Irrigation and aspiration were repeated to remove about 75% of the hematoma volume. Overall, 68% of patients had an end of treatment volume at <15 mL. Following this, the dura and skin were closed as normal [12].

At 1 year, patients who received endoscopic surgery were 12% likelier than medically treated patients to have good functional outcome (mRS 0-3), suggesting this technique may be therapeutic for ICH patients [12]. A limitation to the ICES trial is its small sample size ($n = 20$), which might compromise the ability for statistical comparisons to identify variations in patient traits that might be linked to outcomes. Additionally, the effect of hemorrhage location and size and interruption of white matter tracts on outcome was not addressed and should be further researched in the upcoming ICES phase II trial.

11.2.2 Stereotactic Catheter Aspiration of Clot

Stereotactic aspiration, another minimally invasive procedure, involves clot removal typically with application of fibrinolytic agents through a catheter. This MIS relies on indirect serial imaging to create a three-dimensional roadmap for real-time surgical guidance, allowing the surgeon to identify and immediately address the original bleeding source [5]. A stereotactic frame is attached to the patient's head and a metal cage is placed on the frame. After a CT scan is completed, the surgeon determines the hematoma's coordinates. With the aid of the stereotactic frame, a hollow needle is passed through the burr hole and the brain tissue, directly into the clot (Fig. 11.1c). A large syringe attached to the hollow needle suctions out the contents of the blood clot.

Stereotactic techniques combine hardware access technology with suction liquefaction technology. Studies addressed a variety of fibrinolytic agents, such as urokinase, streptokinase, alteplase, and recombinant tissue plasminogen activator (rtPA), which were injected directly into the hematoma. These agents enhance clot drainage by accelerating lysis rate. Although there are concerns of thrombolytic agents increasing the risk of worsening edema, recent studies support its safety and efficacy [13, 14].

A randomized, controlled clinical trial compared 64 patients treated with minimally invasive stereotactic puncture and thrombolysis therapy (MISPTT) and 58 treated with conventional craniotomy. The MISPTT group had fewer complications and a trend towards improved short-term and long-term outcomes compared to craniotomy patients. Urokinase, the thrombosis agent, did not exacerbate brain edema formation (Fig. 11.3). Additionally, a reduction of the ICH volume seemed to be associated with the reduction of edema volume [13].

Minimally invasive surgery plus recombinant tissue plasminogen activator in intracerebral hemorrhage evacuation (MISTIE) was a randomized, controlled phase II trial that compared stereotactic aspiration with fibrinolytic agents and conservative medical management. The investigators found that this specific procedure had a 14% improvement among people with a mRS of 0-2. This subgroup of patients had 38 fewer days in the hospital. Also, 14% less MISTIE patients were in long-term care over the course of 1 year when compared to patients receiving conservative medical management. For patients with a mRS of 0-3, the treatment effect after 1 year was significant (>10% absolute benefit). These results demonstrate the efficacy and safety of MIS [14]. The investigators of this trial also found an association between hematoma evacuation and reductions in perihematomal edema (PHE) ($\rho = 0.658$; $p < 0.001$). Moreover, PHE is not worsened by rtPA, which was a concern in previous literature. Although mortality remained the same in both groups, a higher incidence of asymptomatic bleeding occurred in the experimental group [14].

Another trial, Stereotactic Aspiration and Thrombolysis of Intracerebral Hemorrhage (SATIH), is an ongoing prospective controlled study that aims to further reduce the rate of bleeding and mortality, as well as improve long-term quality of life. Additionally, a MISTIE phase III trial is currently underway, which will allow for better assessment of the efficacy and safety of MIS plus alteplase. The results from MISTIE III combined with ICES II should compare the effectiveness of endoscopic versus stereotactic techniques: MISTIE relies on a gentle irrigation

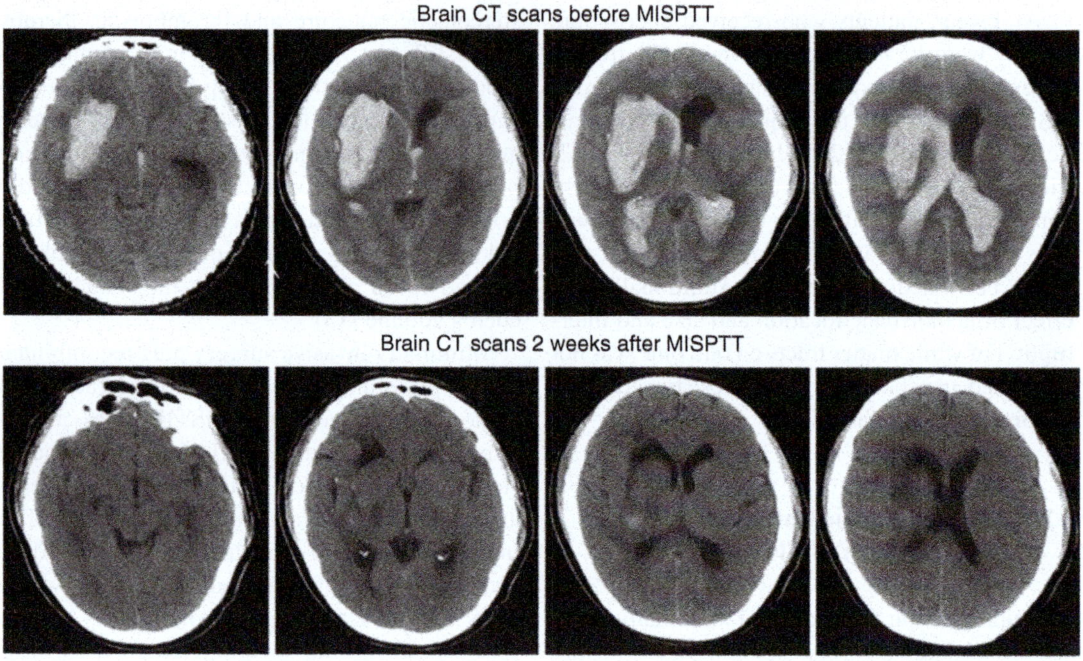

Fig. 11.3 Computed tomography (CT) scans demonstrate the size of the hematoma on serial axial CT images of a patient before and after stereotactic aspiration with thrombolysis. Top images are taken when patient was in a coma (Glasgow Coma Scale (GCS) score 5) with a large hematoma (70 mL before minimally invasive stereotactic puncture and thrombolysis therapy (MISPTT)), and bottom CT scans of the same patient were during consciousness (GCS score 14) 2 weeks after MISPTT. CT scans 2 weeks after MISPTT showed amelioration in hematoma volume and edema in the surrounding brain compared with that prior to MISPTT. The patient was self-sufficient 1 year after onset. Adapted by permission of Journal of Neurology [13]

approach to remove the hematoma by gradual thrombolysis, while ICES illustrates the mechanically aggressive procedure that removes the hematoma right away [12].

11.3 Decompressive Craniectomy

Not all surgical approaches necessarily aim to remove hematoma clot: DC without hematoma evacuation could be beneficial in selected cases of ICH (Fig. 11.1d). Removing a bone flap and opening the underlying dura enables the brain to expand, addressing mass effect and ICP without the additional tissue insult experienced in craniotomies [11]. Though randomized data are still lacking, DC could prevent some deaths; however, many of the people whose deaths are prevented may be left with very serious disability. Concerns around DC also include the increase in PHE that often occurs following surgery [15]. Although an increase in PHE typically results in worse outcome, researchers are uncertain as to whether other not this holds true following DC [15]. DC is suggested to be feasible and may be safe with a specific subset of patients: those with supratentorial ICH [16]. One study illustrated those with conservative treatment were 3.643 times more prone to develop poor outcome than the supratentorial ICH DC group, which was statistically significant (95% CI, 1.040–13.047; p value <0.05) [17]. The AHA/ASA suggest DC might reduce mortality for patients with supratentorial ICH who are in a coma, have large hematomas with significant midline shift, or have elevated ICP refractory to medical management [6]. With promising claims in retrospective studies, investigators agree that randomized controlled trials are justified. Ongoing randomized, controlled trial, SWITCH, is a currently seeking to determine whether decompressive surgery and best medical treatment in patients with spontaneous ICH will improve outcome compared to best medical treatment only.

11.4 Timing

Data on the ideal timing of surgical procedures following ICH remains mixed. Standard care does not recommend routine evacuation of supratentorial ICH in the first 96 h; however, some evidence suggests sooner surgery may be beneficial. STICH II recommends surgery within the first 21 hours post-ictus [10]. Additionally, an individual patient meta-analysis of 2186 patients from 8 trials of surgery for ICH found that surgery improved outcome if performed within 8 hours of hemorrhage [6]. The 2014 guidelines from the European Stroke Organisation state that early surgery may be beneficial for patients with a GCS of 9–12 [5, 6, 18]. Deterioration of consciousness could be due to mass effect from the hematoma or cerebral herniation [6, 11]. No clear evidence at present indicates that ultra-early (within 4 h) removal of the supratentorial ICH improves functional outcome or mortality; a very early craniotomy may be harmful due to increased risk of recurrent bleeding [19]. MIS may facilitate an earlier evacuation of ICH than is possible or practical with conventional craniotomy [20].

Conclusion

Currently, standard care is medical management with delayed surgery if necessary [21]. Surgical procedures are performed to (1) restrict hemorrhage expansion, (2) manage PHE and increased ICP, or (3) address ventricular extension of hemorrhage and hydrocephalus. The latest guidelines for the management of ICH from the AHA/ASA included PubMed searches through August 2013. Since then, new retrospective and prospective studies on surgical indications and developing approaches justified the ongoing randomized, controlled trials in progress. STICH failed to illustrate a significant difference between groups undergoing craniotomy versus conservative treatments, but most recent studies look specifically at MIS, which show promising potential mainly due to its less invasive nature. Standard care can be dramatically altered as new information is published regarding MIS. Controversial data regarding surgical procedures for ICH could be due to the heterogeneity of ICH. Moving forward, very specific studies regarding location and type of hemorrhage would be beneficial.

References

1. van Asch CJ, Luitse MJ, Rinkel GJ, et al. Incidence, case fatality, and functional outcome of intracerebral haemorrhage over time, according to age, sex, and ethnic origin: a systematic review and meta-analysis. Lancet Neurol. 2010;9:167–76.
2. Balami JS, Buchan AM. Complications of intracerebral haemorrhage. Lancet Neurol. 2012;11:101–18.
3. Anderson CS, Chakera TM, Stewart-Wynne EG, et al. Spectrum of primary intracerebral haemorrhage in Perth, Western Australia, 1989-90: incidence and outcome. J Neurol Neurosurg. 1994;57:936–40.
4. Hanley DF. Intracerebral haemorrhage. Lancet. 2011;373:1632–44.
5. Rennert RC, Signorelli JW, Abraham P, et al. Minimally invasive treatment of intracerebral hemorrhage. Expert Rev Neurother. 2015;15:919–33.
6. Hemphill JC, Greenberg SM, Anderson CS, et al. Guidelines for the management of spontaneous intracerebral hemorrhage: a guideline for healthcare professionals from the American Heart Association/American Stroke Association. Stroke. 2015;46:2032–60.
7. Prasad K, Mendelow AD, Gregson B. Surgery for primary supratentorial intracerebral haemorrhage. Cochrane Database Syst Rev. 2008;8:CD000200.
8. Mendelow AD, Gregson BA, Fernandes HM, et al. Early surgery versus initial conservative treatment in patients with spontaneous supratentorial intracerebral haematomas in the International Surgical Trial in Intracerebral Haemorrhage (STICH): a randomised trial. Lancet. 2005;365:387–97.
9. Broderick JP. The STICH trial: what does it tell us and where do we go from here? Stroke. 2005;36:1619–20.
10. Mendelow AD, Gregson BA, Rowan EN, et al. Early surgery versus initial conservative treatment in patients with spontaneous supratentorial lobar intracerebral haematomas (STICH II): a randomised trial. Lancet. 2013;382:397–408.
11. Kim JE, Ko SB, Kang HS, et al. Clinical practice guidelines for the medical and surgical management of primary intracerebral hemorrhage in Korea. J Korean Neurosurg Soc. 2014;56:175–87.

12. Vespa P, Hanley D, Betz J, et al. ICES (Intraoperative Stereotactic Computed Tomography-Guided Endoscopic Surgery) for brain hemorrhage. Stroke. 2016;47:2749–55.
13. Zhou H, Zhang Y, Liu L, et al. Minimally invasive stereotactic puncture and thrombolysis therapy improves long-term outcome after acute intracerebral hemorrhage. J Neurol. 2011;258:661–9.
14. Hanley DF, Thompson RE, Muschelli J, et al. Safety and efficacy of minimally invasive surgery plus alteplase in intracerebral haemorrhage evacuation (MISTIE): a randomised, controlled, open-label, phase 2 trial. Lancet Neurol. 2016;15:1228–37.
15. Fung C, Murek M, Klinger-Gratz PP, et al. Effect of decompressive craniectomy on perihematomal edema in patients with intracerebral hemorrhage. PLoS One. 2016;11:4–12.
16. Fung C, Murek M, Z'Graggen WJ, et al. Decompressive hemicraniectomy in patients with supratentorial intracerebral hemorrhage. Stroke. 2012;43:3207–11.
17. Satter A, Islam M, Haque M, et al. Comparison between decompressive craniectomy with durotomy and conservative treatment in spontaneous supratentorial intracerebral hemorrhage. Mymensingh Med J. 2016;25:316–25.
18. Steiner T, Al-Shahi Salman R, Beer R, et al. European stroke organisation (ESO) guidelines for the management of spontaneous intracerebral hemorrhage. Int J Stroke. 2014;9:840–55.
19. Morgenstern LB, Demchuk AM, Kim DH, et al. Rebleeding leads to poor outcome in ultra-early craniotomy for intracerebral hemorrhage. Neurology. 2001;56:1294–9.
20. Broderick J, Connolly S, Feldmann E, et al. Guidelines for the management of spontaneous intracerebral hemorrhage in adults: 2007 update: a guideline from the American Heart Association/American Stroke Association stroke council, high blood pressure research council, and the quality of care and out. Stroke. 2007;38:2001–23.
21. de Oliveira Manoel AL, Goffi A, Zampieri FG, et al. The critical care management of spontaneous intracranial hemorrhage: a contemporary review. Crit Care. 2016;20:272.

12 Principles and Techniques of Surgical Management of Ruptured Cerebral Aneurysms

Won-Sang Cho and Dae Hee Han

12.1 Introduction

Ruptured aneurysms, if left untreated, have been known to result in dismal clinical outcomes. The mortality rate in these cases is 30–60% within 6 months. Among the risk factors for poor clinical outcomes [1, 2], rebleeding is one of the most influencing factors. Rebleeding occurs most frequently during the first day of initial bleeding in approximately 10–20% of cases, and 50% of ruptured aneurysms rebleed within 6 months, although rebleeding decreases after the first day [3, 4, 5]. Rebleeding is a manageable factor, and management reduces mortality and improves prognoses, and it is therefore a major treatment target. However, there is currently no effective medical treatment for this condition, and surgical or endovascular interventions are the only methods available to prevent rebleeding [6]. In the past century, the chronicle of main events related to these surgical techniques include the following: Dr. Norman Dott performed the first wrapping of a ruptured aneurysm in 1933 [7]; Dr. Walter Dandy performed the first neck clipping of a ruptured posterior communicating artery (PCoA) aneurysm using a silver clip [8]; and the introduction of microscopy in the 1960s was a critical contributor to dramatic improvements in surgical techniques and outcomes [9].

Meanwhile, endovascular intervention became one of major treatment modalities soon after the invention of the detachable platinum coil by Dr. Guido Guglielmi in 1990 and the Food and Drug Administration's approval of the procedure in 1995 [10]. In its first randomized controlled study, the International Subarachnoid Aneurysm Trial in 2002 [11], coil embolization proved comparable to surgical clipping. The one-year morbidity and mortality rates were significantly lower in the coil embolization group than in the surgical clipping group (23.7% vs. 30.6%, $p = 0.0019$) [10], and the results of a midterm follow-up study were the same as the 1-year results (23.5% vs. 30.9%, $p = 0.0001$) [12]. Although there was some criticism regarding the results obtained during the early period, the superiority of coil embolization over surgical clipping in terms of clinical outcomes was acknowledged, even after the lower angiographic outcomes and higher rebleeding rates observed in the coil embolization group were considered. Coil embolization therefore is recommended by clinical guidelines around the world as the first treatment modality if both coil embolization and surgical clipping are available [6, 13–15].

W.-S. Cho
Department of Neurosurgery, Seoul National University Hospital, Seoul, South Korea

D. H. Han (✉)
Department of Neurosurgery, Cerebral and Cardiovascular Disease Center, National Medical Center, Seoul, South Korea
e-mail: daehan@snu.ac.kr

S.-H. Lee (ed.), *Stroke Revisited: Hemorrhagic Stroke*, Stroke Revisited,
https://doi.org/10.1007/978-981-10-1427-7_12

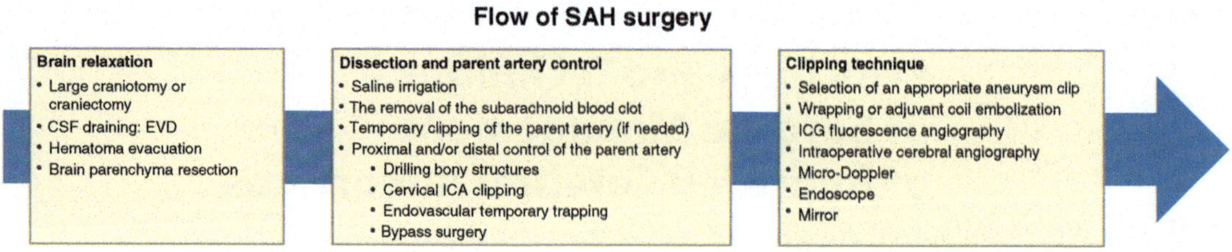

Fig. 12.1 A schematic diagram showing general surgical techniques of subarachnoid hemorrhage (SAH). *CSF* cerebrospinal fluid, *EVD* extraventricular drainage, *ICA* internal carotid artery, *ICG* indocyanine green

Nonetheless, surgical clipping is still recommended as the first line when surgical results are better than coil embolization in certain institutions; in patients younger than 40 years old; in aneurysms with a complex configuration, such as a wide neck or branches arising from the sac, those too small to perform a coil embolization, and those with a mass effect due to size; in hematomas accompanied by high intracranial pressure (ICP); and cases in which an endovascular approach is not feasible because of vessel tortuosity or atherosclerotic vessel wall changes [6, 13, 14]. In this chapter, we examine the surgical techniques used to treat ruptured cerebral aneurysms (Fig. 12.1).

12.2 General and Basic Surgical Techniques

12.2.1 Brain Relaxation

The most important goal during surgery for a ruptured cerebral aneurysm is brain relaxation, which allows enough room to be made for the microscope to view and for surgical instruments to access the affected area. Ruptured aneurysms are always accompanied by variable states of brain swelling, and specific procedures are needed to achieve adequate brain relaxation and space to perform the surgery. These procedures consist of a large craniotomy or craniectomy, draining the cerebrospinal fluid (CSF), evacuating any associated hematoma, and resecting the brain parenchyma. Among these, CSF drainage is the easiest and most effective method for reducing ICP and relaxing brain swelling. Performing a subarachnoid dissection toward the aneurysms can by itself achieve enough CSF drainage and brain relaxation to perform the surgery. However, this procedure usually takes time, and rapid CSF drainage can be more effectively performed using ventricular drainage. Inserting an external ventricular catheter or lumbar catheter to achieve CSF drainage can be performed via a small burr hole in some safety zones or via a lumbar puncture that is made before the craniotomy. In addition, CSF drainage can be achieved through a transcortical puncture, such as Paine's point, after the craniotomy and dural opening have been performed or through an opening in the lamina terminalis or cisterna magna during an approach to the aneurysm through the subarachnoid dissection.

12.2.2 Dissection and Parent Artery Control

Because subarachnoid hemorrhage (SAH) itself makes it difficult to identify vessels and cranial nerves, surgeons should be familiar with structures of intracranial vessels and should carefully dissect the subarachnoid space to avoid injuring them. Saline irrigation and the removal of the subarachnoid blood clot are helpful for identifying and dissecting neurovascular structures. Major vessels are not as difficult to identify and safely dissect. However, it is easy to damage small perforators during the dissection. Therefore, dissection should be performed through the bare side of the major vessels, from which perforators do not arise. For example, perforators from the anterior (ACA) and middle cerebral (MCA) arteries usually arise from the posterosuperior wall of the parent artery facing the brain parenchyma, and dissections performed through the anteroinferior wall should therefore be safe. As the ruptured aneurysm closes during the subarachnoid dissection, temporary clipping of the parent artery could be needed to achieve proximal or distal control. Marking the clipping point on the parent artery is sometimes helpful because it allows for prompt and appropriate temporary clipping without causing perforator damage in a situation such as rebleeding.

Proximal and/or distal control of the parent artery is essential in a surgery for ruptured aneurysms in order to prevent rebleeding or minimize the amount of bleeding. One of the important factors to consider when choosing a surgical approach is the convenience of controlling the parent artery. Proximal control of the parent artery is usually enough to perform permanent clipping of the ruptured aneurysm. However, temporarily trapping the parent artery is sometimes needed in cases in which a considerable amount of bleeding has occurred, such as aneurysms arising from the internal carotid artery (ICA) and those with retrograde flow via collaterals or in cases requiring the surgeon to precisely dissect large/giant aneurysms or complex structures under a clear microscopic view. Proximal control is not easy to achieve in paraclinoid ICA and posterior circulation aneurysms because of bony structures, such as the anterior and posterior clinoid process, jugular tubercle, and petrous bone. Hence, drilling in these bony structures is needed to achieve proximal control. When drilling bony structure is not enough for proximal control, other alternatives, such as temporary clipping at the cervical ICA and endovascular temporary trapping, can be considered. For large or giant paraclinoid ICA aneurysms, in which drilling the anterior clinoid process is not enough to expose the proximal ICA, exposing the cervical ICA is a good alternative. Recently, it has been shown that transient endovascular trapping of the parent artery can be performed using a balloon catheter in a hybrid operating room.

Clipping of complex aneurysms, such as dissecting, giant thrombosed and atherosclerotic aneurysms, is more time-consuming and difficult than clipping normal aneurysms. Therefore, bypass surgery could be required for flow restoration and to prevent ischemic insult during the temporary clipping of complex aneurysms. Preoperative balloon test occlusion and intraoperative methods, such as intraoperative physiologic monitoring, indocyanine green (ICG) angiography, cerebral angiography, and micro-Doppler, are helpful for evaluating perfusion status and determining whether bypass surgery is needed.

12.2.3 Clipping Techniques

A general practice during aneurysm clipping is to clip the neck through the closure line and parallel to the long axis of the neck along the parent artery using a clip blade that is 1.5 times longer than the aneurysm neck. Some considerations should be taken into account when selecting an appropriate aneurysm clip. These include the size and shape of the aneurysm itself in addition to the spatial relationships among the aneurysm, parent artery, and brain and the clip. Clipping perpendicular to the long axis of the neck can compromise the parent artery, the neck remnant or sac, and the neck tear. However, when clipping perpendicular to the long axis of the neck is unavoidable because of the surgical approach and the geometry of the aneurysm and parent artery, the clipping should be carefully performed using the following technical tips in order to prevent neck tearing and bleeding: lowering aneurysmal pressure by proximally or distally controlling the parent artery using temporary clips and intentionally retaining a small piece of the neck.

When rebleeding occurs before the adjacent neurovascular structures are identified and before complete clipping has been performed, hasty clipping without identifying the exact rupture point should be avoided because inaccurate clipping can make the rupture point larger and result in a more severe situation. In such a situation, the surgeons should calmly perform a temporary clipping combined with suction using multiple suction catheters or compression with cottonoid over the rupture point until the rupture point and essential adjacent anatomy are clarified.

Some aneurysms are difficult to completely clip because of their fusiform configuration and aneurysmal changes that occur in the parent artery itself. Retaining a small part of the aneurysm is better than symptomatically compromising the parent artery. Wrapping and adjuvant coil embolization are good alternatives. However, a wrapped remnant or a coil embolization should be routinely followed up because of the possibility of regrowth or recurrence and rebleeding [22].

Although aneurysms with atherosclerotic walls appear complete after clipping, some such situations are problematic. These include persistent inflow into the sac and a compromised parent artery. When the atherosclerosis is not even, the aneurysm walls are completely occluded in some sections and incompletely occluded in the others, through which intra-aneurysmal flow continues. Therefore, ICG fluorescence angiography and intraoperative cerebral angiography are helpful, and additional clips can be considered selectively or routinely based on the findings. Complete clipping of the atherosclerotic aneurysm on the microscopic view is sometimes accompanied by stenosis or occlusion of the parent artery because of intraluminal atheroma. Hence, performing redundant clipping while leaving a little space at the neck is advisable, and some tools, such as micro-Doppler and intraoperative angiography, are helpful for detecting changes in flow and identifying intraluminal stenosis.

Clip slippage sometimes occurs in large aneurysms or those with atherosclerotic walls. For example, high intra-aneurysmal pressure within the sac can push out the clip. Therefore, using a reinforcing clip, using clips with a higher closing force, or using multiple clips can be useful. When a thick atheroma involves a part of the aneurysm, clipping the softer wall without parent artery compromise can be considered because the thick and hard atherosclerotic wall has a very low risk of rupturing.

Even when completely clipping the ruptured aneurysm is considered, a close inspection of the region around the clipped aneurysm using ICG fluorescence angiography, intraoperative angiography, micro-Doppler, an endoscope, and a mirror is recommended because incomplete structures, such as a remnant aneurysm or a compromised perforator or parent artery, are commonly observed when treating ruptured aneurysms.

As the role of endovascular intervention has become larger and surgical roles have become smaller, difficult cases that cannot be treated using endovascular interventions have tended to be increasingly referred to surgical teams. In addition to the previously mentioned routine clipping techniques, other surgical techniques that require a great deal of skill, such as bypass and trapping, aneurysmorrhaphy, and direct puncture/suction decompression and reconstructive clipping, are needed to treat rare but complex aneurysms, including dissecting, blood blister-like, large or giant, thrombosed and atherosclerotic aneurysms. Hence, while the roles of surgeons are decreasing, the training of key surgeons should continue.

12.3 Specific Considerations [16–21]

12.3.1 Aneurysms Arising from the ICA

Among ICA aneurysms, in extradural aneurysms, conservative observation is recommended unless the aneurysm causes a mass effect or ruptures because the extradural origin is associated with too low a risk of bleeding [23]. The treatment indications in ICA aneurysms include intradural paraclinoid ICA aneurysms with ophthalmic involvement, superior hypophyseal artery aneurysms, PCoA aneurysms, anterior choroidal artery (AChA) aneurysms, and blood blister-like aneurysms. Most paraclinoid ICA aneurysms can be treated using endovascular interventions. However, surgical treatment is considered in cases with a high probability of ophthalmic artery compromise and no collaterals and those with aggravation of cranial neuropathy caused by a mass effect on adjacent cranial nerves. Precautions, such as temporary clipping or trapping, multiple suction, and temporary cardiac arrest, should be always taken in consideration to combat intraprocedural rebleeding because bleeding from the ICA is quite substantial. When there is little room to place a clip to achieve proximal control, drilling into the anterior clinoid process or exposing the cervical ICA are needed. When a long temporary clipping time is expected, whether collateral flow via the anterior communicating artery (ACoA) and PCoA is possible should be checked, and a donor artery for bypass surgery should be prepared in case it is needed to prevent ischemic injury during temporary flow interruption. When clipping an aneurysm arising from the superior hypophyseal artery, preserving the artery is important because it supplies the inferior part of the optic nerve, and an injury in this location can cause partial visual defects on the superior part of the affected side. The direction of the aneurysm is one of the determinants that should be considered when selecting the surgical approach and clip design because the proximal ICA is trapped within the anterior clinoid process, and there is little opportunity to deviate and manipulate the ICA (Fig. 12.2). Wide-necked paraclinoid ICA aneurysms that grow toward the true medial side are very difficult to clip via a routine pterional approach because of the way conventional clips are designed. In these cases, fenestrated clips with a blade rotated toward the aneurysm neck or a craniotomy that exposes the more inferior part of the middle cranial fossa should be considered to make clipping more convenient and to reduce the risk of neck tear and neck remnant.

When clipping aneurysms arising from the PCoA and AChA, preserving these arteries is the most important goal. Some tactics should be taken into consideration, such as clip direction and the distance between the clip and aneurysm neck or branching arteries because clip torsion or slippage caused by brain expansion/swelling and high blood pressure in the ICA can cause delayed compromise of the parent artery and neck remnant. Sometimes, a few branches of the PCoA and AChA arise from the ICA, and these should be closely inspected and preserved without injury. When an aneurysm adheres to the oculomotor nerve, meticulous dissection and detachment is important to prevent additional oculomotor injury. Certain aneurysms that arise from the PCoA and AChA are hard to identify because they are located on the side opposite to the microscopic

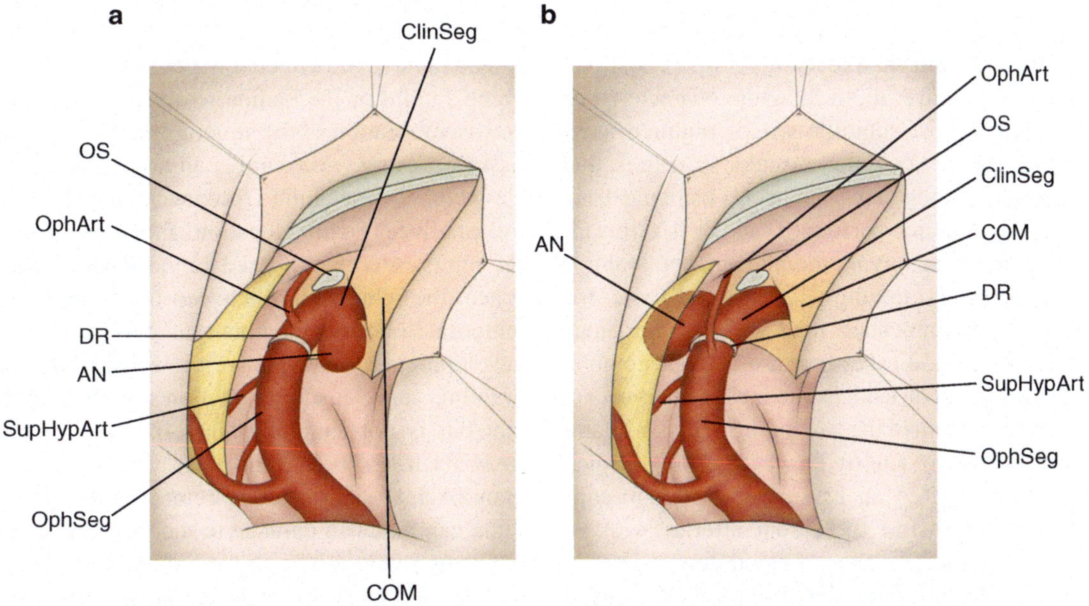

Fig. 12.2 Operative views of clinoidal segment aneurysms. (**a**) Anterolateral variant. (**b**) Medial variant. *OS* optic strut, *OphArt* ophthalmic artery, *DR* dural ring, *AN* aneurysm, *SupHypArt* superior hypophyseal artery, *OphSeg* ophthalmic segment, *ClinSeg* clinoidal segment, *COM* carotid-oculomotor membrane

view. In addition, branches, such as the PCoA and AChA, and perforators, such as the medial lenticulostriate artery and superior hypophyseal artery that arise from the medio-inferior wall of the ICA, are also difficult to identify. In such cases, a mirror or endoscope is useful and sometimes essential for preventing compromise of the branching arteries and rebleeding during blind clipping.

In cases of ICA bifurcation aneurysms, posteriorly directed cases are difficult to clip because they are in the space opposite to the microscopic view and the medial lenticulostriate arteries arising from the posterosuperior wall of ICA. It is not easy to detach the perforators from the sac to make a room for a clip blade. In addition, incomplete clipping and clipping in compromised perforators are frequent. Therefore, closely inspecting the region using a mirror, endoscope, ICG fluorescence angiography, and intraoperative angiography is essential for complete and safe clipping.

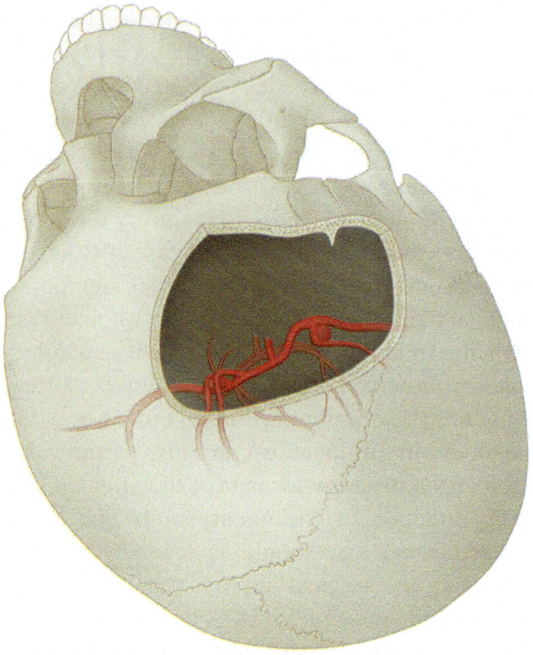

Fig. 12.3 Pterional craniotomy for approach to middle cerebral artery and anterior communicating artery aneurysms

12.3.2 Aneurysms Arising from the MCA

MCA aneurysms consist primarily of M1, MCA bifurcation, and M2 aneurysms (Fig. 12.3). MCA aneurysms have the following characteristics: this is the most common site of ruptured aneurysms, they are complex vascular structures, they develop draining veins, the lateral lenticulostriate artery is a major perforator, and it is clinically important to supplying the major functional cortex. Surgical clipping is relatively more frequently recommended than endovascular intervention in these cases because of their complex vascularity, their tendency to have a wide-necked configuration, and the lack of difficulty in finding a surgical approach [6]. However, during surgical clipping of MCA aneurysms, it is easy to compromise or distort the parent arteries with the clip. Therefore, the state of blood flow and neurological function should always be checked using micro-Doppler, ICG angiography, intraoperative physiological monitoring, and angiography.

Because brain swelling generally accompanies an SAH, CSF drainage is very important to make room for the dissection and to control the ICP. A sylvian dissection is not sufficient for achieving effective CSF drainage and brain relaxation. Instead, ventricular catheter insertion can be rapidly and effectively performed through Paine's point or the lamina terminalis. A preoperative evaluation of the structures of the sylvian fissure using cerebral angiography and T2-weighed magnetic resonance imaging is informative. The final location of the sylvian dissection is determined based on the subarachnoid space, the relationship between the frontal and temporal lobes, the amount of SAH, and the development of sylvian veins. Preserving the draining veins during dissection is very important but is not easy to achieve because of the SAH itself. Especially in cases with thick sylvian SAH, too meticulously removing the hematoma can result in damage to the draining veins and consequentially exaggerated brain swelling. Compression is better than coagulation for controlling venous bleeding. Intermittent releasing the retractor is important because long-term retraction can cause brain swelling as a result of retraction injury and venous compromise.

Retracting the temporal lobe is usually better than retracting the frontal lobe because of probable parenchymal injury and neurological sequelae.

When clipping M1 aneurysms, preserving the lenticulostriate artery is the most important goal. Aneurysms embedded in the frontal lobe and those positioned high or posteriorly directed should be carefully dissected, and the surrounding structures should be checked to avoid, as much as possible, injuring the brain parenchyma and perforators.

Except for proximal M2 aneurysms, sylvian dissection is difficult because the subarachnoid space is very narrow and the frontal and temporal lobes are usually tightly adhered at this location. In addition, locating these aneurysms is not easy because MCA branches are complex and the aneurysms are embedded within the deep insular cortex. Hence, preoperative angiographic findings should be carefully reviewed, and intraoperative navigation systems are recommended because they are very useful for locating these aneurysms.

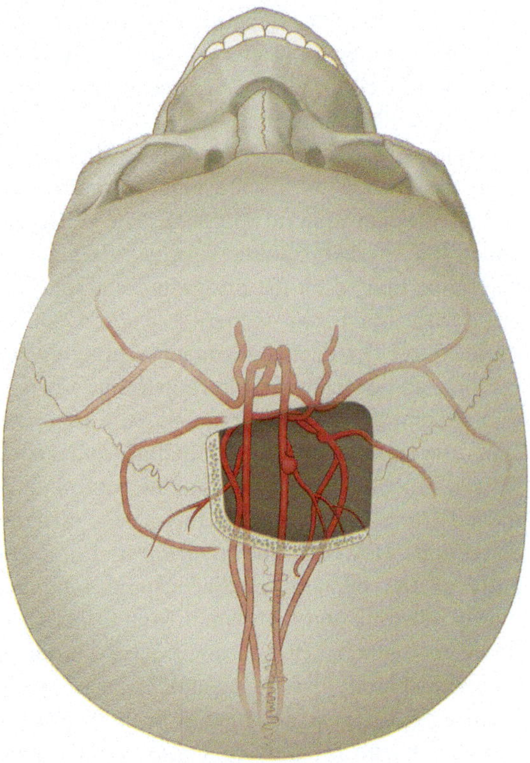

Fig. 12.4 Interhemispheric approach for aneurysms in the distal anterior cerebral artery

12.3.3 Aneurysms Arising from the ACA

Aneurysms arising from the ACA include those most frequently located at the ACoA and distal ACA. ACoA aneurysms are usually clipped via the lateral approach, such as conventional pterional (Fig. 12.3) and supraorbital keyhole craniotomy, or an anterior interhemispheric approach (Fig. 12.4). The approach side is determined based on the laterality of the dominant proximal ACA, the aneurysmal geometry (e.g., its size, direction, and associated perforators), hemispheric non-dominance, and the location of associated hematoma. Most affected cases can be treated via the lateral approach. However, an anterior interhemispheric approach would be advantageous for high-positioned and posteriorly directed cases in order to preserve perforators and secure a clear surgical view (Fig. 12.4). An anterior interhemispheric approach has an advantage in that it can be used to identify the H-complex and posteriorly hidden perforators. However, it also has a disadvantage in that it can result in frontal lobe injury during dissection, bilateral olfactory nerve injury, and a deep surgical field. When using a pterional approach, CSF can be effectively drained after the lamina terminalis is opened, and focal aspiration of the nonfunctioning rectus gyrus is helpful for exposing deep or high-positioned large aneurysms. Minimizing frontal lobe retraction with bone exposure as close to the skull base as possible is important, and dissecting the olfactory nerve is sometimes needed to prevent nerve injury. Preserving the perforators from the ACA and ACoA, including the recurrent artery of Heubner and the medial lenticulostriate artery, is very important because these vessels supply the hypothalamus, fornix, caudate nucleus, and anterior limb of the internal capsule. Because ischemic changes in such areas cannot be detected using intraoperative physiological monitoring, it is important to use direct visual inspection with the assistance of ICG or intraoperative angiography and micro-Doppler. Because the vessels surrounding the ACoA are complex and their perforators well developed, it is necessary to use a variety of shapes of clips.

Distal ACA aneurysms are usually clipped via a bicoronal incision, a parasagittal craniotomy, and an interhemispheric approach. The side from which the interhemispheric approach is made is determined based on the bridging veins that traverse the brain and superior sagittal sinus. Preoperative magnetic resonance imaging or cerebral angiography and intraoperative navigation systems are useful for choosing the approach side. The superior part of the medial frontal lobe is loosely adhered to the falx and the contralateral medial frontal lobe, making this a less difficult dissection. However, the anterior and inferior parts of the bilateral medial frontal lobe are tightly adhered, and the medial frontal lobes are prone to damage. Hence, anterior and inferior interhemispheric dissections should be carefully performed because the medial frontal lobe is associated with memory functions. Unlike ruptured aneurysms located in other parent arteries, it is very possible to reach the ruptured sac before exposing the proximal parent artery because of the anatomical characteristics of the interhemispheric approach. Therefore, when the aneurysm is nearly exposed, a careful dissection should be performed, and the surgeons should try to identify the proximal part of the parent artery in order to exert proximal control. The distal ACA is frequently smaller in size than the aneurysm, and the ACA is therefore easily compromised after clipping. The use of a mini-clip is advantageous in such situations. During the dissection, it is advisable to preserve and avoid compromising the perforators from the distal ACA to the corpus callosum or medial frontal lobe and the callosomarginal artery that supplies the motor cortex.

12.3.4 Aneurysms Arising from the Posterior Circulation

Posterior circulation aneurysms account for approximately 10% of cerebral aneurysms, relatively frequently have a fusiform shape and are dissecting type. Endovascular intervention is usually recommended as the first-line treatment option because of the difficulty of accessing the deep skull base, close proximity to the brainstem and lower cranial nerves, variable vascular anatomy, high rebleeding risk, and surgical complication rate. However, a surgical approach would be appropriate for giant and thrombosed aneurysms with a mass effect and those with major branches or perforators arising from the sac.

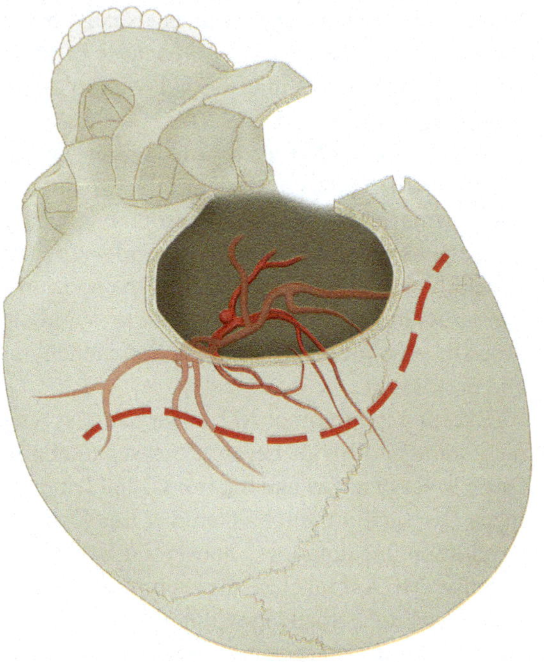

Fig. 12.5 Orbitozygomatic approach for aneurysms in the basilar bifurcation, superior cerebellar and posterior cerebral arteries. *Red line*: skin incision

Aneurysms at the basilar bifurcation (BB), posterior cerebral artery (PCA), and superior cerebellar artery (SCA) can be surgically managed using routine pterional trans-sylvian, orbitozygomatic trans-sylvian, and subtemporal transtentorial approaches. An orbitozygomatic approach is suitable for highly positioned BB aneurysms (Fig. 12.5), and a subtemporal approach is recommended for BB aneurysms located below the posterior clinoid process. The trans-sylvian approach has some advantages in that it reveals both proximal PCAs and makes a relatively lager amount of space for the procedure. However, it also has a disadvantage in that it is difficult to inspect posteriorly directed perforators and clip blades, and clipping an anteriorly or posteriorly directed cerebral aneurysm is therefore not easy. On the other hand, when using a subtemporal approach, perforators are easy to identify, and clipping anteriorly or posteriorly directed aneurysms is more feasible than when using another approach. However, the contralateral proximal PCA is difficult to see, and the exposed space is narrow, especially in ruptured aneurysms, and the basal temporal lobe and adjacent nerves, such as the oculomotor and trochlear nerves, are therefore vulnerable to damage.

When using a trans-sylvian approach to reach BB aneurysms, the following structures are sequentially passed through: windows made by the optic nerve, ACA, ICA, and PCoA; the Liliequist membrane; and the interpeduncular cistern harboring the BB aneurysms. The accessible windows consist of the optico-carotid triangle (made by the lateral margin of the optic nerve, the medial margin of the ICA, and the inferior margin of the ACA), the supra-carotid triangle (made by the superior margin of the ACA, the lateral margin of the optic nerve, and the medial margin of the MCA), and the carotico-oculomotor triangle (made by the lateral margin of the ICA, the anterior clinoid process, and the medial margin of the oculomotor nerve with a traversing PCoA). Among these, the carotico-oculomotor triangle is frequently used because it is a wider space than the others and has a lower risk of injuring the optic nerve, ICA and ICA perforators than an approach via the optico-carotid triangle and a lower risk of injuring the medial lenticulostriate perforators than an approach via the supra-carotid triangle.

SCA aneurysms can be approached via the trans-sylvian and subtemporal routes, and the latter is usually advantageous because SCA aneurysms are located below the posterior clinoid process. Making a tentorial incision and opening the crural and ambient cisterns exposes the SCA aneurysm. The trochlear nerve is prone to injury during a tentorial incision. Because it is located within the subarachnoid space under the arachnoid membrane, preserving the arachnoid membrane while making a tentorial incision can protect the nerve. Aneurysms that occur in the P1, P2, and P3 segments of the PCA can be accessed by opening the crural and ambient cisterns using a subtemporal approach, and those that occur in the P3 and P4 segments can be approached by opening the quadrigeminal cistern using a posterior interhemispheric approach.

Aneurysms arising from the basilar trunk, anterior inferior cerebellar artery, and vertebra-basilar junction are the rarest. However, this space is very narrow and deep, and the perforators originating from the parent arteries and lower cranial nerves are very complex. Hence, more than 90% of them are treated using an endovascular intervention rather than surgery. According to the location, which can range from the BB via the mid-basilar artery to the vertebra-basilar junction, the type of approach is selected in the following order: trans-sylvian, extradural temporo-polar, subtemporal, anterior petrosal, trans-facial trans-clival, combined supratentorial and infratentorial, retro-labyrinthine trans-sigmoid, and far lateral. Recently, advancements in the endonasal endoscopic approach have gradually made it possible to access deep-seated aneurysms located at the basilar trunk, SCA, anterior inferior cerebellar artery, vertebra-basilar junction, proximal posterior inferior cerebellar artery (PICA), and proximal PCA, ACoA, and paraclinoid ICA in a less invasive manner [24].

Aneurysms located in the PICA and vertebral arteries are generally accessible via the far lateral approach (Fig. 12.6), and distal PICA aneurysms can be accessed via the midline sub-

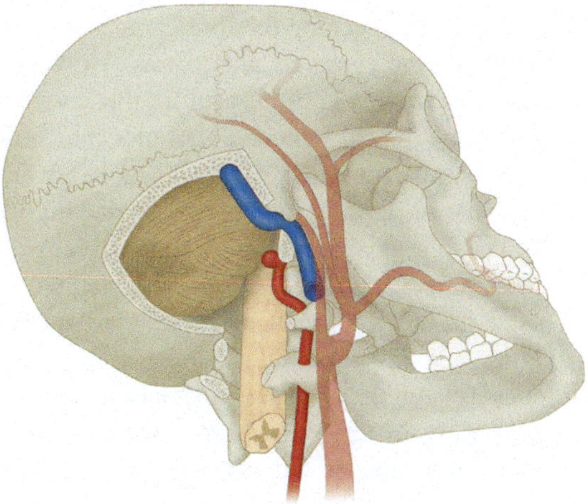

Fig. 12.6 Far lateral transcondylar approach for vertebral artery aneurysm

occipital or retromastoid suboccipital approaches. When performing the far lateral approach, the lower cranial nerves are prone to damage because the aneurysms can be manipulated by passing the cranial nerves. During the procedure used to approach proximal PICA aneurysms, surgeons should be careful not to injure the perforators when approaching from the distal vertebral artery and proximal PICA because there could be lateral medullary syndrome. When the jugular tubercle disturbs the surgical view, drilling the jugular tubercle and the medial one-third of the occipital condyle should be considered. In cases in which the aneurysm involves the PICA itself, sacrificing the involved portion of the PICA is sometimes considered. In such a situation, preserving the perforators originating from the PICA and restoring flow with bypass surgery, such as occipital artery-PICA or PICA-PICA microanastomoses, should be considered. When the preservation of the perforators cannot be guaranteed, performing a PICA segment occlusion without bypass surgery may be a good less invasive option because the territory of the distal PICA is usually supplied by the leptomeningeal collaterals, and the clinical symptoms caused by the infarction of the unilateral PICA territory can be recovered.

Conclusion

As the devices and techniques of endovascular intervention rapidly develop, endovascular approach has become the first choice of treatment for the ruptured aneurysms. However, surgical clipping is still useful for those which cannot be treated with endovascular intervention or those for which surgery is more advantageous, and complex cases that needed highly skilled surgical techniques are relatively increasing. Advanced support systems are used in order to reduce surgical complications, and less invasive surgical approaches such as keyhole or endoscopic approaches are increasing in order to shorten the operation time and achieve the satisfactory cosmetic results. As the surgical cases are decreasing, experienced neurovascular surgeons are also decreasing. So, it is considered to organize the international training system and share the surgical experience in order to maintain rare but experienced surgeons.

References

1. Winn HR, Richardson AE, Jane J. The assessment of the natural history of single aneurysms that have ruptured. In: Hopkins LN, Long DM, editors. Clinical management of intracranial aneurysms. New York: Raven Press; 1982. p. 1–10.
2. Locksley HB. Natural history of subarachnoid hemorrhage, intracranial aneurysms and arteriovenous malformations. J Neurosurg. 1966;25:321–68.
3. Jane JA, Kassel NF, Torner JC, et al. The natural history of aneurysms and arteriovenous malformations. J Neurosurg. 1985;62:321–3.
4. Hijdra A, Vermeulen M, van Gijn J, et al. Rerupture of intracranial aneurysms: a clinicoanatomic study. J Neurosurg. 1987;67:29–33.
5. Ohkuma H, Tsurutani H, Suzuki S. Incidence and significance of early aneurysmal rebleeding before neurosurgical or neurological management. Stroke. 2001;32:1176–80.
6. Cho WS, Kim JE, Park SQ, et al. Korean clinical practice guidelines for aneurysmal subarachnoid hemorrhage. J Kor Neurosurg Soc. 2018;61:127–66.
7. Dott NM. Intracranial aneurysms cerebral arterio-radiography and surgical treatment. Edinb Med J. 1933;40:219–34.
8. Dandy WE. Intracranial aneurysm of the internal carotid artery cured by operation. Ann Surg. 1938;107:654–9.
9. Krayenbuhl HA, Yasargil MG, Flamm ES, et al. Microsurgical treatment of intracranial saccular aneurysms. J Neurosurg. 1972;37:678–86.
10. Guglielmi G, Viñuela F, Dion J, Duckwiler G. Electrothrombosis of saccular aneurysms via endovascular approach. Part 2: preliminary clinical experience. J Neurosurg. 1991;75:8–14.
11. Molyneux A, Kerr R, Stratton I, et al. International subarachnoid aneurysm trial (ISAT) of neurosurgical clipping versus endovascular coiling in 2143 patients with ruptured intracranial aneurysms: a randomised trial. Lancet. 2002;360:1267–74.
12. Molyneux AJ, Kerr RS, Yu LM, et al. International subarachnoid aneurysm trial (ISAT) of neurosurgical clipping versus endovascular coiling in 2143 patients with ruptured intracranial aneurysms: a randomised comparison of effects on survival, dependency, seizures, rebleeding, subgroups, and aneurysm occlusion. Lancet. 2005;366:809–17.
13. Connolly ES Jr, Rabinstein AA, Carhuapoma JR, et al. Guidelines for the management of aneurysmal subarachnoid hemorrhage: a guideline for

healthcare professionals from the American heart association/American stroke association. Stroke. 2012;43:1711–37.
14. Steiner T, Juvela S, Unterberg A, et al. European stroke organization guidelines for the management of intracranial aneurysms and subarachnoid haemorrhage. Cerebrovasc Dis. 2013;35:93–112.
15. Committee for guidelines for management of aneurysmal subarachnoid hemorrhage. Japanese society on surgery for cerebral stroke. Evidence-based guidelines for the management of aneurysmal subarachnoid hemorrhage. English edition. Neurol Med Chir (Tokyo). 2012;52:355–429.
16. Cho WS, Kim JE, Kang HS, et al. Keyhole approach and neuroendoscopy for cerebral aneurysms. J Korean Neurosurg Soc. 2017;60:275–81.
17. Cho WS, Kim JE, Kang HS, et al. Dual-channel endoscopic indocyanine green fluorescence angiography for clipping of cerebral aneurysms. World Neurosurg. 2017;100:316–24.
18. Cho WS, Kim JE, Kim SH, et al. Endoscopic fluorescence angiography with indocyanine green: a preclinical study in the swine. J Korean Neurosurg Soc. 2015;58:513–7.
19. Macdonald RL, editor. Neurosurgical operative atlas. Vascular neurosurgery, 2nd edn. New York: Thieme; 2009.
20. Britz GW, et al. Surgical approaches to intracranial aneurysms. In: Winn HR, editor. Youmans and Winn neurological surgery, 7th edn. Philadelphia: Elsevier; 2017. p. 3289–97.
21. Lawton MT. Seven aneurysms: tenets and techniques for clipping. New York: Thieme; 2011.
22. Jabbarli R, Pierscianek D, Wrede K, et al. Aneurysm remnant after clipping: the risks and consequences. J Neurosurg. 2016;125:1249–55.
23. Thompson BG, Brown RD Jr, Amin-Hanjani S, et al. Guidelines for the management of patients with unruptured intracranial aneurysms: a guideline for healthcare professionals from the American Heart Association/American Stroke Association. Stroke. 2015;46:2368–400.
24. Szentirmai O, Hong Y, Mascarenhas L, et al. Endoscopic endonasal clip ligation of cerebral aneurysms: an anatomical feasibility study and future directions. J Neurosurg. 2016;124:463–8.

13 Angiographic Intervention in Hemorrhagic Stroke

Chae Wook Huh, Duk Ho Gho, and Sung-Chul Jin

13.1 General Principles

13.1.1 Overview

Angiographic intervention has an important role in the diagnosis and treatment of hemorrhagic stroke. In terms of diagnostic tools, conventional cerebral angiography remains the gold standard for the diagnosis of ruptured vascular lesions, such as intracranial aneurysms, arteriovenous malformations (AVMs), and dural arteriovenous fistulas (dAVF). In addition, for intracerebral hematomas in young patients or those without identifiable risk factors, conventional cerebral angiography should also be performed to exclude the possibility of occult vascular lesions. Furthermore, substantial advancements in endovascular surgery are accelerated by various factors, including rapid advances in imaging technology, continued medical device development, and technical improvements. As a result, the competence of angiographic intervention in the management of hemorrhagic stroke has progressed from an alternative to surgery for inaccessible intracranial lesions or inoperable patients to frontline treatment tools. Previously inaccessible neurovascular lesions have become treatable with these minimally invasive techniques, with reduced morbidity and mortality using the angiographic intervention.

The most notable field in angiographic intervention is the treatment of intracranial aneurysms. Surgical treatment of intracranial aneurysms can, in most cases, achieve complete elimination of the aneurysm without compromising the parent vessel or adjacent perforators. However, several risk factors might increase the risk of morbidity and mortality. These factors include the aneurysm size, morphology, and location. The age, neurological status, and medical comorbidities of the patient also play a role. According to the International Subarachnoid Aneurysm Trial (ISAT), patients with subarachnoid hemorrhage fare better with coil embolization than with surgical clipping [1]. More recently, the Barrow Ruptured Aneurysm Trial also showed better outcomes of coil embolization compared with those of surgical clippings [2]. In recent decades, endovascular coiling was also limited by the aneurysm morphology and adjacent vascular structure, and the introduction of balloon- or stent-assisted techniques reduced the area of the "uncoilable" aneurysm. More recently, a new generation of endovascular devices – the flow diverter – became available. Wide-necked large, giant, and blood-blister aneurysms are treated with the flow diverter by mechanisms of

C. W. Huh · S.-C. Jin (✉)
Department of Neurosurgery, Inje University Haeundae Paik Hospital, Busan, South Korea

D. H. Gho
Department of Neurosurgery, Seodaegu Hospital, Busan, South Korea

S.-H. Lee (ed.), *Stroke Revisited: Hemorrhagic Stroke*, Stroke Revisited,
https://doi.org/10.1007/978-981-10-1427-7_13

flow redirection and neoendothelialization across the aneurysmal neck [3–5].

In the field of AVM and dAVF, endovascular surgery can be used individually or as part of multimodal treatments with stereotactic radiosurgery and surgical resection. While surgical resection remains the most definite treatment option, embolization can achieve total AVM occlusion in selected AVM patients with deep located small-sized AVMs [6]. In addition, for carotid-cavernous fistula and other forms of dAVF, endovascular surgery is a good treatment option. Several embolic materials are available, including n-butyl cyanoacrylate, polyvinyl alcohol, and Onyx, which are appropriate embolic materials that can be used in individual cases.

13.1.2 Preoperative Evaluation

The operators should identify the patient's general and neurological status. A review of the medical records, including medical comorbidities (hypertension, diabetes mellitus, cardiac disease, chronic kidney disease, and allergic history), history of antiplatelet and anticoagulant medications, and previous computed tomography (CT) and magnetic resonance image (MRI), is necessary. Laboratory evaluation including kidney function (BUN/creatinine) is essential. If impaired renal function is identified, the use of nonionic contrast agents, procedural hydration, and pretreatment with sodium bicarbonate or oral N-acetylcysteine should be considered. The operator should also be in a position to recognize and manage acute hydrocephalus and intracranial hypertension.

13.1.3 Preparation for Endovascular Surgery

During the perioperative period of hemorrhagic stroke, an emergent situation can often be encountered. To control blood pressure, inotropic agents (dopamine or phenylephrine) or antihypertensive agents should be prepared. Anticoagulant status is critically important for successful endovascular surgery, with systemic heparinization needed. Likewise, protamine sulfate for rapid reversal of the heparin effect also should be prepared in case of intraprocedural rupture. If an adjuvant procedure (balloon or stent-assisted techniques) is expected, 300 mg of clopidogrel can be administered, with intravenous aspirin considered on a case-by-case manner.

13.1.4 Anesthesia and Monitoring

Most endovascular surgeries are performed under general anesthesia. In some circumstances, such as a high risk of general anesthesia, conscious sedation may be acceptable. An arterial line is placed in the radial artery to closely monitor the patient's blood pressure, and anesthesiologist is aware of the need to avoid blood pressure fluctuation. Arterial oxygen saturation and cardiac rhythm are monitored during the procedure. For the early detection of neurological deterioration, neuro-monitoring such as somatosensory-evoked potential (SSEP) and motor-evoked potential (MEP) can be prepared.

13.1.5 Conventional Cerebral Angiography (Fig. 13.1)

All endovascular surgery should be performed in the angiography suite with biplane digital subtraction and fluoroscopic imaging capabilities. Many vascular neurosurgical diseases that were previously treated as high risk in the operating room can now be safely treated in the angiography suite. However, prior to endovascular surgery of hemorrhagic stroke, satisfactory cerebral angiography should be performed.

Conventional cerebral angiography is critical to determine the optimal treatment for hemorrhagic stroke. For planned coil embolization of ruptured intracranial aneurysm, three-dimensional rotational reconstructive image is necessary to accurately assess the aneurysm morphology and location, including its size, geometry, dome to neck ratio, and relationship to

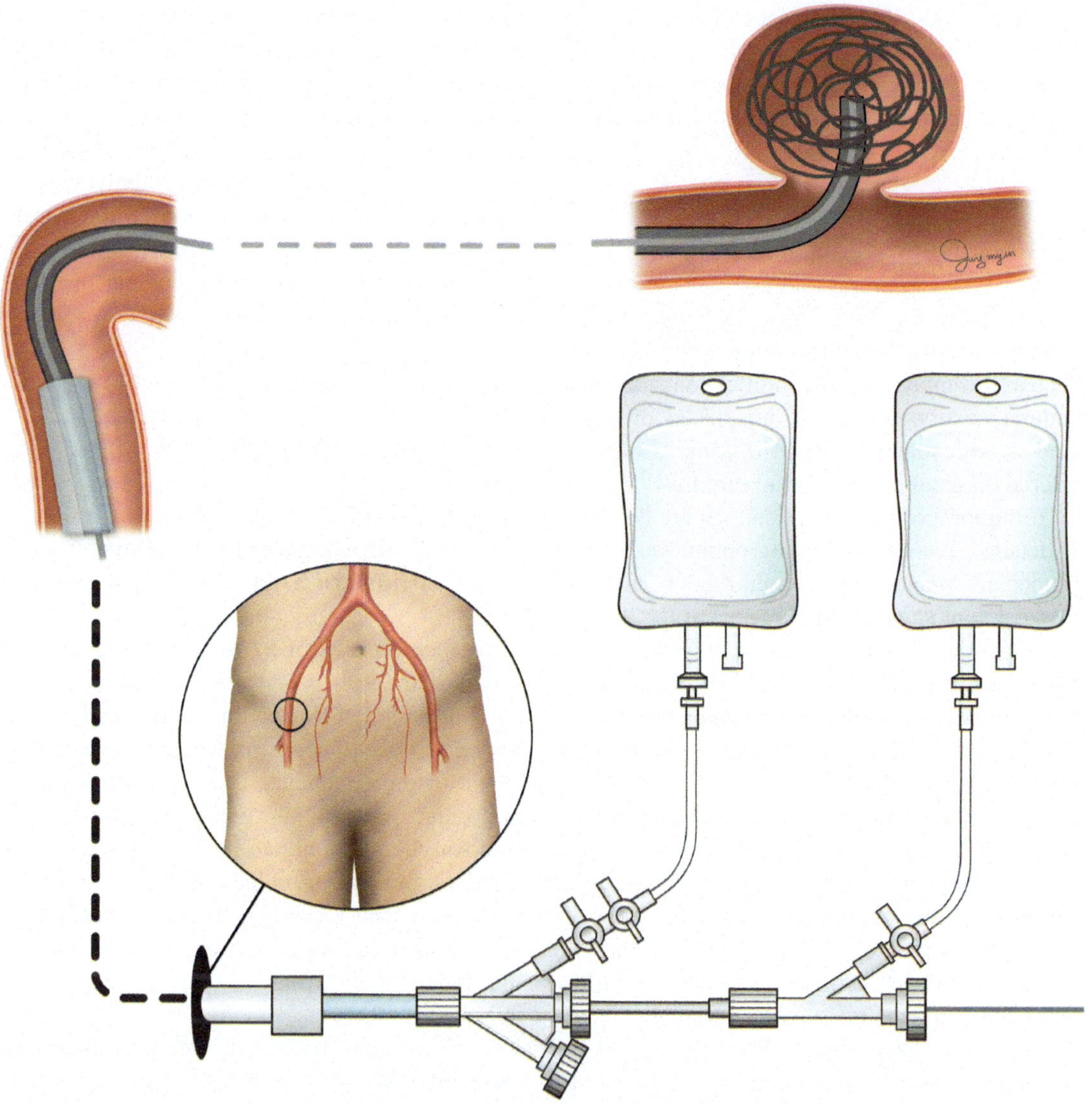

Fig. 13.1 A schematic representation of the coil embolization system

the parent vessel and involved arterial branches, so that working views can be planned appropriately. Furthermore, for the treatment of AVM or dAVF, conventional cerebral angiography can also provide highly detailed information regarding the anatomic features in all phases, including points of fistulous connections, associated aneurysms, nidus size, and arterial and venous flow patterns necessary for utilizing the Spetzler-Martin grading scale, but they can also provide important hemodynamic information regarding dominant arterial filling and pedicle arrangements. Therefore, preoperative conventional cerebral angiography should be of sufficient quality to characterize vascular lesions. In the case of large and giant aneurysms, AVM, and dAVF, it is essential to evaluate both external carotid arteries.

Furthermore, the operator makes the overall technical decision based on the angiographic details. Selection of the diameter and system of guiding catheter, angle and number of microcatheters, and planned adjuvant technique (balloon or stent assist) are planned carefully.

Ultimately, if endovascular surgery is planned, an immediate preoperative angiography is necessary to evaluate the vascular anatomy and to ensure the appropriateness of the planned procedure.

13.1.6 Intraprocedural Management

The operator should be aware and prepared to acutely manage intraprocedural complications, such as thromboembolic complications, intraprocedural aneurysm rupture, misplaced or herniated embolic materials, flow-limiting vasospasm, arterial dissection, and arterial rupture.

If intraprocedural complications are detected, a detailed review of angiographic image and immediate management should be performed. Pretreatment angiographic images of the lesions, parent vascular tree, and capillary blush are mandatory to evaluate intraprocedural complications. Emergency cross-sectional imaging must be available if a procedure-related complication occurs or is suspected.

A thromboembolic event is major complication of endovascular surgery, so systemic heparinization is necessary. With any endovascular surgery, it is crucial to employ proper anticoagulation to minimize the risk of thromboembolic complications, but heparin may not be administered for hemorrhagic stroke, especially in the situation of aneurysmal SAH due to risk of rebleeding. Systemic heparin is usually withheld until at least the framing coil has been deployed into the ruptured aneurysm [7]. A continuous catheter flushing system is also important for prevention of flow stasis and thromboembolism. A commonly used system for continuous flushing is the Tuohy-Borst Y-valve setup, which provides a constant stream of heparinized flush (3000–6000 units per liter) using a pressurized bag at rate of 150–200 mL minimum per hour. The operator should check the patient's anticoagulant status and maintenance of the flushing system.

Intraprocedural aneurysm rupture and arterial perforation during endovascular surgery have continued to be devastating complications. If such complications occur, immediate management should be performed, including rapid heparin reversal, use of a temporary occlusion balloon to tamponade the bleeding site, and rapid aneurysm occlusion. In the case of massive intracranial hematoma or acute hydrocephalus, emergency computed tomographic imaging should be used to identify the problem, and emergent ventriculostomy may be performed in a case-by-case manner [8].

13.2 Principles of Angiographic Intervention in SAH

13.2.1 Brief Concept of Coil Embolization in the Acute Phase of SAH

In the acute phase of SAH, urgent treatment of ruptured aneurysms is recommended because of the high risk of rebleeding associated with a poor prognosis. Therefore, therapeutic occlusion of the ruptured aneurysm is one of the most important treatment goals of SAH [9]. Endovascular techniques offer the prospect of reducing the risk of rebleeding without the need for craniotomy [10]. The ruptured aneurysm is packed with various coils that block the circulating blood flow from the parent arteries and induce thrombosis.

Endovascular techniques are classified into reconstructive and deconstructive treatments according to the occlusion of parent artery. Reconstructive endovascular techniques include simple coil embolization, balloon-assisted coil embolization, stent-assisted coil embolization, and flow diversion. These techniques reduce the risk of rebleeding by blocking the aneurysm from the circulating blood flow without occlusion of the parent artery. Deconstructive endovascular technique is used to occlude the parent artery containing the aneurysm and is a viable and durable solution for certain intracranial aneurysms. In particular, it has been used for the treatment of aneurysm involving the vertebrobasilar junction and posterior cerebral artery when adequate collateral flow is present.

13.2.2 Simple Coil Embolization

Since Dr. Guglielmi first introduced electrolytically detachable platinum microcoils in 1990, the coil embolization technique has been continuously developed with advancements of endovascular devices. Simple coil embolization is the mainstream technique in endovascular treatment. Under fluoroscopic guidance, various catheter systems are navigated from the arterial circulation entrance to the parent artery containing the ruptured aneurysm. A microcatheter is placed in the aneurysm and progressively filled with various types of detachable coils that are suitable for the shape of the aneurysm. The aneurysm cavity is first filled with a framing coil. Additional coils of various sizes, shapes, and softness are filled until a sufficient packing density is obtained. The filled coils isolate the aneurysm from the circulating blood flow, and the remaining space is filled with a thrombus (Fig. 13.2a–d). It is well known that packing the coils as tightly as possible is important to avoid recanalization. However, excessive coil packing may result in intraprocedural ruptures, and appropriate packing is required. It is controversial, but a packing density (coil volume/aneurysm volume × 100%) of 20–25% has been reported to be effective for avoiding recanalization [11]. Simple coil embolization is feasible for aneurysms that have narrow neck or favorable dome to neck ratio (generally defined as a neck less than 4 mm in diameter or a dome to neck ratio greater than 2) (Fig. 13.3), to hold the coils within the aneurysm cavity.

The multiple catheter technique (Fig. 13.4a) is a method for treating aneurysms with an unfavorable anatomy using two or more catheters. Neck remodeling techniques, such as the balloon- or stent-assisted technique, are widely used to treat aneurysms with a less favorable anatomy. However, there are some technical difficulties in performing these techniques. The introduction of additional devices into small intracranial vessels may increase the risk of vascular injury, and these

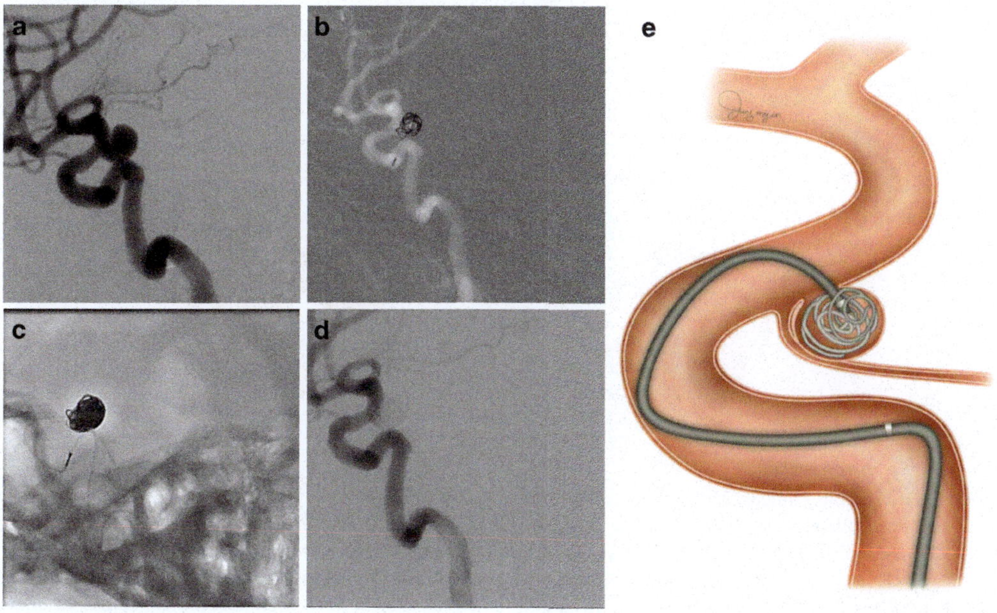

Fig. 13.2 Simple coil embolization technique. Case. Simple coil embolization technique for the posterior communicating artery (PcomA) aneurysm. (**a**) Initial digital subtraction angiography (DSA) shows an aneurysm arising from the origin of PcomA. (**b**) The frame coil and subsequent coils were deployed through a microcatheter located in the aneurysm cavity. (**c**) Complete occlusion of the aneurysm was achieved. (**d**) Post-procedural DSA shows the treatment result. (**e**) An illustration of simple coil embolization. The frame coil is deployed through a microcatheter located in the aneurysm cavity

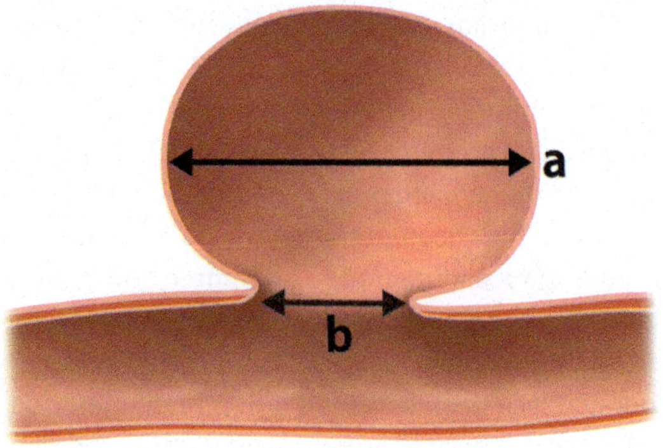

Fig. 13.3 A schematic representation of the dome to neck ratio (a/b). An aneurysm with a less favorable anatomy is usually defined as having a neck larger than 4 mm or a dome to neck ratio of 2 or less

neck remodeling techniques may be unsuitable for use in aneurysms, such as those with important branches arising from the fundus [12]. Baxter et al. described a double microcatheter technique for the detachable coil treatment of large, wide-necked intracranial aneurysms in 1998. In this technique, the initial coil frame is stabilized with two coils by interlocking them with each, and it is based on the concept of securely bracing the coils adjacent to one another to achieve a stable configuration [12, 13]. The multiple catheter technique might be helpful when there is evidence of coil instability or parent vessel compromise during embolization of an aneurysm with a wide neck or unfavorable dome to neck ratio [13].

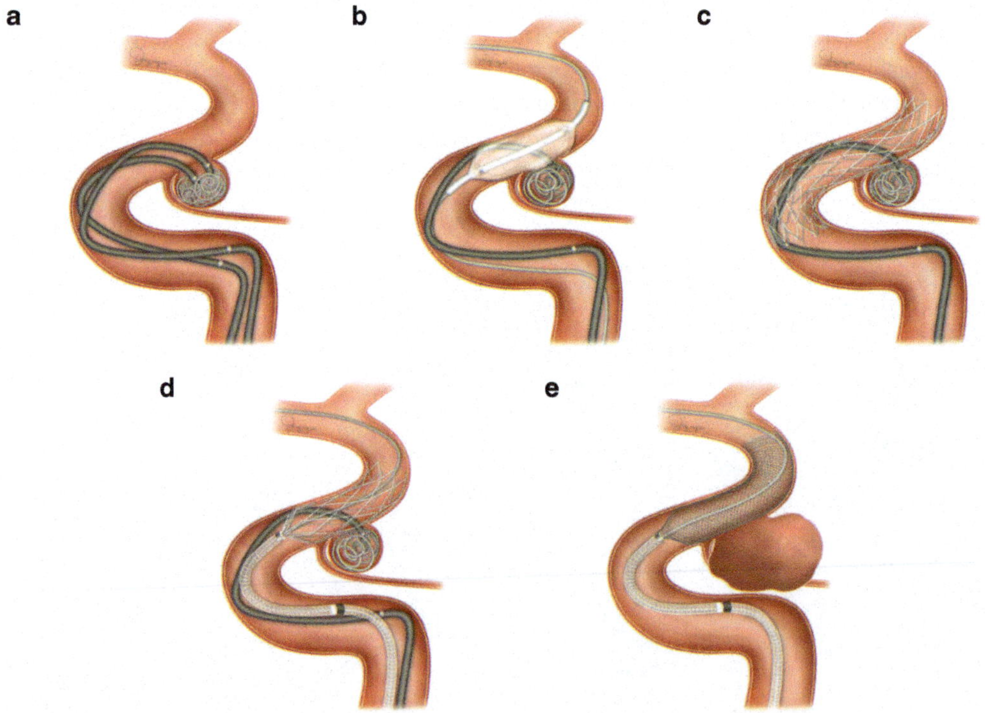

Fig. 13.4 (**a**) Multiple catheter coil embolization technique. Two microcatheters are located in the aneurysm cavity. The frame coils from each microcatheters interlock with each other, stabilizing the initial coil frame. (**b**) Balloon-assisted coil embolization technique. The balloon is located across the aneurysm neck and serves as a temporary supportive scaffold. (**c**) Stent-assisted coil embolization technique. The stent is placed across the aneurysm neck. The stent provides a permanent supportive scaffold for stabilization of the coil mass. (**d**) A schematic representation of stent-assisted coil embolization use by the jailing technique. Aneurismal catheterization is performed before deployment of a self-expandable stent across the aneurysm neck. Thus, the microcatheter is "jailing" between the stent and the parent vessel wall. (**e**) A schematic representation of the flow diversion device across the aneurysm neck

13.2.3 Balloon-Assisted Coil Embolization

In the case of aneurysms with a wide neck or unfavorable dome to neck ratio, simple coil embolization may jeopardize the patency of the parent artery because the filled coils cannot be stabilized in the aneurysm cavity. Moret et al. first described balloon-assisted coil embolization in 1997, a technique that provides temporary supportive scaffolding to the neck of these aneurysms by inflation of a compliant microballoon (Fig. 13.4b) [14]. It prevents the coils from protruding into the parent artery and leads to higher packing densities and more effective parent vessel reconstruction [15]. Balloon-assisted coil embolization has gained popularity for the treatment of ruptured aneurysms with a less favorable anatomy (wide neck or unfavorable dome to neck ratio) because it does not require the routine use of antiplatelet agents [16]. Moreover, balloon inflation allows control of the extravasation and prevents devastating consequences for the patient [17]. The stent-assisted technique does not provide side branch protection from coil herniation or proximal control during an intraprocedural rupture. Thus, when a side branch is in close proximity to the neck of an aneurysm, the balloon-assisted technique can be an effective and safe modality.

However, there are some concerns about the potential morbidity associated with this technique, especially the high risk of thromboembolic complications [18] related to the use of two microcatheters and hemodynamic stasis due to balloon inflation [17]. Sluzewski et al. reported that compared with simple coil embolization, balloon-assisted coil embolization techniques were associated with higher thromboembolic complications and intraprocedural rupture [19]. Several studies have suggested that the balloon-assisted technique should be reserved for cases in which the conventional coil embolization technique is inappropriate, but there is no consensus concerning this issue.

13.2.4 Stent-Assisted Coil Embolization

Endovascular strategies for managing aneurysms with a less favorable anatomy, such as a wide neck and unfavorable dome to neck ratio, have previously included the balloon remodeling technique [20]. However, many aneurysms still cannot be guaranteed based on the technical feasibility and the long-term durability of the balloon remodeling technique. Unlike the balloon-assisted technique, stent-assisted coil embolization provides permanent supportive scaffolding via the deployment of an intracranial stent for stabilization of the coil mass (Fig. 13.4c). This procedure reduces the rate of aneurysm recanalization by redirecting the blood flow reducing the intra-aneurysmal flow and promoting endothelialization at the level of the aneurysm neck [21–24].

In the early days of the stent-assisted technique, the stents for coronary and peripheral vascular embolization were experimentally applied to the cerebral vessel. However, the characteristics of balloon-expandable coronary stents have limited their use in cerebral aneurysm therapy. They lack sufficient flexibility such that excessive force during deployment could damage the vessel wall [20]. The ideal stent for cerebral vessels should have a low profile, be flexible, and consist of self-expandable material to accommodate the complex geometry of the intracranial arteries [20]. Since the first US Food and Drug Administration (FDA) approval of the Neuroform stent (Stryker Inc.) in 2002, a variety of stents have been developed and applied.

There are two types of stents depending on their design: open-cell (in which not all struts are interrelated) and closed-cell (in which all stent struts are interconnected). The aforementioned Neuroform stent is an open-cell designed stent with relatively fewer thromboembolic complications in the form of procedure-related transient ischemic attack (TIA) and stroke [25]. In contrast, the Enterprise stent (Codman Inc.) is the first closed-cell designed stent to treat intracranial aneurysms, and the advantages of the closed-cell stent include the ability of the stent to be partially deployed, recaptured, and redeployed [21, 25]. It is also easier to deploy than the open-cell stent and enables the treatment of additional aneurysms, but the closed-cell design of the stent has a greater tendency to slightly alter the normal vascular anatomy owing to its design [21, 26].

When performing stent-assisted coil embolization, aneurismal catheterization is performed before deployment of a self-expandable stent across the aneurysm neck (Jailing technique) (Fig. 13.4d). Following deployment of the stent, embolization coils are delivered with the microcatheter positioned within the aneurysm dome and wedged between the stent and the aneurysm dome [27]. This technique prevents the situation in which a stent is deployed but the aneurysm cannot be subsequently catheterized [28]. In particular cases, such as dissection of the aneurysm or basilar top aneurysm, the stent-assisted technique may be applied as an overlapping or Y-stenting technique.

There is reluctance to deploy stents in the setting of SAH because of the risk of thromboembolic complications in patients who are not prepared with antiplatelet agents, and fear of the use of antiplatelet agents during the acute phase of SAH may increase the risk of rebleeding. There is no clear consensus about the use of antiplatelet agents, but in several recent studies, a proper antiplatelet therapy regimen did not increase intracerebral hemorrhage during the acute phase of SAH treated with stent-assisted coil embolization [16].

13.2.5 Flow Diversion Devices

Flow diversion is the placement of a low-porosity, high-pore-density device in the parent vessel at the aneurysm neck to decrease flow into the aneurysm and redirect the flow to the distal part of the parent vessel [29]. The lower the porosity, the better are the chances of occluding the aneurysm, but excessive low porosity would lead to occlusion of any branch covered by the device. Most flow diversion devices have a porosity of approximately 70%, whereas conventional intracranial stents have a porosity of approximately 90%. The pore density is the number of metal-enclosed pores per unit surface area [30]. A higher pore density can increase the uniform coverage across the aneurysm neck and potentially limit the perforator occlusion. A lower porosity and increased pore density are design goals for flow diversion devices aimed at occluding aneurysms.

Accordingly, flow diversion devices promote endothelialization of the flow diversion device and subsequently block the aneurysm from the circulating blood flow over time, while there is no occlusion of the covered adjacent branches (Fig. 13.4e). The main hemodynamic effects that lead to aneurysm thrombosis without the placement of intra-aneurysmal material are the decrease in velocity of intra-aneurysmal flow, reduction in flow turbulence, and reduction of wall shear stress [31, 32]. After the Pipeline for Uncoilable or Failed Aneurysm Study (PUFS) was completed, the Pipeline embolization device (Medtronic) was first approved for use by the US FDA in 2011.

The use of flow diversion devices without adequate antiplatelet therapy can be associated with serious thrombotic complications such as in-stent thrombosis and thromboembolism. Current flow diverters necessitate 3 months of dual antiplatelet agents and lifelong aspirin to avoid in-stent thrombosis [29]. However, the use of antiplatelet agents in the acute phase of SAH is controversial due to potential bleeding complications. In addition, compared with conventional coil embolization or surgical clipping, flow diversion does not achieve immediate aneurysm obliteration and does not decrease the risk of immediate rebleeding. Thus, flow diversion after aneurysmal SAH is not preferred as the primary therapeutic option. Natarajan et al. recommended that flow diversion is not the primary treatment of choice after aneurysmal SAH, but it is a reasonable final option if other, safer options are not available to treat the aneurysm [29].

13.2.6 Limitation

Since the ISAT, endovascular coil embolization has become a favorable therapeutic option for patients with SAH. However, there are questions about the durability and long-term efficacy of coil embolization. Aneurysm remnants or recurrences and the need for retreatment are more common after endovascular coiling than after clipping. Therefore, follow-up imaging is mandatory.

13.3 Other Indications Including Dural AV Fistula and AVM

Intracranial dural AV fistula and AVM are abnormal arteriovenous channels without a capillary bed. The difference between AV fistula and AVM is the presence or not of a nidus. Both diseases present with intracerebral hemorrhage.

In dural AV fistula, leptomeningeal reflux is related to venous hypertension and will be a predisposing factor for intracerebral hemorrhage. The goal of endovascular treatment obliterates abnormal fistulous channels without interfering with normal venous drains. Endovascular treatment can be accessed via the transvenous, trans-arterial route or direct puncture of the affected dural sinus. Advances have been achieved in embolic material and devices for trans-arterial endovascular treatment rather than transvenous endovascular treatment. Endovascular treatment is a primary treatment for dural AVF presenting with intracerebral hemorrhage (Fig. 13.5a).

In AVM, combined dural AVF and prenidal, intranidal, or flow-related aneurysms are predisposing factors for AVM rupture. Endovascular treatment has not been a primary treatment modality for ruptured AVM because low complete angiographic obliteration rate in endovascular treatment will increase rebleeding of the ruptured AVM. In general, endovascular treatment is performed before microsurgical resection to enhance the surgical accessibility. In ruptured small AVM that are not feasible for surgical resection, endovascular treatment demonstrated a high complete angiographic obliteration rate and will be considered a primary treatment option (Fig. 13.5b).

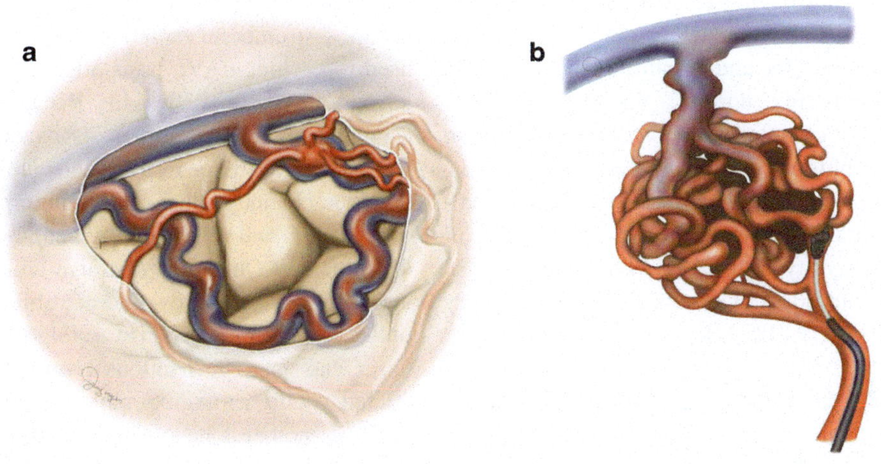

Fig. 13.5 (**a**) A schematic representation of the dural arteriovenous fistula (dAVF). This figure shows the connection between the meningeal arteries and cortical vein. There is retrograde blood flow into the superior sagittal sinus and the engorged cortical vein. (**b**) A schematic representation of the arteriovenous malformation (AVM). The microcatheter is placed in one feeding artery, and Onyx is allowed to occlude the proximal parts of the draining veins and nidus

13.3.1 Endovascular Treatment for Dural Arteriovenous Fistula

13.3.1.1 Definition of Dural Arteriovenous Fistula and Classifications

A dural arteriovenous fistula is defined as an abnormal arteriovenous malformation without a nidus between dural arteries and adjacent venous sinuses with occasional reflux into the cortical veins [33]. They represent 10–15% of all cerebral vascular malformations [34]. dAVF have been classified as a benign type with a dural sinus drain or an aggressive type with a leptomeningeal drain and/or reflux, which may be associated with hemorrhage or nonhemorrhagic neurologic deficits [35]. The classification systems defined by Cognard et al. [36] and Borden et al. [37], which are designed to grade the risks and natural course of dAVF, have been widely used.

13.3.1.2 Target of Endovascular Treatment of Ruptured dAVF

With the advancement of embolic materials and devices in the field of neurointervention, endovascular treatment is now regarded as the primary treatment option, especially in high-risk dAVF such as hemorrhagic presentation. The primary objective of endovascular treatment is to obliterate occlusion of the entire fistulous channels with preservation of normal venous channels. However, in complex dAVF with an expectation to avoid obliteration of total fistulous channels, the goal of endovascular treatment is an intentional partial treatment strategy with reversal of the aggressive type of dAVF to a benign type to facilitate subsequent Gamma Knife radiosurgery or neurosurgery [38, 39].

13.3.1.3 Endovascular Access Routes

Conventionally, transvenous endovascular treatment that occludes fistulous channels and the adjacent affected sinus has been widely used. However, transvenous endovascular treatment is not always possible for the isolated affected sinus or stenotic dural sinus. With the development of liquid embolic materials such as Onyx or PHIL, trans-arterial endovascular treatments that occlude feeding arteries and fistulous channels have been attempted and gradually increased. In cases of small-calibered, tortuous feeding arteries, trans-arterial endovascular treatment may be challenging. Additionally, embolization of feeding arteries that are at risk for anastomosis in the internal carotid or vertebral artery may cause cerebral/cerebellar infarction or cranial nerve palsy. In dAVF that are challenging or inaccessible via trans-arterial or transvenous access, direct puncture of the affected sinus via transorbital or craniotomy has provided good results [40–42].

13.3.1.4 Embolic Materials

Embolic materials are classified into detachable fibered/non-fibered coils, particles (polyvinyl alcohol, PVA), and liquid embolic materials. The liquid embolic materials that are currently used include n-butyl-2-cyanoacrylate (NBCA; Codman, Raynham, MA, USA), Onyx (eV3; Neurovascular Inc., Irvine, CA, USA), and PHIL (MicroVention-Terumo; Tustin, CA, USA). Coils are mainly used for transverse occlusion of the affected sinus. PVA is not a durable treatment option, and it has not been recently applied. It was previously used for benign dAVF as a palliative treatment or for residual fistulous channels as an alternative treatment. NBCA named “glue” is a cheap, fast embolic material, and it was widely used to occlude dAVF trans-arterially before the advent of Onyx or PHIL [43]. Because NBCA is a liquid adhesive, its major disadvantages are a short injection time, insufficient glue casting of fistulous channels, unexpected gluing of normal drain veins, and a low cure rate (30–50%) [44, 45]. Because Onyx is a cohesive liquid embolic agent, it provides a slow and controlled injection unlike NBCA, resulting in a larger amount of Onyx cast into the fistulous channels, which is related to a higher angiographic cure rate [46, 47]. PHIL is another cohesive liquid embolic material composed of hydroxyethyl methacrylate (PHEMA) and dimethyl sulfoxide. Accordingly, PHIL also provides a slow and controlled injection. Additionally, computed CT or MRA after PHIL embolization showed fewer artifacts and good delineation of the embolic cast due to the absence of a metal component such as tantalum.

Endovascular treatment using PHIL showed a similar angiographic cure rate compared with that of Onyx [48].

In conclusion, endovascular treatment of dAVF includes a number of options with varying risks and effectiveness for individual lesions. Endovascular treatment of dAVF is a proven safe and effective method for treating these complex cerebrovascular lesions.

13.3.2 Endovascular Treatment for Arteriovenous Malformation

13.3.2.1 Definition of AVM and Natural History

Arteriovenous malformations (AVMs) are direct connections between arteries and veins without a capillary bed and consist of anomalous entangled vessels defined as a nidus. Approximately 2% of hemorrhagic strokes are caused by AVMs [49]. Hemorrhagic stroke is the most common symptom of AVMs, ranging from 53 to 65% [49, 50]. The annual risk of hemorrhage ranges from 1.3 to 4% per year [49, 51], increasing to 6–7% during the first year after the first hemorrhagic stroke [51, 52]. AVF and prenidal, intranidal, or flow-related aneurysms have been reported to increase the risk of AVM rupture [53, 54]. The morbidity of ruptured AVMs has been reported to be half or two-thirds of ruptured AVMs [55, 56]. Mortality has been reported to be approximately one to two-tenths of ruptured AVMs.

13.3.2.2 Objectives of Endovascular Treatment for Ruptured AVMs

Endovascular treatment of ruptured AVM may have varying goals. The first goal of endovascular treatment is mainly to decrease the arterial supply or the AVM size to resect AVM easily before surgery. By decreasing the AVM size as well as its blood flow, endovascular treatment has been reported to shorten the operation time and reduce blood loss [57]. Endovascular treatment and subsequent microsurgery can treat AVM in a staged manner, resulting in a reduction of blood flow to the nidus that will prevent normal pressure perfusion syndrome such as postoperative hemorrhage [58].

Another goal of endovascular treatment is to reduce the AVM size or to eliminate high-risk features for radiosurgery. Outcomes of combined endovascular treatment and subsequent radiosurgery have shown varying degree of complete occlusion ranging from 14 to 90% [59]. Endovascular treatment before radiosurgery was found to be most effective for AVM with a size of 4–6 cm for which approximately 90% were reduced to a size that was amendable to radiosurgery [60].

For small-sized ruptured AVM positioned in a deep location, endovascular treatment may be the primary treatment option to obliterate AVM angiographically. The selection of patients should be a cardinal rule for endovascular treatment to cure AVMs. Small AVMs with few feeding arteries, a compact rather than a diffuse nidus, and an absence of perinidal angiogenesis are positive factors for curing AVMs primarily by endovascular treatment [61, 62].

For AVMs that are not amenable to treatment, palliative or targeted treatment of high-risk features such as associated aneurysms or fistula is considered. However, partial endovascular treatment is not recommended because the outcome of partial endovascular treatment seems to be worse than the natural history [63, 64].

In conclusion, endovascular treatment of ruptured AVMs may play a pivotal role in obliterating AVM completely for microsurgery or radiosurgery. Endovascular treatment should be carefully considered as a primary treatment option for carefully selected AVMs with a favorable profile for complete AVM obliteration.

References

1. Molyneux A, Kerr R, Stratton I, et al. International subarachnoid aneurysm trial (ISAT) of neurosurgical clipping versus endovascular coiling in 2143 patients with ruptured intracranial aneurysms: a randomised trial. Lancet. 2002;360:1267–74.
2. Mcdougall CG, Spetzler RF, Zabramski JM, et al. The barrow ruptured aneurysm trial. J Neurosurg. 2012;116:135–44.
3. Rouchaud A, Brinjikji W, Cloft HJ, et al. Endovascular treatment of ruptured blister-like

aneurysms: a systematic review and meta-analysis with focus on deconstructive versus reconstructive and flow-diverter treatments. AJNR Am J Neuroradiol. 2015;36:2331–9.
4. Pierot L. Flow diverter stents in the treatment of intracranial aneurysms: where are we? J Neuroradiol. 2011;38:40–6.
5. Kallmes DF, Ding YH, Dai D, et al. A new endoluminal, flow-disrupting device for treatment of saccular aneurysms. Stroke. 2007;38:2346–52.
6. Mendes GA, Silveira EP, Caire F, et al. Endovascular management of deep arteriovenous malformations: single institution experience in 22 consecutive patients. Neurosurgery. 2016;78:34–41.
7. Raymond J, Roy D. Safety and efficacy of endovascular treatment of acutely ruptured aneurysms. Neurosurgery. 1997;41:1235–45. discussion 1245-1236
8. Sluzewski M, Bosch JA, Van Rooij WJ, et al. Rupture of intracranial aneurysms during treatment with Guglielmi detachable coils: incidence, outcome, and risk factors. J Neurosurg. 2001;94:238–40.
9. Janssen H, Berlis A, Lutz J, et al. State of practice: endovascular treatment of acute aneurysmal SAH in Germany. AJNR Am J Neuroradiol. 2017;38:1574–9.
10. Molyneux AJ, Kerr RS, Yu LM, et al. International subarachnoid aneurysm trial (ISAT) of neurosurgical clipping versus endovascular coiling in 2143 patients with ruptured intracranial aneurysms: a randomised comparison of effects on survival, dependency, seizures, rebleeding, subgroups, and aneurysm occlusion. Lancet. 2005;366:809–17.
11. Sadato A, Adachi K, Hayakawa M, et al. Effects of anatomic characteristics of aneurysms on packing density in endovascular coil embolization: analysis of a single center's experience. Neurosurg Rev. 2016;39:109–14. discussion 114
12. Kwon OK, Kim SH, Oh CW, et al. Embolization of wide-necked aneurysms with using three or more microcatheters. Acta Neurochir. 2006;148:1139–45. discussion 1145
13. Baxter BW, Rosso D, Lownie SP. Double microcatheter technique for detachable coil treatment of large, wide-necked intracranial aneurysms. AJNR Am J Neuroradiol. 1998;19:1176–8.
14. Moret J, Cognard C, Weill A, et al. Reconstruction technic in the treatment of wide-neck intracranial aneurysms. Long-term angiographic and clinical results. Apropos of 56 cases. J Neuroradiol. 1997;24:30–44.
15. Kurre W, Berkefeld J. Materials and techniques for coiling of cerebral aneurysms: how much scientific evidence do we have? Neuroradiology. 2008;50:909–27.
16. Cai K, Zhang Y, Shen L, et al. Comparison of stent-assisted coiling and balloon-assisted coiling in the treatment of ruptured wide-necked intracranial aneurysms in the acute period. World Neurosurg. 2016;96:316–21.
17. Chalouhi N, Jabbour P, Tjoumakaris S, et al. Single-center experience with balloon-assisted coil embolization of intracranial aneurysms: safety, efficacy and indications. Clin Neurol Neurosurg. 2013;115:607–13.
18. Ross IB, Dhillon GS. Balloon assistance as a routine adjunct to the endovascular treatment of cerebral aneurysms. Surg Neurol. 2006;66:593–601. discussion 601-592
19. Sluzewski M, Van Rooij WJ, Beute GN, et al. Balloon-assisted coil embolization of intracranial aneurysms: incidence, complications, and angiography results. J Neurosurg. 2006;105:396–9.
20. Akpek S, Arat A, Morsi H, et al. Self-expandable stent-assisted coiling of wide-necked intracranial aneurysms: a single-center experience. AJNR Am J Neuroradiol. 2005;26:1223–31.
21. Muto M, Giurazza F, Ambrosanio G, et al. Stent-assisted coiling in ruptured cerebral aneurysms: multi-center experience in acute phase. Radiol Med. 2017;122:43–52.
22. Kim M, Levy EI, Meng H, et al. Quantification of hemodynamic changes induced by virtual placement of multiple stents across a wide-necked basilar trunk aneurysm. Neurosurgery. 2007;61:1305–12. discussion 1312-1303
23. Vanninen R, Manninen H, Ronkainen A. Broad-based intracranial aneurysms: thrombosis induced by stent placement. AJNR Am J Neuroradiol. 2003;24:263–6.
24. Bendok BR, Parkinson RJ, Hage ZA, et al. The effect of vascular reconstruction device-assisted coiling on packing density, effective neck coverage, and angiographic outcome: an in vitro study. Neurosurgery. 2007;61:835–40. discussion 840-831
25. Kadkhodayan Y, Rhodes N, Blackburn S, et al. Comparison of Enterprise with Neuroform stent-assisted coiling of intracranial aneurysms. AJR Am J Roentgenol. 2013;200:872–8.
26. Higashida RT, Halbach VV, Dowd CF, et al. Initial clinical experience with a new self-expanding nitinol stent for the treatment of intracranial cerebral aneurysms: the Cordis Enterprise stent. AJNR Am J Neuroradiol. 2005;26:1751–6.
27. Pearl M, Gregg L, Gailloud P. Endovascular treatment of aneurysmal subarachnoid hemorrhage. Neurosurg Clin N Am. 2010;21:271–80.
28. Rong-Bo Q, Hua J, Kai W, et al. Stent-jail technique in endovascular treatment of wide-necked aneurysm. Turk Neurosurg. 2013;23:179–82.
29. Natarajan SK, Shallwani H, Fennell VS, et al. Flow diversion after aneurysmal subarachnoid hemorrhage. Neurosurg Clin N Am. 2017;28:375–88.
30. Makoyeva A, Bing F, Darsaut TE, et al. The varying porosity of braided self-expanding stents and flow diverters: an experimental study. AJNR Am J Neuroradiol. 2013;34:596–602.
31. Fiorella D, Hsu D, Woo HH, et al. Very late thrombosis of a pipeline embolization device construct: case report. Neurosurgery. 2010;67:onsE313–4. discussion onsE314
32. Sadasivan C, Cesar L, Seong J, et al. An original flow diversion device for the treatment of intracranial

aneurysms: evaluation in the rabbit elastase-induced model. Stroke. 2009;40:952–8.
33. Vinuela F, Fox AJ, Debrun GM, et al. Spontaneous carotid-cavernous fistulas: clinical, radiological, and therapeutic considerations. Experience with 20 cases. J Neurosurg. 1984;60:976–84.
34. Newton TH, Cronqvist S. Involvement of dural arteries in intracranial arteriovenous malformations. Radiology. 1969;93:1071–8.
35. Lasjaunias PBA. Surgical neuroangiography: endovascular treatment of craniofacial lesions. Berlin: Springer; 1987.
36. Cognard C, Gobin YP, Pierot L, et al. Cerebral dural arteriovenous fistulas: clinical and angiographic correlation with a revised classification of venous drainage. Radiology. 1995;194:671–80.
37. Borden JA, Wu JK, Shucart WA. A proposed classification for spinal and cranial dural arteriovenous fistulous malformations and implications for treatment. J Neurosurg. 1995;82:166–79.
38. Friedman JA, Pollock BE, Nichols DA, et al. Results of combined stereotactic radiosurgery and transarterial embolization for dural arteriovenous fistulas of the transverse and sigmoid sinuses. J Neurosurg. 2001;94:886–91.
39. Bertalanffy A, Dietrich W, Kitz K, et al. Treatment of dural arteriovenous fistulae (dAVF's) at the superior sagittal sinus (SSS) using embolisation combined with micro- or radiosurgery. Minim Invasive Neurosurg. 2001;44:205–10.
40. Luo CB, Teng MM, Chang FC, et al. Transorbital direct puncture of the posterior cavernous sinus through the internal carotid artery for embolization of isolated cavernous sinus dural arteriovenous fistula. J Neurointerv Surg. 2013;5:e1.
41. Luo CB, Chang FC, Wu HM, et al. Transcranial embolization of a transverse-sigmoid sinus dural arteriovenous fistula carried out through a decompressive craniectomy. Acta Neurochir. 2007;149:197–200. discussion 200
42. Houdart E, Saint-Maurice JP, Chapot R, et al. Transcranial approach for venous embolization of dural arteriovenous fistulas. J Neurosurg. 2002;97:280–6.
43. Rabinov JD, Yoo AJ, Ogilvy CS, et al. ONYX versus n-BCA for embolization of cranial dural arteriovenous fistulas. J Neurointerv Surg. 2013;5:306–10.
44. Kim DJ, Willinsky RA, Krings T, et al. Intracranial dural arteriovenous shunts: transarterial glue embolization--experience in 115 consecutive patients. Radiology. 2011;258:554–61.
45. Nelson PK, Russell SM, Woo HH, et al. Use of a wedged microcatheter for curative transarterial embolization of complex intracranial dural arteriovenous fistulas: indications, endovascular technique, and outcome in 21 patients. J Neurosurg. 2003;98:498–506.
46. Maimon S, Nossek E, Strauss I, et al. Transarterial treatment with Onyx of intracranial dural arteriovenous fistula with cortical drainage in 17 patients. AJNR Am J Neuroradiol. 2011;32:2180–4.
47. Cognard C, Januel AC, Silva NA Jr, et al. Endovascular treatment of intracranial dural arteriovenous fistulas with cortical venous drainage: new management using Onyx. AJNR Am J Neuroradiol. 2008;29:235–41.
48. Lamin S, Chew HS, Chavda S, et al. Embolization of intracranial Dural arteriovenous fistulas using PHIL liquid embolic agent in 26 patients: a multicenter study. AJNR Am J Neuroradiol. 2017;38:127–31.
49. Brown RD Jr, Wiebers DO, Torner JC, et al. Frequency of intracranial hemorrhage as a presenting symptom and subtype analysis: a population-based study of intracranial vascular malformations in Olmsted country, Minnesota. J Neurosurg. 1996;85:29–32.
50. Hofmeister C, Stapf C, Hartmann A, et al. Demographic, morphological, and clinical characteristics of 1289 patients with brain arteriovenous malformation. Stroke. 2000;31:1307–10.
51. Ondra SL, Troupp H, George ED, et al. The natural history of symptomatic arteriovenous malformations of the brain: a 24-year follow-up assessment. J Neurosurg. 1990;73:387–91.
52. Fleetwood IG, Steinberg GK. Arteriovenous malformations. Lancet. 2002;359:863–73.
53. Kim EJ, Halim AX, Dowd CF, et al. The relationship of coexisting extranidal aneurysms to intracranial hemorrhage in patients harboring brain arteriovenous malformations. Neurosurgery. 2004;54:1349–57. discussion 1357-1348
54. Redekop G, Terbrugge K, Montanera W, et al. Arterial aneurysms associated with cerebral arteriovenous malformations: classification, incidence, and risk of hemorrhage. J Neurosurg. 1998;89:539–46.
55. Graf CJ, Perret GE, Torner JC. Bleeding from cerebral arteriovenous malformations as part of their natural history. J Neurosurg. 1983;58:331–7.
56. Perret G NH. Arteriovenous malformations: an analysis of 545 cases of cranio-cerebral arteriovenous malformations and fistulae reported to the cooperative study. In: Sahs A, Perret G, Locksley H, Nishioka H, eds. Intracranial Aneurysms and Subarachnoid Hemorrhage: A Cooperative Study. JB Lippincott, Philadelphia; 1969.
57. Jafar JJ, Davis AJ, Berenstein A, et al. The effect of embolization with N-butyl cyanoacrylate prior to surgical resection of cerebral arteriovenous malformations. J Neurosurg. 1993;78:60–9.
58. Strozyk D, Nogueira RG, Lavine SD. Endovascular treatment of intracranial arteriovenous malformation. Neurosurg Clin N Am. 2009;20:399–418.
59. Izawa M, Chernov M, Hayashi M, et al. Combined management of intracranial arteriovenous malformations with embolization and gamma knife radiosurgery: comparative evaluation of the long-term results. Surg Neurol. 2009;71:43–52. discussion 52-43
60. Yashar P, Amar AP, Giannotta SL, et al. Cerebral arteriovenous malformations: issues of the interplay between stereotactic radiosurgery and endovascular surgical therapy. World Neurosurg. 2011;75:638–47.

61. Siddiqui AH, Chen PR, Rosenwasser RH. Endovascular therapy: indications, complications, and outcome. Informa Healthcare, New York; 2007.
62. Crowley RW, Ducruet AF, Mcdougall CG, et al. Endovascular advances for brain arteriovenous malformations. Neurosurgery. 2014;74(Suppl 1):S74–82.
63. Heros RC. Embolization of arteriovenous malformations. J Neurosurg. 2004;100:807–9. discussion 809
64. Han PP, Ponce FA, Spetzler RF. Intention-to-treat analysis of Spetzler-Martin grades IV and V arteriovenous malformations: natural history and treatment paradigm. J Neurosurg. 2003;98:3–7.

Management of Antithrombotic-Related Intracerebral Hemorrhage

14

Tarun Girotra, Wuwei Feng, and Bruce Ovbiagele

14.1 Epidemiology

14.1.1 Incidence

Intracerebral hemorrhage (ICH) accounts for about 10–20% of all strokes worldwide. The overall global annual incidence of ICH is estimated to be 24.6 per 100,000 (95% CI 19.7–30.7) [1].

Ethnic differences in incidence of ICH are striking. The annual incidence of ICH is 48.9 per 100,000 in black population and 26.6 per 100,000 population in white population [2]. Hispanics have also been observed to have a greater risk of ICH compared to non-Hispanic white population (OR 2.6, 95% CI 1.4–6.1) [3]. Asian population appears to be at a greater risk of ICH compared to other populations. A meta-analysis found that Asian populations have a higher proportion of ICH compared to white populations [28.0% (95% CI 23.6–32.6%) vs. 12.4% (95% CI 10.2–14.7%)] [4].

Age is another important non-modifiable risk factor for ICH. Population over 85 years of age has an almost tenfold yearly increase in risk of ICH compared to population between 45 and 54 years of age. Female gender has been associated with lower risk of ICH, although large-scale observation studies have found this to be statistically non-significant (RR 0.85, 95% CI 0.61–1.18) [5].

14.1.2 Antithrombotic-Related ICH

Long-term use of aspirin has been noted to have an increased risk of ICH compared to placebo with a RR of 1.65 (95% CI 1.05–5.99) per one meta-analysis [6]. AC-related ICH is estimated to be 2–9 cases per 100,000 population/year. This number is expected to rise as the global average life expectancy and the incidence of conditions requiring AC use such as atrial fibrillation increase. The use of warfarin carries a 0.3–3.7% annual risk of ICH. New oral anticoagulants (NOACs) have become more popular in recent years as they have several advantages: fewer interactions with food and other drugs, rapid onset, and freedom from the need to have periodic blood test monitoring and relatively shorter half-life. The rates of major bleedings, GI bleeding, and ICH from the three pivotal trials have been summarized in Table 14.1 [7–10]. Several recent meta-analyses showed that the use of NOACs is associated with a lower risk of ICH compared to warfarin use with RR varying from 0.46 (95% CI 0.33–0.65) to 0.48 (95% CI 0.39–0.59) [11, 12]. Postmarketing studies have also shown consistent benefit of NOACs in terms of

T. Girotra · W. Feng
Medical University of South Carolina,
Charleston, SC, USA

B. Ovbiagele (✉)
Department of Neurology, Medical University of South Carolina, Charleston, SC, USA
e-mail: ovibes@musc.edu

S.-H. Lee (ed.), *Stroke Revisited: Hemorrhagic Stroke*, Stroke Revisited,
https://doi.org/10.1007/978-981-10-1427-7_14

Table 14.1 Risk of bleedings in major non-vitamin K antagonist oral anticoagulant (NOAC) trials [7–10]

	RELY			ARISTOTLE		ROCKET-AF		ENGAGE-AF		
Event	Dabigatran 110 mg	Dabigatran 150 mg	Warfarin	Apixaban	Warfarin	Rivaroxaban	Warfarin	Edoxaban 60 mg	Edoxaban 30 mg	Warfarin
Major bleedings (% per year)	2.71[a]	3.11	3.36	2.13[a]	3.09	3.6	3.4	2.75[a]	1.61[a]	3.43
GI bleeding (% per year[b])	1.12	1.51[a]	1.02	0.76	0.86	3.2[a,b]	2.2[b]	1.51	0.82[a]	1.23
ICH (% per year)	0.23[a]	0.3[a]	0.74	0.33[a]	0.80	0.5[a]	0.7	0.39[a]	0.26[a]	0.85

GI gastrointestinal, *ICH* intracerebral hemorrhage
[a]$p < 0.05$ compared to warfarin
[b]GI bleeding rate reported as frequency in ROCKET-AF trial

lower risk of ICH compared to warfarin [13]. Warfarin-related ICH also seems to be greater in Asian population compared to white populations (hazard ratio 4.06, 95% CI 2.06–6.67) [14]. Lowering of ICH risk with NOACs is amplified in Asian populations as a recent meta-analysis found that Asians have lower odds or developing ICH associated with NOAC (OR 0.33, 95% CI 0.22–0.5) than non-Asians (OR 0.52, 95% CI 0.42–0.64) compared to warfarin [15].

Cilostazol is commonly used in Asian countries as an antiplatelet agent in place of aspirin. The phase 3, non-inferiority trial, cilostazol for prevention of secondary stroke (CSPS 2), compared 100 mg twice a day cilostazol to 81 mg daily aspirin in 2757 Asian patients. The criterion of non-inferiority was met, and the primary end point of any stroke was 2.76% in cilostazol group and 3.76% in the aspirin group (HR 0.74, 95% CI 0.64–0.98) after a mean follow-up of 29 months [16]. The frequency of ICH was significantly lower in cilostazol group (8/1337) compared to aspirin (27/1335) (p = 0.0027). A subsequent meta-analysis noticed an insignificant decrease of stroke recurrence with cilostazol compared to aspirin in chronic phase (RR 0.82, 95% CI 0.62–1.08, p = 0.15), but the risk of hemorrhagic stroke was still significantly lower with cilostazol (RR 0.29, 95% CI 0.15–0.56, p = 0.0002) [17].

A Cochrane database review observed that the risk of ICH with clopidogrel is not statistically different from aspirin (OR 0.89, 95% CI 0.59–1.35) [18]. Genetic polymorphism in the CYP2C19 gene has been an area of interest. There is a greater prevalence of CYP2C19*2 and CYP2C19*3 allele in Asian population which is associated with decreased activation of clopidogrel to the active metabolite resulting in decreased effectiveness of clopidogrel. A different allele, CYP2C19*17, has been recently noted to be prevalent in European and African populations [19]. This allele is associated with rapid metabolism of clopidogrel and has been observed with greater risk of hemorrhagic complications (HR 1.26, 95% CI 1.05–1.50) [20]. Clinical implication of this increased risk is unclear however.

14.2 Pharmacology of Antithrombotics

A detailed discussion on the pharmacology of various antiplatelets and anticoagulants is beyond the scope of this chapter, but Fig. 14.1a, b demonstrates the mechanism of action of various commonly used antiplatelets and anticoagulants (Fig. 14.2).

14.3 Management of ICH

14.3.1 General Management

ICH presents clinically with acute focal neurological deficits. With small hemorrhages, the clinical symptoms progress and evolve over minutes to hours depending on the rate of hematoma expansion and subsequent peri-hematoma edema. Larger hemorrhages typically present more dramatically with decreased level of awareness, vomiting, headache, and, in severe cases, signs of herniation. Seizure is a common complication after ICH, especially lobar hemorrhage. The basic principles of management of ICH are similar to that of spontaneous ICH and are detailed in other chapters.

14.3.2 Treatment of Antiplatelet-Related ICH

Observational studies have yielded mixed results regarding hematoma expansion and outcomes in patients on antiplatelet therapy treated with platelet transfusion [22–24]. Recently concluded randomized, open-label controlled trial (platelet transfusion versus standard care after acute stroke due to spontaneous cerebral hemorrhage associated with antiplatelet use or the "PATCH" trial) aimed to identify the effects of platelet transfusion in patients with supratentorial ICH and antiplatelet agent use for at least 7 days prior to ICH. They enrolled 190 patients and found that treatment arm receiving platelet transfusion had a higher rate of dependence and death (modified Rankin scale, mRS 4–6) at 3 months (OR 2.04, 95% CI

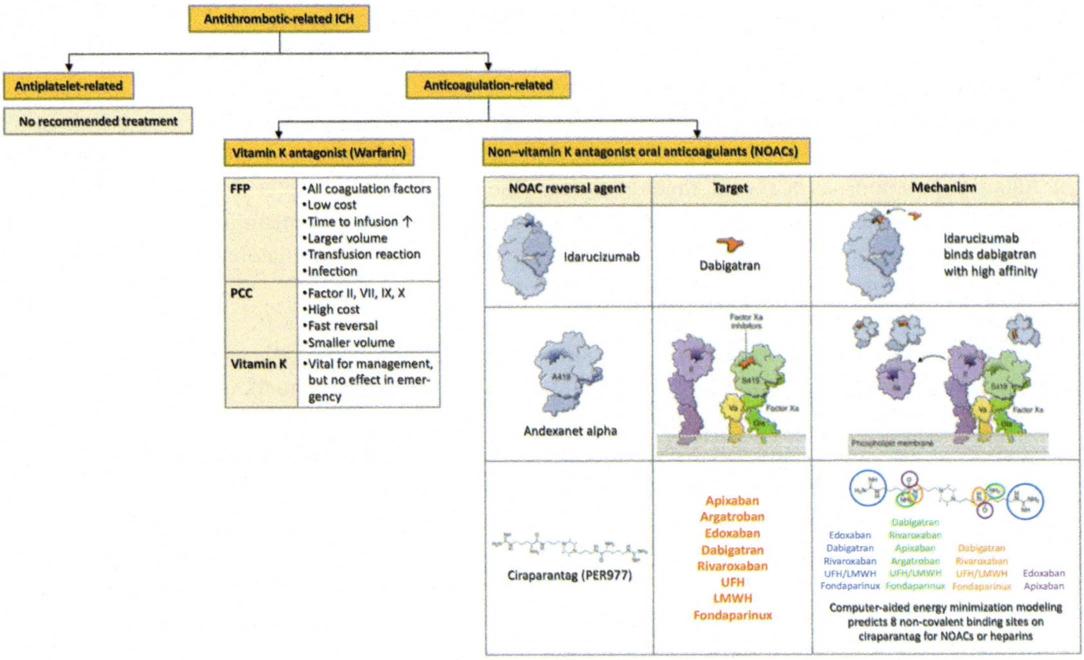

Fig. 14.1 Summary of treatment for antithrombotic-related intracerebral hemorrhage (ICH). The table for treatment of non-vitamin K antagonist oral anticoagulant (NOAC)-related ICH was reproduced by permission of Circulation [21]. *ICH* intracerebral hemorrhage, *FFP* fresh frozen plasma, *PCC* prothrombin complex concentrate

1.12–3.74, $p = 0.0195$) compared to the placebo arm [25]. No difference was noted in median ICH growth at 24 h or adverse events between the two groups. Because of lack of definitive data, routine use of platelet transfusion in patients with ICH while on an antiplatelet agent without thrombocytopenia is not recommended.

14.3.3 Treatment of Vitamin K Antagonist (Warfarin)-Related ICH

Warfarin inhibits vitamin K epoxide reductase leading to decreased synthesis of factors II, VII, IX, and X. The first step is to immediately stop warfarin and/or antiplatelet if patients take both. Reinstating these factors is the physiological basis of VKA reversal agents. Four agents have been used to reverse the warfarin, including fresh frozen plasma (FFP), prothrombin complex concentrate (PCC), recombinant factor VII (rFVII), and vitamin K.

14.3.3.1 Fresh Frozen Plasma

Historically, FFP was the most commonly used agent to reverse anticoagulation effect of warfarin. It contains all coagulation factors, including those inhibited warfarin, in a non-concentrated form. Despite its widespread availability and low cost, there are several important limitations which make PCC a more preferred option for reversing warfarin-related anticoagulation in ICH patients. Firstly, FFP needs to be thawed and crossmatched before it can be administered in a patient which leads to devastating delays. Secondly, because it is not concentrated, patients typically end up receiving large volumes of FFP to correct INR which leads to fluid overload in patients with chronic cardiac, renal, and hepatic diseases. Lastly, patients receiving FFP are at risk of developing transfusion reactions and infections.

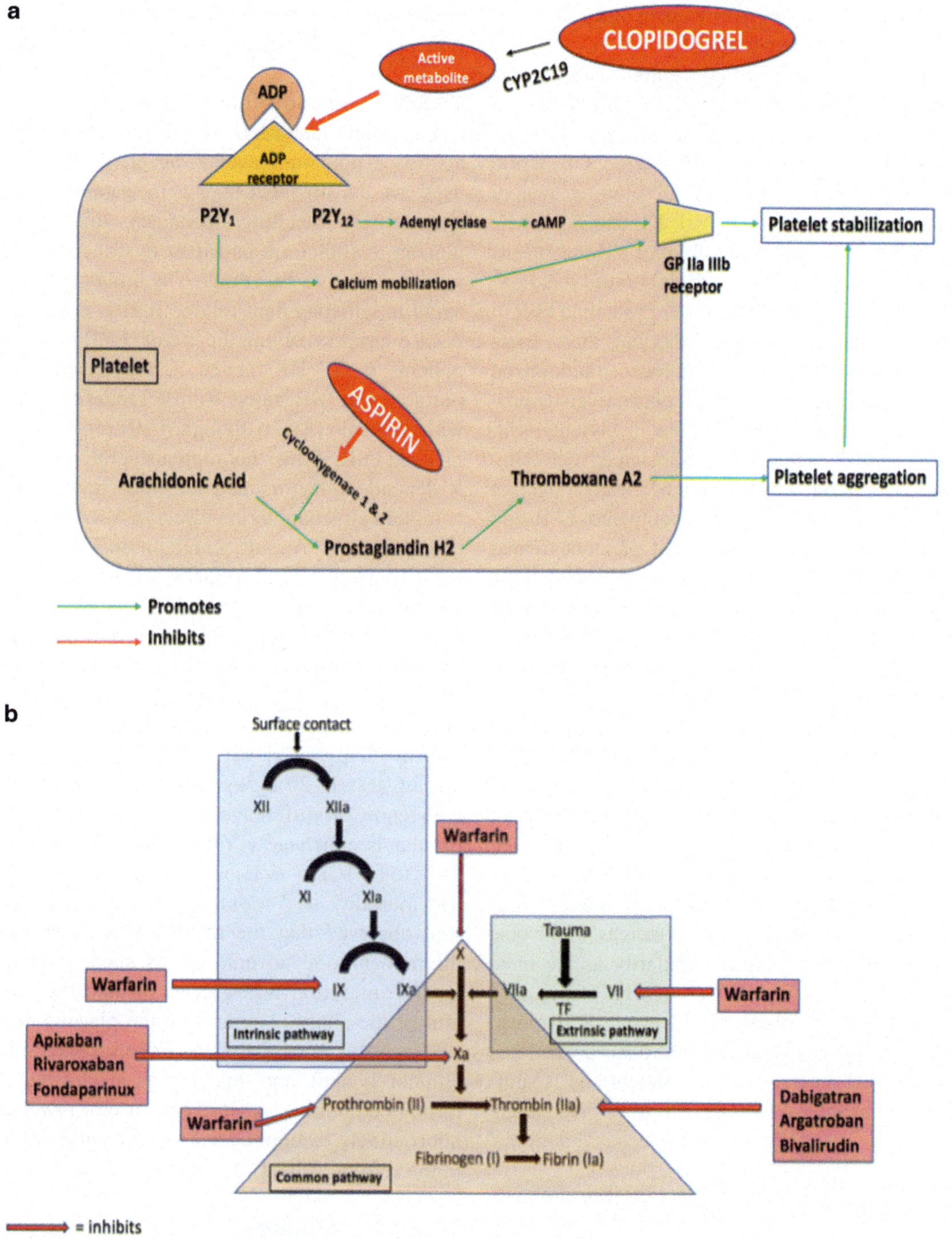

Fig. 14.2 (**a**) Mechanism of action of antiplatelet agents. (**b**) Coagulation cascade and mechanism of action of anticoagulants. *ADP* adenosine diphosphate, *CYP* cytochrome P450, *cAMP* cyclic adenosine monophosphate, *GP* glycoprotein

14.3.3.2 Prothrombin Complex Concentrate

Prothrombin complex concentrate (PCC) has emerged as the most attractive alternative to FFP. PCC comes in two preparations, four-factor (4PCC) and three-factor PCC (3PCC). While both formulations contain all clotting factors inhibited by warfarin (II, VII, IX, and X), 4PCC contains a larger amount of factor VII than available 3PCC agents. Earlier trials showed that PCC normalizes INR at a much faster rate than FFP in patients with major bleeding, but these trials lacked patients with ICH. A recent randomized controlled trial (fresh frozen plasma versus prothrombin complex concentrate in patients with intracerebral hemorrhage associated with vitamin K antagonist or the "INCH" trial) looked at 50 patients with ICH and compared FPP and 4PCC. The study showed that patients treated with 4PCC had a much faster reversal of INR (INR of <1.3 within 3 h, 67% with PCC and 9% with FPP, OR 30.6, 95% CI 4.7–197.9, $p = 0.0003$) and decreased hematoma expansion at 3 and 24 h [26]. There was no significant benefit in survival and functional independence at 90 days, but it was noted that the five deaths occurring in the first 48 h had notable hematoma expansion and were exclusively in the FFP arm. The rate of thromboembolic events was observed to be similar between FPP and PCC arms in all the studies mentioned above. Due to quicker normalization of INR without increased adverse events, PCC has gained popularity as the most preferred agent for VKA-related ICH. The dose of 4PCC to be used for reversal of warfarin depends on the first international normalized ratio (INR) on arrival of the patient and is summarized in Table 14.2. PCC has to be given along with vitamin K. The disadvantages are high cost, limited availability, and potential prothrombotic.

Table 14.2 Recommended dose of prothrombin complex concentrate (PCC) for vitamin K antagonist (VKA) reversal

INR level	Dose of 4PCC
2–4	25 IU/kg (maximum 2500 IU)
4–6	35 IU/kg (maximum 3500 IU)
>6	50 IU/kg (maximum 5000 IU)

INR international normalized ratio, *4PCC* four-factor prothrombin complex concentrate

14.3.3.3 Recombinant Factor VII

Recombinant factor VII (rFVII) has been evaluated as a potential reversal agent. It has been used as an off-label agent in patients with uncontrolled bleeding secondary to trauma, platelet dysfunction, and liver dysfunction and in perioperative bleeding. The utility of this agent in anticoagulant-related ICH is not clear. A case series involving the use of rFVII in seven patients with VKA-related ICH decreased the pretreatment INR (range from 1.7 to 6.6) to <1.6 within 10 min [27]. Although rFVII rapidly normalized INR, it does not replenish other vitamin K-dependent factors and may not reverse the complete anticoagulation effect of VKA as efficiently as PCC. A multicenter, phase 3, randomized controlled trial ("factor seven in acute hemorrhagic stroke" or "FAST" trial) administered rFVII (20 μg/kg or 80 μg/kg) or placebo in 841 patients with spontaneous ICH within 4 h of symptom onset. Compared to placebo, increase in ICH volume at 24 h from baseline was 3.8 mL less in 80 μg/kg rFVII arm ($p < 0.001$) and 2.6 mL less in 20 μg/kg rFVII arm ($p = 0.08$). No significant difference was noted in intraventricular hemorrhage (IVH) volume increase at 24 h, total (ICH + IVH) volume increase at 72 h, and mortality at 3 months, however [28]. The trial observed that the rate of serious arterial thromboembolic adverse events such as myocardial infarction was greater in the 80 μg/kg arm of the study compared to the placebo arm (8% vs. 4%, $p = 0.04$). Due to lack of definite clinical benefit and increase risk of arterial thromboembolic adverse events, use of rFVII is not routinely recommended for reversal of VKA in the setting of ICH.

14.3.3.4 Vitamin K

Intravenous vitamin K administration itself is not sufficient as an emergent reversal agent, but it is a vital part of managing a VKA-associated bleeding complication. It is generally administered in a high dose of 5–10 mg intravenously. The onset of action begins about 2 h post administration and peaks about 24 h after administration. The advantage of this delayed action is that it provides a sustained reversal; however, the disadvantage is that ICH may continue to grow before its peak time. High dose of vitamin K can result in a variable period of refractoriness to warfarin if warfarin needs to be resumed. Other advantages of vitamin K are low cost and wide availability.

14.3.4 New Oral Anticoagulant (NOAC)-Related ICH

NOACs offer a distinct advantage over VKA regarding reliable pharmacodynamics and pharmacokinetics, rapid onset and offset of action, lack of dietary interactions, and lack of routine coagulation parameter monitoring. As mentioned earlier, the NOACs are associated with a lower risk of ICH compared to VKA. For those patients that do end up with ICH associated with NOACs such as apixaban and dabigatran, the mortality and outcomes are similar to those associated with VKA [29].

Validation of blood coagulation tests for NOACs and incorporation of these in clinical practice are missing currently. Thrombin time (TT) is the most sensitive test for dabigatran, and a normal TT excludes the clinically relevant action of dabigatran. Activated partial thromboplastin time (aPTT) is less reliable than TT for dabigatran but is more readily available across hospitals and emergency departments and is often used as a surrogate marker of anticoagulant activity. Prothrombin time (PT) has poor sensitivity for dabigatran.

Partial thromboplastin time demonstrates insufficient sensitivity and linearity with factor X inhibitors such as apixaban, rivaroxaban, and edoxaban. PT can be elevated with factor X inhibitors but cannot be relied on to exclude the clinically relevant anticoagulant effect of these medications in the setting of a normal PT. Chromogenic anti-factor X inhibitor assays have been developed for rivaroxaban, apixaban, and edoxaban, but they are not yet validated to be included in management guidelines.

14.3.4.1 Non-specific Agents

Among non-specific hemostatic agents, PCC has limited data from three small randomized, placebo-controlled studies involving healthy volunteers. These studies showed a dose-dependent reversal of the anticoagulant effect of rivaroxaban and edoxaban but not dabigatran [30–32]. An in vitro study using human plasma exposed to rivaroxaban obtained from healthy donors found that rFVII was superior to a 4PCC at normalizing laboratory coagulation studies [33]. Other in vitro studies involving healthy human volunteers have shown that activated PCC (also known as factor VIII inhibitor bypassing activity or FEIBA) corrected more coagulation parameters than PCC [34, 35]. There was a recent small prospective study evaluating the administration of FEIBA 50 U/kg dose in 127 patients with ICH, which included 5 patients on NOACs (3 on rivaroxaban, 1 on apixaban, and 1 on dabigatran) presenting within 48 h of the last dose and receiving FEIBA. None of these patients were noted to have hematoma expansion or thrombotic complications [36].

As mentioned above, reversal of these blood coagulation parameters does not necessarily indicate reversal of the complete anticoagulant effect of these medications. Finally, whether reversal of coagulation parameters lead to improved clinical outcomes has not yet been shown in a randomized clinical trial. In the absence of convincing clinical data, the European Heart Rhythm Association (EHRA) has recommended 50 U/kg dose of PCC or aPCC (FEIBA) in severe life-threatening hemorrhages associated with NOACs. A recent statement from AHA has endorsed PCC use for ICH with use of the factor X inhibitors until a more specific antidote becomes available [37].

FFP is of unclear utility, and vitamin K supplementation is not recommended. Activated charcoal can be used if the most recent NOAC dose is within 2 h. Hemodialysis can remove 49–57% dabigatran within 4 h and may be considered for chronically low creatinine clearance (<30 mL/min) or in a setting of acute kidney injury. Factor X inhibitors are highly protein bound making hemodialysis not effective in the emergent setting.

14.3.4.2 Specific Reversal Agents

Idarucizumab

Idarucizumab is a humanized monoclonal antibody fragment that binds to dabigatran with 350-fold higher affinity than thrombin and is cleared via kidneys. Several preclinical trials showed the effective reversal of anticoagulation parameters associated with dabigatran. Recently concluded multicenter, phase 3 trial (Reversal Effects of Idarucizumab on Active Dabigatran or the REVERSE-AD trial) achieved primary end point of median maximum percentage reversal of dilute TT (dTT) and ecarin clotting time (ECT) within 4 h in 100% of the 504 dabigatran-treated patients who suffered from uncontrolled bleeding including ICH (group A) or had to undergo emergent surgery (group B) [38]. All patients were given two 2.5 g boluses of the medication 15 min apart. There were 98 patients with ICH analyzed in this study, and 30-day mortality in this group was noted to be 16.4%. By comparison, the mortality rates in the RELY study were noted to be 41% and 35% with dabigatran 110 mg and 150 mg, respectively [39]. This should be interpreted with caution as it was a single-arm study, but the utilization of this agent is recommended by AHA in patients with ICH who are taking dabigatran in the attempts to reverse the anticoagulation effect [37]. Since the approval of idarucizumab, there have been case reports of successful use of intravenous tissue plasminogen activator (tPA) in patients presenting with an acute ischemic stroke while on dabigatran [40, 41]. There has not been an official statement from any of the regulatory bodies regarding the reversal of dabigatran with idarucizumab for the purpose of acute ischemic stroke treatment, and further studies are required to assess the overall risk of hemorrhagic conversion and outcomes in such scenarios.

Andexanet Alfa

Andexanet alfa is a modified human recombinant factor Xa decoy protein developed as a reversal agent for factor Xa inhibitors such as apixaban, rivaroxaban, and edoxaban. It is also considered to have an action against indirect factor X inhibitors such as low molecular weight heparin which acts through antithrombin. Several phase 2 studies, including andexanet alfa, a Novel Antidote to the Anticoagulation Effects of FXA Inhibitors Apixaban (ANNEXA-A) and Rivaroxaban (ANNEXA-R), have shown anticoagulant reversal effect of andexanet by measuring anti-FXa activity and mean FXa inhibitor concentration within few minutes of intravenous administration [42]. An ongoing phase 3, nonrandomized, open-label, single-arm study called ANNEXA-4 trial (ClinicalTrials.gov Identifier: NCT02329327) is assessing the efficacy and safety of andexanet in patients presenting with major acute bleed while on direct FXa inhibitors and low molecular weight heparin. The protocol from the trial dictates that patients were given 800 mg intravenous bolus followed by infusion of 960 mg over 12 h if the anticoagulant was taken within 7 h from the event. If the anticoagulant was taken over 7 h before the event, a decreased dose of 400 mg IV bolus followed by 480 mg IV infusion over 12 h is given. The preliminary data analysis from the study showed results from 47 patients out of which 20 (43%) had an intracranial hemorrhage. There was a relative decrease in the mean anti-FXa activity in 89% of patients on rivaroxaban ($n = 20$) and 93% of patients on apixaban ($n = 20$) after the initial bolus. Eighty percent of patients among the ICH group were reported to have excellent (<20% increase in ICH volume from baseline) or good (20–30% increase in ICH volume from baseline) hemostasis based on hematoma growth on CT scan at 1 and 12 h after infusion. The preliminary safety analysis in ANNEXA-4 showed thrombotic event rate of 18% ($n = 12$) within 30 days of antidote [43]. Preclinical trials had shown neutralizing antibodies developing in 17% of patients given andexanet, but the clinical significance of this is unknown [42]. This agent is currently under review for approval by several regulatory agencies.

Ciraparantag

Ciraparantag (PER977) is another agent which binds to unfractionated heparin, low molecular weight heparin, and NOAC such as dabigatran, apixaban, rivaroxaban, and edoxaban. In healthy volunteers, this agent shortens the whole blood evaluated. For instance, a randomized controlled trial is assessing whether left atrial appendage closure is a safe and effective alternative to NOAC in patients with ICH (ClinicalTrials.gov Identifier: NCT03243175).

Conclusion

Antithrombotic (anticoagulant and antiplatelet)-induced ICH is a serious complication associated with high mortality and morbidity. With an aging world population, increasingly more people will require anticoagulants due to greater prevalence atrial fibrillation, a condition with a frequency which strongly correlated with rising age. As such, it is envisioned that an expected surge in the presence of atrial fibrillation in the population will be accompanied by an increase in the absolute number of hemorrhagic complications. An astute knowledge of agents necessary for the reversal of the anticoagulants becomes critical for all providers involved in the care of antithrombotic-related ICH. The NOACs are associated with a decreased risk of hemorrhagic complications compared to traditional VKA like warfarin, and efforts are ongoing to develop agents that can reverse the pharmacological effects of NOAC on the coagulation cascade quickly and safely. Recently approved idarucizumab is gaining popularity across the world, and more reversal agents are in the process of development.

References

1. Ikram MA, Wieberdink RG, Koudstaal PJ. International epidemiology of intracerebral hemorrhage. Curr Atheroscler Rep. 2012;14:300–6.
2. Flaherty ML, Woo D, Haverbusch M, et al. Racial variations in location and risk of intracerebral hemorrhage. Stroke. 2005;36:934–7.
3. Labovitz DL, Halim A, Boden-Albala B, et al. The incidence of deep and lobar intracerebral hemorrhage in whites, blacks, and Hispanics. Neurology. 2005;65:518–22.
4. Tsai C-F, Thomas B, Sudlow CLM. Epidemiology of stroke and its subtypes in Chinese vs white populations: a systematic review. Neurology. 2013;81:264–72.
5. Van Asch CJ, Luitse MJ, Rinkel GJ, et al. Incidence, case fatality, and functional outcome of intracerebral haemorrhage over time, according to age, sex, and ethnic origin: a systematic review and meta-analysis. Lancet Neurol. 2010;9:167–76.
6. Mcquaid KR, Laine L. Systematic review and meta-analysis of adverse events of low-dose aspirin and clopidogrel in randomized controlled trials. Am J Med. 2006;119:624–38.
7. Connolly SJ, Ezekowitz MD, Yusuf S, et al. Dabigatran versus warfarin in patients with atrial fibrillation. N Engl J Med. 2009;361:1139–51.
8. Granger CB, Alexander JH, Mcmurray JJ, et al. Apixaban versus warfarin in patients with atrial fibrillation. N Engl J Med. 2011;365:981–92.
9. Patel MR, Mahaffey KW, Garg J, et al. Rivaroxaban versus warfarin in nonvalvular atrial fibrillation. N Engl J Med. 2011;365:883–91.
10. Giugliano RP, Ruff CT, Braunwald E, et al. Edoxaban versus warfarin in patients with atrial fibrillation. N Engl J Med. 2013;369:2093–104.
11. Gomez-Outes A, Terleira-Fernandez AI, Calvo-Rojas G, et al. Dabigatran, rivaroxaban, or apixaban versus warfarin in patients with nonvalvular atrial fibrillation: a systematic review and meta-analysis of subgroups. Thrombosis. 2013;2013:640723.
12. Ruff CT, Giugliano RP, Braunwald E, et al. Comparison of the efficacy and safety of new oral anticoagulants with warfarin in patients with atrial fibrillation: a meta-analysis of randomised trials. Lancet. 2014;383:955–62.
13. Villines Todd CT. Safety of direct oral anticoagulants: insights from postmarketing studies. Am J Med. 2016;129:S41.
14. Shen AY, Yao JF, Brar SS, et al. Racial/ethnic differences in the risk of intracranial hemorrhage among patients with atrial fibrillation. J Am Coll Cardiol. 2007;50:309–15.
15. Wang K-L, Lip GYH, Lin S-J, et al. Non-vitamin K antagonist oral anticoagulants for stroke prevention in Asian patients with nonvalvular atrial fibrillation: meta-analysis. Stroke. 2015;46:2555–61.
16. Shinohara Y, Katayama Y, Uchiyama S, et al. Cilostazol for prevention of secondary stroke (CSPS 2): an aspirin-controlled, double-blind, randomised non-inferiority trial. Lancet Neurol. 2010;9:959–68.
17. Shi L, Pu J, Xu L, et al. The efficacy and safety of cilostazol for the secondary prevention of ischemic stroke in acute and chronic phases in Asian population—an updated meta-analysis. BMC Neurol. 2014;14:251.
18. Sudlow CL, Mason G, Maurice JB, et al. Thienopyridine derivatives versus aspirin for preventing stroke and other serious vascular events in high vascular risk patients. Cochrane Database Syst Rev. 2009;4:CD001246.
19. Li-Wan-Po A, Girard T, Farndon P, et al. Pharmacogenetics of CYP2C19: functional and clinical implications of a new variant CYP2C19*17. Br J Clin Pharmacol. 2010;69:222–30.

20. Zabalza M, Subirana I, Sala J, et al. Meta-analyses of the association between cytochrome CYP2C19 loss- and gain-of-function polymorphisms and cardiovascular outcomes in patients with coronary artery disease treated with clopidogrel. Heart. 2012;98:100–8.
21. Ruff CT, Giugliano RP, Antman EM. Management of bleeding with non-vitamin K antagonist oral anticoagulants in the era of specific reversal agents. Circulation. 2016;134:248–61.
22. Sansing LH, Messe SR, Cucchiara BL, et al. Prior antiplatelet use does not affect hemorrhage growth or outcome after ICH. Neurology. 2009;72:1397–402.
23. Naidech AM, Jovanovic B, Liebling S, et al. Reduced platelet activity is associated with early clot growth and worse 3-month outcome after intracerebral hemorrhage. Stroke. 2009;40:2398–401.
24. Naidech AM, Bernstein RA, Levasseur K, et al. Platelet activity and outcome after intracerebral hemorrhage. Ann Neurol. 2009;65:352–6.
25. Baharoglu MI, Cordonnier C, Al-Shahi Salman R, et al. Platelet transfusion versus standard care after acute stroke due to spontaneous cerebral haemorrhage associated with antiplatelet therapy (PATCH): a randomised, open-label, phase 3 trial. Lancet. 2016;387:2605–13.
26. Steiner T, Poli S, Griebe M, et al. Fresh frozen plasma versus prothrombin complex concentrate in patients with intracranial haemorrhage related to vitamin K antagonists (INCH): a randomised trial. Lancet Neurol. 2016;15:566–73.
27. Sorensen B, Johansen P, Nielsen GL, et al. Reversal of the International Normalized Ratio with recombinant activated factor VII in central nervous system bleeding during warfarin thromboprophylaxis: clinical and biochemical aspects. Blood Coagul Fibrinolysis. 2003;14:469–77.
28. Mayer SA, Brun NC, Begtrup K, et al. Efficacy and safety of recombinant activated factor VII for acute intracerebral hemorrhage. N Engl J Med. 2008;358:2127–37.
29. Wilson D, Seiffge DJ, Traenka C, et al. Outcome of intracerebral hemorrhage associated with different oral anticoagulants. Neurology. 2017;88:1693–700.
30. Eerenberg ES, Kamphuisen PW, Sijpkens MK, et al. Reversal of rivaroxaban and dabigatran by prothrombin complex concentrate: a randomized, placebo-controlled, crossover study in healthy subjects. Circulation. 2011;124:1573–9.
31. Levi M, Moore KT, Castillejos CF, et al. Comparison of three-factor and four-factor prothrombin complex concentrates regarding reversal of the anticoagulant effects of rivaroxaban in healthy volunteers. J Thromb Haemost. 2014;12:1428–36.
32. Zahir H, Brown KS, Vandell AG, et al. Edoxaban effects on bleeding following punch biopsy and reversal by a 4-factor prothrombin complex concentrate. Circulation. 2015;131:82–90.
33. Perzborn E, Heitmeier S, Laux V, et al. Reversal of rivaroxaban-induced anticoagulation with prothrombin complex concentrate, activated prothrombin complex concentrate and recombinant activated factor VII in vitro. Thromb Res. 2014;133:671–81.
34. Marlu R, Hodaj E, Paris A, et al. Effect of non-specific reversal agents on anticoagulant activity of dabigatran and rivaroxaban: a randomised crossover ex vivo study in healthy volunteers. Thromb Haemost. 2012;108:217–24.
35. Escolar G, Fernandez-Gallego V, Arellano-Rodrigo E, et al. Reversal of apixaban induced alterations in hemostasis by different coagulation factor concentrates: significance of studies in vitro with circulating human blood. PLoS One. 2013;8:e78696.
36. Dibu JR, Weimer JM, Ahrens C, et al. The role of FEIBA in reversing novel oral anticoagulants in intracerebral hemorrhage. Neurocrit Care. 2016;24:413–9.
37. Raval AN, Cigarroa JE, Chung MK, et al. Management of patients on non-vitamin K antagonist oral anticoagulants in the acute care and periprocedural setting: a scientific statement from the American Heart Association. Circulation. 2017;135:e604–33.
38. Pollack CVJ, Reilly PA, Van Ryn J, et al. Idarucizumab for dabigatran reversal—full cohort analysis. N Engl J Med. 2017;377:431–41.
39. Steiner T, Weitz JI, Veltkamp R. Anticoagulant-associated intracranial hemorrhage in the era of reversal agents. Stroke. 2017;48:1432–7.
40. Tireli D, He J, Nordling MM, et al. Systemic thrombolysis in acute ischemic stroke after dabigatran etexilate reversal with idarucizumab—a case report. J Stroke Cerebrovasc Dis. 2017;26:e123–5.
41. Vosko MR, Bocksrucker C, Drwiła R, et al. Real-life experience with the specific reversal agent idarucizumab for the management of emergency situations in dabigatran-treated patients: a series of 11 cases. J Thromb Thrombolysis. 2017;43:306–17.
42. Siegal DM, Curnutte JT, Connolly SJ, et al. Andexanet alfa for the reversal of factor Xa inhibitor activity. N Engl J Med. 2015;373:2413–24.
43. Connolly SJ, Milling TJJ, Eikelboom JW, et al. Andexanet alfa for acute major bleeding associated with factor Xa inhibitors. N Engl J Med. 2016;375:1131–41.
44. Ansell JE, Bakhru SH, Laulicht BE, et al. Use of PER977 to reverse the anticoagulant effect of edoxaban. N Engl J Med. 2014;371:2141–2.
45. Goldstein JN, Fazen LE, Wendell L, et al. Risk of thromboembolism following acute intracerebral hemorrhage. Neurocrit Care. 2009;10:28–34.
46. Paciaroni M, Agnelli G, Venti M, et al. Efficacy and safety of anticoagulants in the prevention of venous thromboembolism in patients with acute cerebral hemorrhage: a meta-analysis of controlled studies. J Thromb Haemost. 2011;9:893–8.
47. Eckman MH, Rosand J, Knudsen KA, et al. Can patients be anticoagulated after intracerebral hemorrhage? A decision analysis. Stroke. 2003;34:1710–6.

from increasing in size because of this pressure, but it may enter a secondary growth phase when the expanding force is greater than the surrounding hemostatic pressure. The model that best explains this phenomenon is called the "avalanche model," in which secondary hematoma growth occurs due to the rupture of multiple vessels surrounding the initial hematoma [6]. The clinical definition of hematoma growth has not yet been settled, but it is often considered that hematoma growth has occurred when the ICH volume increases by more than 33%. According to this definition, hematoma growth occurs in about 32% of ICH patients [7]. Inevitably, this growth causes additional physical injury to the brain tissue and leads to further neurological deterioration.

There are some neuroimaging markers that would predict hematoma growth. The most representative marker is the "spot sign," the clinical usefulness of which has now been widely accepted. Spot sign refers to extravasated contrast visualized as highly attenuated foci inside the ICH lesion, in enhanced computed tomography (CT). The relative risk of hematoma growth with the presence of a spot sign was about 2.8 times greater compared to its absence, and patients with a spot sign showed a greater number of early neurological deterioration events and also higher mortality rates [7]. The ICH guidelines of the American Stroke Association indicated that contrast-enhanced CT may be considered to help identify patients at risk for hematoma expansion [8]. It is not necessary to take contrast-enhanced CT in all ICH patients, but physicians in a stroke center in which contrast-enhanced CT is available may get useful information with it. In addition to the spot sign, there are other neuroimaging markers, such as noncontrast CT hypodensities and the black hole sign [9, 10].

As noted above, because hematoma expansion has a negative impact on ICH patients, recombinant factor VIIa has been noted as a hemostatic agent that can halt expansion. However, in a phase 3 clinical trial, recombinant factor VIIa succeeded in decreasing hematoma volume but did not decrease mortality rates [11]. This result should never be interpreted as suggesting that hematoma growth is not critical to clinical outcome. The study results may have been affected by a number of factors, including whether the dose of recombinant factor VIIa was sufficient to demonstrate a benefit, whether the administration time of the drug was appropriate, and whether there were differences in patient ethnicities. Therapeutics to prevent hematoma expansion should continue to be explored in the future.

15.1.1.3 Perihematomal Edema

Perihematomal edema is the result of secondary sterile, noninfectious inflammation following ICH. Basically, extravasated blood is a foreign material from the standpoint of neural tissue, so components of blood cause neural toxicity and promote sterile inflammation. Perihematomal edema consists of three phases. In the early phase during the first several hours following ICH, edema forms by hydrostatic pressure and clot retraction. In the second phase (continuing for 2 days after onset of ICH), thrombin, produced from the coagulation cascade of the blood, causes neural toxicity, resulting in perihematomal edema. Interestingly, in warfarin-induced ICH, the hematoma volume is generally greater than with spontaneous ICH, but the volume of perihematomal edema may be reduced, because thrombin production is inhibited by warfarin. In the third phase after 3 days after onset, hemoglobin and heme are released by the lysis of red blood cells, and heme is further degraded into iron, carbon monoxide, and biliverdin, by heme oxygenase. Each of these components becomes a major source of toxicity and oxidative stress to the neural tissue. As such, perihematomal edema inevitably occurs in most ICH cases. Even when patients with ICH survive the period of initial ictus, neurological deterioration often occurs due to perihematomal edema, leading to death in some cases. The greater the edema, relative to the hematoma volume, the worse the functional outcome is likely to be. In particular, in the case of a small ICH, less than 30 mL in size, edema volume affects patient outcome more than the hematoma volume [12]. Because perihematomal edema is as important as the hematoma volume itself in prognosis following ICH, many attempts have been made to reduce secondary injury by inhibiting oxidative stress and inflammatory response in the perihematomal area.

15.1.1.4 Intraventricular Hemorrhage (IVH) and Hydrocephalus Induced by IVH

IVH occurs when a hemorrhage extends to the ventricles: 30–50% of ICH patients have combined IVH [13]. In the presence of IVH, mortality rates increase to 50–75% [13]. There are two main mechanisms of brain injury following IVH. First, blood from the IVH flows into the subarachnoid space through the cerebrospinal fluid circulation, causing irritation of the cerebral cortex, which is similar to SAH. Second, IVH may impede the flow of cerebrospinal fluid, leading to obstructive hydrocephalus.

In terms of location, ICH adjacent to a ventricle may more easily lead to IVH. Accordingly, IVH is most commonly caused by thalamic hemorrhage, followed by caudate hemorrhage, and rarely occurs following lobar hemorrhage. However, IVH does not always have a negative impact. In some cases of thalamic ICH, when the hemorrhage extends to the ventricle before involving the internal capsule, local tissue pressure might be released due to the drainage of blood, resulting in preserved motor function.

In about half of the cases of IVH, obstructive hydrocephalus occurs due to obstruction of the third or fourth ventricle by a blood clot, which may result in an extremely poor outcome. Obstructive hydrocephalus frequently develops after IVH with thalamic hemorrhage, due to the high likelihood of blocking the cerebral aqueduct. In addition, as IVH volume increases, the risk for the development of hydrocephalus also increases. Acute obstructive hydrocephalus is an emergency situation that requires surgical intervention, such as extraventricular drainage.

15.1.2 Protective Factors

Even in the same ICH, the prognosis may vary according to the individual brain condition or health, which may provide resistance power against the ICH. In this chapter, we refer to factors associated with individual innate brain conditions as "protective factors." The mechanisms by which these protective factors affect prognosis are explained in two ways. First, vulnerable brain tissue has less physical resistance to the expanding force of a hematoma. Second, when neuronal circuits have already been damaged due to previous brain lesions, the neural reserve may be in a reduced state, and in such cases, functional deterioration may be severe even with small hemorrhages, as compared to similar cases with no previous lesion. These protective factors generally reflect the degree of brain function or health and may be visualized as radiological markers such as white matter lesions (or leukoaraiosis), cerebral microbleeds (CMBs), and previous stroke lesions that may show vulnerability of the white matter. Here, the prognostic role of white matter lesions and CMBs will be discussed in detail.

15.1.2.1 White Matter Lesions

White matter lesions are aroused by long-standing hypoperfusion within the white matter area. Pathologically, it is characterized as "incomplete infarction," which refers to selective neuronal necrosis, with relative preservation of the glial element, and "edema-related gliosis" which refers to local disruption of the blood-brain barrier (BBB) with parenchymal leakage of plasma constituents and resultant cumulative neuronal and glial damage. In short, this is a radiological biomarker suggesting chronic ischemic damage of the brain and usually occurs in the centrum semiovale, the internal border zone, which is the most hypoperfused area. Functionally, white matter lesions may weaken both physical constituents and functional cortical-subcortical neuronal circuits in the brain and, in turn, are associated with vascular dementia, gait disorder, and poststroke cognitive dysfunction. Because the BBB was weakened by white matter lesions, hematoma size may become larger, causing more severe neurological deterioration. In a multicenter clinical study evaluating the association of ICH with white matter lesions, Lee et al. showed that white matter lesions are closely related to immediate

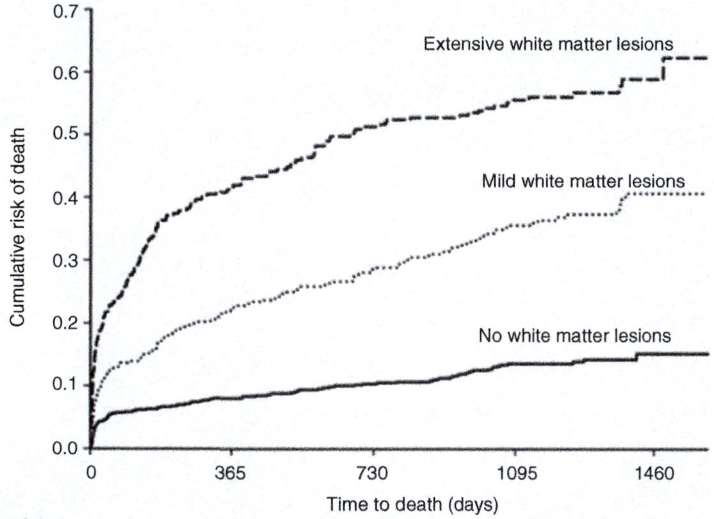

Numbers at risk

	0	365	730	1095	1460
No WMLs	665	611	596	444	50
Mild WMLs	386	302	277	192	30
Extensive WMLs	270	158	132	101	14

Fig. 15.2 Mortality curve of the study population according to the severity of white matter lesions (WMLs). Kaplan-Meier curves are shown for mortalities over 4 years of follow-up. $P < 0.001$ for overall comparisons across WML severities. Adapted by permission, from Neurology [14]

neurologic severity, 30-day mortality, and long-term mortality, in a dose-dependent manner (Fig. 15.2) [14]. In addition, patients with extensive white matter lesions showed a 2.8-fold increase in long-term mortality risk, as compared to patients with no, or only mild, lesions. These poor outcomes are likely to be associated with increased hematoma size, decreased neural activity reserve, and the occurrence of IVH due to white matter lesions. Considering that white matter lesions are present in approximately 50% of ICH patients, identification of white matter lesions may be useful in predicting the prognosis of the ICH patient at the bedside.

15.1.2.2 CMBs

CMBs refer to small, rounded, low-density lesions observed in gradient echo sequence or susceptibility-weighted imaging sequence of magnetic resonance imaging (MRI) (Fig. 15.3). Pathologically, these are small extravasations of blood due to tiny ruptures of penetrating arteries which have become arteriosclerotic by long-standing hypertension. These are visualized with exaggeration due to the paramagnetic effect of hemosiderin deposits, resulting in a "blooming artifact." Most lesions are asymptomatic but share the same underlying pathophysiology, and the same location, with ICH [15], except for the amount of bleeding that occurs. In this context, CMBs have been widely accepted as the most useful biomarker for the prediction of ICH. CMBs have been reported to be associated with the occurrence of both new incident ICH [16] and recurrent ICH [17], and the predictive power of CMBs is much greater than any other clinical variable or imaging biomarker, such as white matter lesions. In addition, CMBs were shown to have a strong association with both aspirin-related [18] and warfarin-related ICH [19]. Furthermore, the presence of CMBs is positively correlated to hematoma volume and also related to poor outcomes in ICH patients [20]. However, its clinical usefulness remains limited because there is no general consensus on the number or location of CMBs, or standard MRI sequences, for the prediction of ICH.

15.1.3 Systemic and Neurological State

Not all prognostic factors for ICH are present within the brain. Since the patient's brain state is closely related to the body response, the systemic and neurological state is likely to have a

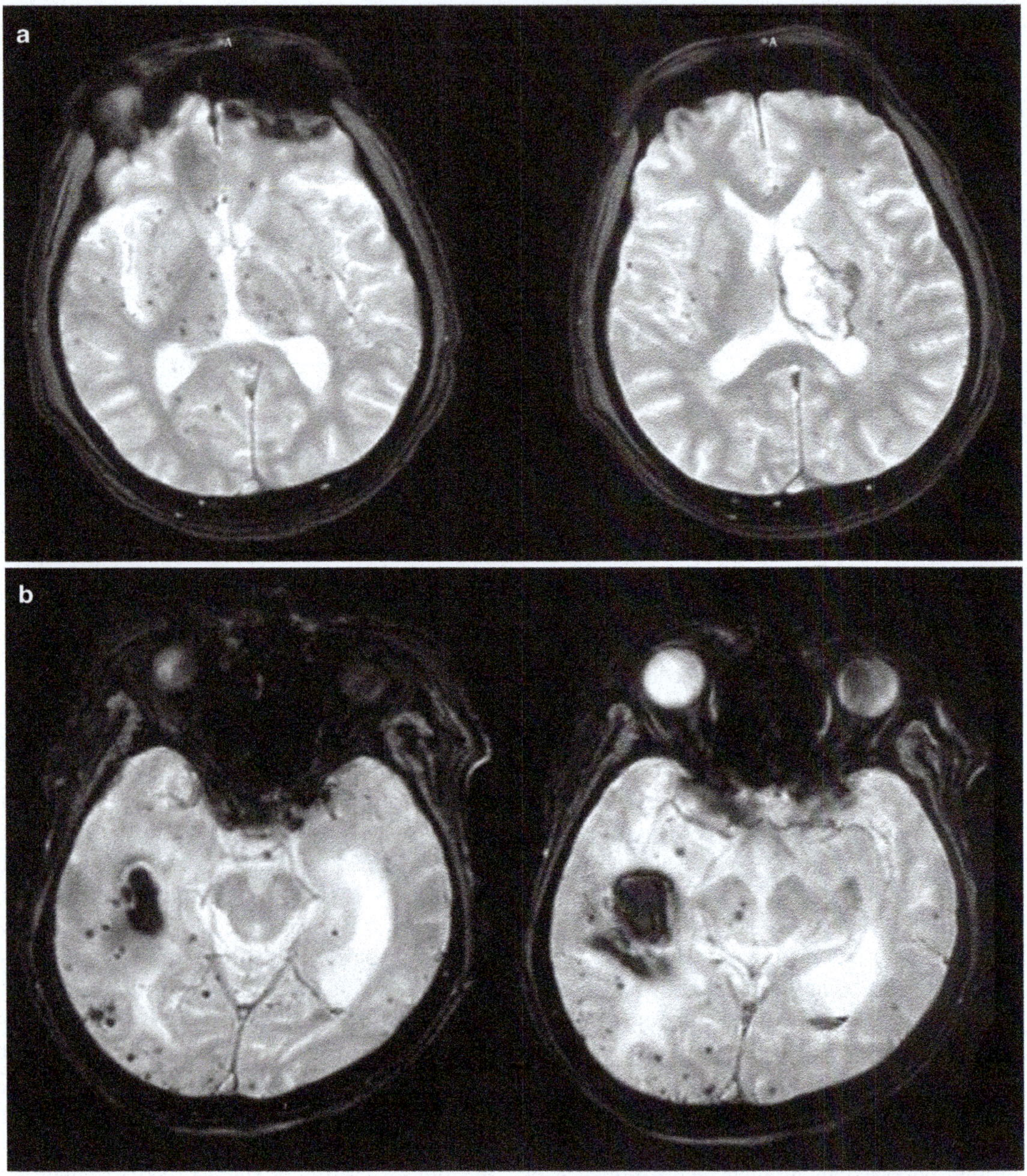

Fig. 15.3 Cerebral microbleeds (CMBs) visualized on gradient echo image (GRE). (**a**) Thalamic ICH occurred in a patient with multiple CMBs in deep gray matters. (**b**) Lobar ICH occurred in a patient with multiple lobar CMBs

considerable impact on the prognosis. Here, we describe how systemic factors, such as age, comorbidity, complications of ICH, and the systemic response to ICH, affect prognosis of ICH.

15.1.3.1 Age

Old age is one of the most important prognostic factors in almost all diseases. This is because the likelihood of comorbidities increases and the impact of risk factors on ICH is greater. However, age per se is one of the most independent and poor prognostic factors for ICH. In one study, mortality was increased by about 2.85 times when age is ≥65 compared to age <65 [21]. This is due to the fact that older patients have age-related changes in the cardiovascular system and the brain, and physiological changes occur in other systemic organs as well. In the brain, vascular density decreases, microembolic brain injury occurs, and vessel basement membranes thicken, while endothelial dysfunction and BBB permeability increase [22]. All of these age-related changes make the brain more susceptible to injury. In systemic organs, physiologic reserve decreases with age. Specifically, response to sympathetic stimulation is reduced, pulmonary function decreases, and medications might have different pharmacological effects. In addition, sarcopenia, the loss of skeletal muscle mass and function, occurs with age. When sarcopenia occurs, muscle mass is reduced and fat mass is increased, resulting in a marked weakness of muscle power. Thus, such organ system dysfunctions make patients more vulnerable to complications, such as sepsis and cognitive decline, and also increase hospital stays.

15.1.3.2 Level of Consciousness

The level of consciousness in ICH patients decreases when the ascending reticular activating system is involved, which can occur in the following situations: (1) in a supratentorial hemorrhage where the reticular activating system is widely spread, when the lesion is so large that it affects the function of the contralateral hemisphere, (2) when ICH occurs in the thalamus or brain stem where the reticular formation is compact, (3) when the brain stem is compressed by a mass effect resulting from the ICH, and (4) when metabolic insults, such as sepsis, affect the whole brain function. The level of consciousness is related to the "attack factors," but it has greater impact on the patient's prognosis in its own right. A decreased level of consciousness is a major obstacle to treatment because (1) the patient could more easily be exposed to infections, such as aspiration pneumonia and pressure sores, and (2) it becomes difficult to detect further neurological deterioration. For these reasons, the level of consciousness on admission is an important prognostic factor in patients with ICH.

15.1.3.3 Blood Glucose

In patients with diabetes, acute diseases generally become more severe than in patients without diabetes, because diabetes induces a systemic pro-inflammatory state [23]. In addition, diabetic patients frequently have combined diseases in other organs or systems, such as the kidneys and the autonomic nervous system, which may lead to an attenuation of appropriate protective responses to ICH. Systemic hyperglycemia is more commonly induced in stress conditions, such as ICH, in diabetic patients, which promotes lactic acidosis and free radical production, and could lead to a pro-inflammatory response in the brain. Therefore, it is important to adjust the blood glucose level appropriately in diabetic patients with ICH, and intensive glucose lowering should be performed from the beginning. However, in nondiabetic patients with ICH, hyperglycemia is usually caused by a stress response, so controversy exists regarding whether it should be controlled in these patients. In a multicenter observation study conducted in Korea, hyperglycemia has been reported to be associated with early and long-term mortality in nondiabetic patients [24], but this result has not achieved a broad consensus. Regardless of the presence of diabetes, careful blood glucose monitoring is required in patients with ICH.

15.1.3.4 Fever and Infection

Acute ICH is frequently accompanied by fever. This is because (1) patients become vulnerable to infection after ICH and (2) noninfectious fevers may occur due to systemic inflammatory response syndrome or to the involvement of thermoregulatory centers in the hypothalamus or brain stem (central hyperthermia) [25]. Fever often accompanies IVH. A clinical observation study reported that 91% of ICH patients experienced a fever ≥37.5 °C, and 42% experienced a fever ≥38.5 °C, during 72 h of body temperature monitoring, in 196 acute ICH patients. Fever persisted for more than 24 h in 57% of patients [26]. When the fever persisted for 24–48 h, the likelihood of a poor outcome (Glasgow Outcome Scale of 1 or 2, equivalent to death or a vegetative state) increased about 8-fold and increased about 13-fold for patients experiencing a fever for 48 h or more [26]. Fever is associated with increased intracranial pressure, decreased cerebral blood flow, and increased inflammatory cytokines and axonal death, which may have a deleterious effect on prognosis [27]. However, simply controlling the fever, without treatment of infection, did not improve the prognosis of ICH [28]. Since patients become vulnerable to indolent infections after ICH, it is helpful to find the source of infections and to treat them with appropriate antibiotics.

15.1.3.5 Antithrombotics

Thrombosis is required in order to inhibit expansion of the hematoma during the initial stages of ICH. Accordingly, the use of antithrombotics prior to the onset of ICH, including antiplatelets and anticoagulants, inhibits thrombosis in the hematoma and, in turn, leads to a larger hematoma, producing poorer outcomes. A population-based study indicated that ICH mortality increased about 2.5-fold in patients with regular aspirin use prior to ICH, compared to those not using aspirin regularly [29]. In a prospective multicenter study, 141 patients with warfarin-related ICH were treated with prothrombin complex concentrate (PCC), and in-hospital mortality remained high at 42.3%, although a prolonged prothrombin time was corrected in a majority of the patients [30]. Taken together, these data suggest that prior use of antithrombotics is a strong, poor prognostic factor in ICH.

15.2 SAH

It is well understood that aneurysmal SAH is the most devastating form of stroke. Nevertheless, 6–17% of SAH patients achieve functional independence and return to their previous occupations [31]. Thus, the prediction of outcome in SAH patients is also essential for individualized care. Basically, since the condition of patients with SAH is likely to be grave from the outset, the amount of hemorrhage and the neurological severity at the initial stage are the most powerful factors for determining outcomes. This information can be easily investigated with neurologic examinations and a CT scan at the time of presentation. Other systemic factors, including age, comorbidity, and fever, may also affect prognosis in SAH patients. More importantly, a variety of complications following SAH (e.g., rebleeding, edema, hydrocephalus, SAH-induced cardiac dysfunction, and systemic hyperthermia) may seriously influence the prognosis, depending on the severity. For example, delayed territorial infarction induced by vasospasm may be more devastating in some cases. Therefore, it is of paramount importance to identify and closely monitor patients at high risk for poor outcomes.

15.2.1 Clinical and Radiological Grading Systems

15.2.1.1 Hunt and Hess Scale, Fisher Scale, WFNS Scale, and Other Prediction Models

In case of SAH, the clinical and radiological grading at presentation is strongly correlated to the overall prognosis. The three most commonly used grading systems in SAH are the Fisher scale (or the modified Fisher scale), the Hunt and Hess scale, and the World Federation of Neurological Surgeons (WFNS) scale (Table 15.1) [32–34]. The Fisher (or modified Fisher) scale is graded by radiological findings, and WFNS is graded by the Glasgow Coma Scale and by focal neurological deficits. The Hunt and Hess scale is graded by the level of consciousness and by the neurological deficit. These grading systems are used not only to standardize patient assessments among medical centers and to guide treatment decisions but also to predict prognosis. Despite their common use in clinical practice, these grading systems have intrinsic limitations of high inter- and intra-rater variability [35]. Because of these limitations, many efforts have been made to develop new prediction models, although none have been found to be sufficiently accurate [36]. Recently, the SAHIT (Subarachnoid Hemorrhage International Trialists) multinational cohort study group has developed and validated an outcome prediction model of aneurysmal SAH by pooling data from more than 10,000 records [37]. This prediction model is categorized into a core, neuro, and full model. The core model includes age, premorbid hypertension, and WFNS grade, while the neuro model includes aneurysmal size, location, and the Fisher scale, in addition to the core model components. The full model includes

Table 15.1 The Fisher scale, Hunt and Hess scale, and World Federation of Neurological Surgeons (WFNS) scale [32–34]

	Fisher scale	Hunt and Hess scale	WFNS scale
1	No blood visualized	Asymptomatic or minimal headache and slight nuchal rigidity	GCS 15, no motor deficit
2	A diffuse deposition or thin layer with all vertical layers (interhemispheric fissure, insular cistern, ambient cistern) <1 mm thick	Moderate-to-severe headache, nuchal rigidity, no neurological deficit other than cranial nerve palsy	GCS 13–14, no motor deficit
3	Localized clots and/or vertical layers ≥1 mm thickness	Drowsy, confusion, or mild focal deficit	GCS 13–14, with motor deficit
4	Diffuse or no subarachnoid blood, but with intracerebral or intraventricular clots	Stupor, moderate-to-severe hemiparesis, possibly early decerebrate rigidity and vegetative disturbances	GCS 7–12, with or without motor deficit
5		Deep coma, decerebrate rigidity, moribund appearance	GCS 3–6, with or without motor deficit

repair modality (surgical clipping, endovascular coiling, or conservative management), in addition to the neuro model. This model is the most comprehensive prediction model to date, although it requires further validation in additional independent research groups.

Since SAH is a rapidly deteriorating disease requiring quick decision-making, it is evident that these three grading systems are useful and practical. In most studies examining prediction models for SAH, the WFNS, the Fisher scale, and the Hunt and Hess scales appear to be better predictive factors than any other parameters. Taken together, these three grading systems are the most useful tools for prediction of aneurysmal SAH outcomes, despite some intrinsic limitations, which suggests how toxic the blood component of the hemorrhage is, within the subarachnoid space.

15.2.1.2 Aneurysmal Size and Location

Aneurysmal size is a well-known poor prognostic factor. The size of the aneurysm is not inherently important, but the amount of bleeding may be greater when a larger aneurysm is ruptured. It was reported that a poor outcome after 12 months was five times more likely to occur when the aneurysmal size is ≥13 mm [38]. In another study, aneurysmal size was graded into three groups (≤12 mm, 13–24 mm, and ≥25 mm), and poor outcome was observed in the ≥25 mm group [39].

In terms of the aneurysmal location, aneurysms on the internal carotid artery showed the best clinical outcome, followed by aneurysms on the anterior cerebral artery, middle cerebral artery, and the posterior circulation system [39]. Poorer outcomes associated with aneurysms of the posterior circulation system are due to the fact that such ruptures may extensively affect the brain stem and the circle of Willis, while aneurysms in other locations may affect more limited regional brain areas.

15.2.1.3 Age and Premorbid Hypertension

Among the clinical variables other than those related to the SAH severity, age must be considered first for prediction models [36, 37]. With age, the brain, as well as the cardiovascular system and other systemic organs, naturally undergo degenerative changes. Consequently, brain structure and functions are more vulnerable to SAH-induced injury in older patients, and systemic organs are also susceptible to complications, such as infection and metabolic dysfunctions.

In addition, premorbid hypertension should be regarded as significant prognostic factors for SAH outcome. In patients with long-standing hypertension, the brain may have cumulative arteriolosclerotic changes, which are more vulnerable to brain damage after SAH.

15.2.2 Prediction of Complications After SAH

As mentioned above, the overall outcome of SAH is largely determined by the initial severity of the SAH event. However, for physicians or intensivists who care for SAH patients, it may be more important to predict complications following SAH. SAH patients are at risk of experiencing further clinical deterioration due to various complications, such as delayed cerebral ischemia, rebleeding, and hydrocephalus during hospitalization. If a prediction of the complications is possible, physicians could apply various preventive strategies, as well as more appropriate immediate treatments (see also Chap. 10).

15.2.2.1 Vasospasm and Delayed Cerebral Ischemia

Vasospasm is one of the most disastrous complications following SAH, resulting in a delayed infarction. There has been a great deal of interest regarding the predictive factors of vasospasm after SAH. It was reported that the incidence of vasospasm may be associated with a large SAH amount and also the presence of combined IVH. However, the Fisher scale as a conventional radiological grading was not able to predict vasospasm, which may be because it does not grade the presence of IVH in detail. Thus, it was suggested that the modified Fisher scale would better predict vasospasm and delayed cerebral ischemia [40]. With respect to the prediction of vasospasm, the modified Fisher scale may be more useful than the original Fisher scale. Other SAH scales, such as the WFNS and the Hunt and Hess scale, as well as clinical variables such as cigarette smoking, preexisting hypertension, diabetes mellitus, and cocaine use, have also been reported to have predictive values for vasospasm to some extent [41–45].

15.2.2.2 Rebleeding

Rebleeding occurs in 8–23% of ruptured aneurysmal SAH within 72 h [46]. According to a meta-analysis, high systolic blood pressure, poor Hunt and Hess scale scores (3–4), intracerebral or intraventricular hematomas, posterior circulation aneurysms, and aneurysms >10 mm in size were risk factors for rebleeding [47]. In a single-center trial, the modified Fisher scale (3–4) and the external drain of cerebrospinal fluid were associated with the incidence of rebleeding [48]. When rebleeding occurs in the initial survivor of SAH, the mortality rate increases to 20–60% [46]. Given that approximately 50–90% of rebleeding occurs in the first 6 h, ultra-early obliteration of the aneurysm should be conducted in high-risk patients [46].

15.2.2.3 Hydrocephalus

Hydrocephalus occurs following SAH in about 20–30% of patients [49]. About 20% of hydrocephalus occurs during the acute phase (first 3 days), while the remainder occurs during the subacute (4–14 days) or chronic phases (after 14 days) [49]. With hydrocephalus, cognitive dysfunction or other focal neurological deficits are further developed, and proper intervention, such as external ventricular drainage, lumbar drainage, or ventriculoperitoneal shunt, must be immediately considered.

Hydrocephalus is caused by a sudden mechanical obstruction of the circulation of the cerebrospinal fluid by blood clots either at the ventricles or around arachnoid granulations. Accordingly, hydrocephalus is likely to develop with large amounts of blood after SAH. In a meta-analysis study on shunt dependency after SAH-induced hydrocephalus, high Fisher grade, acute hydrocephalus, in-hospital complications, presence of intraventricular blood, high Hunt and Hess scale, rebleeding, posterior circulation location of the aneurysm, and age ≥60 years were shown to be risk factors [50].

Conclusions

In this chapter, factors determining the prognosis of ICH and SAH were thoroughly discussed. In ICH, the prognostic factors were divided into three categories: attack factors, protective factors, and systemic and neurological state. Except for some extreme cases, the outcome of ICH is not determined by a single category of prognostic factors but by a combination of all three categories, which are closely inter-related. In SAH, a devastating neurological emergency, the overall outcome depends on the SAH grade and neurological severity at symptom onset. However, even when a poor outcome is predicted on admission, it is fundamental for physicians to recognize the risks of complications and monitor their patients closely. Physicians should focus on converting a high-risk patient into a better outcome through timely intervention. Through this chapter, we hope the reader will logically categorize the predictive factors of hemorrhagic stroke at the bedside, predict the outcomes of patients, and use this information for appropriate decision-making.

References

1. Mayer SA, Sacco RL, Shi T, et al. Neurologic deterioration in noncomatose patients with supratentorial intracerebral hemorrhage. Neurology. 1994;44:1379–84.
2. Weimar C, Weber C, Wagner M, et al. Management patterns and health care use after intracerebral hemorrhage. A cost-of-illness study from a societal perspective in Germany. Cerebrovasc Dis. 2003;15:29–36.
3. Rost NS, Smith EE, Chang Y, et al. Prediction of functional outcome in patients with primary intracerebral hemorrhage: the FUNC score. Stroke. 2008;39:2304–9.
4. Zia E, Engstrom G, Svensson PJ, et al. Three-year survival and stroke recurrence rates in patients with primary intracerebral hemorrhage. Stroke. 2009;40:3567–73.
5. Davis SM, Broderick J, Hennerici M, et al. Hematoma growth is a determinant of mortality and poor outcome after intracerebral hemorrhage. Neurology. 2006;66:1175–81.
6. Schlunk F, Greenberg SM. The pathophysiology of intracerebral hemorrhage formation and expansion. Transl Stroke Res. 2015;6:257–63.
7. Demchuk AM, Dowlatshahi D, Rodriguez-Luna D, et al. Prediction of haematoma growth and outcome in patients with intracerebral haemorrhage using the CT-angiography spot sign (PREDICT): a prospective observational study. Lancet Neurol. 2012;11:307–14.
8. Hemphill JC 3rd, Greenberg SM, Anderson CS, et al. Guidelines for the management of spontaneous intracerebral hemorrhage: a guideline for healthcare professionals from the American Heart Association/American Stroke Association. Stroke. 2015;46:2032–60.
9. Boulouis G, Morotti A, Brouwers HB, et al. Association between hypodensities detected by computed tomography and hematoma expansion in patients with intracerebral hemorrhage. JAMA Neurol. 2016;73:961–8.
10. Li Q, Zhang G, Xiong X, et al. Black hole sign: novel imaging marker that predicts hematoma growth in patients with intracerebral hemorrhage. Stroke. 2016;47:1777–81.
11. Mayer SA, Brun NC, Begtrup K, et al. Efficacy and safety of recombinant activated factor VII for acute intracerebral hemorrhage. N Engl J Med. 2008;358:2127–37.
12. Murthy SB, Moradiya Y, Dawson J, et al. Perihematomal edema and functional outcomes in intracerebral hemorrhage: influence of hematoma volume and location. Stroke. 2015;46:3088–92.
13. Balami JS, Buchan AM. Complications of intracerebral haemorrhage. Lancet Neurol. 2012;11:101–18.
14. Lee SH, Kim BJ, Ryu WS, et al. White matter lesions and poor outcome after intracerebral hemorrhage: a nationwide cohort study. Neurology. 2010;74:1502–10.
15. Lee SH, Bae HJ, Kwon SJ, et al. Cerebral microbleeds are regionally associated with intracerebral hemorrhage. Neurology. 2004;62:72–6.
16. Soo YO, Yang SR, Lam WW, et al. Risk vs benefit of anti-thrombotic therapy in ischaemic stroke patients with cerebral microbleeds. J Neurol. 2008;255:1679–86.
17. Greenberg SM, Eng JA, Ning M, et al. Hemorrhage burden predicts recurrent intracerebral hemorrhage after lobar hemorrhage. Stroke. 2004;35:1415–20.
18. Wong KS, Chan YL, Liu JY, et al. Asymptomatic microbleeds as a risk factor for aspirin-associated intracerebral hemorrhages. Neurology. 2003;60:511–3.
19. Lee SH, Ryu WS, Roh JK. Cerebral microbleeds are a risk factor for warfarin-related intracerebral hemorrhage. Neurology. 2009;72:171–6.
20. Lee SH, Kim BJ, Roh JK. Silent microbleeds are associated with volume of primary intracerebral hemorrhage. Neurology. 2006;66:430–2.
21. Celikbilek A, Goksel BK, Zararsiz G, et al. Spontaneous intra-cerebral hemorrhage: a retrospective study of risk factors and outcome in a Turkish population. J Neurosci Rural Pract. 2013;4:271–7.
22. Camacho E, Lopresti MA, Bruce S, et al. The role of age in intracerebral hemorrhages. J Clin Neurosci. 2015;22:1867–70.
23. Devaraj S, Dasu MR, Jialal I. Diabetes is a proinflammatory state: a translational perspective. Expert Rev Endocrinol Metab. 2010;5:19–28.
24. Lee SH, Kim BJ, Bae HJ, et al. Effects of glucose level on early and long-term mortality after intracerebral haemorrhage: the acute brain bleeding analysis study. Diabetologia. 2010;53:429–34.
25. Deogaonkar A, De Georgia M, Bae C, et al. Fever is associated with third ventricular shift after intracerebral hemorrhage: pathophysiologic implications. Neurol India. 2005;53:202–6.
26. Schwarz S, Hafner K, Aschoff A, et al. Incidence and prognostic significance of fever following intracerebral hemorrhage. Neurology. 2000;54:354–61.
27. Rossi S, Zanier ER, Mauri I, et al. Brain temperature, body core temperature, and intracranial pres-

sure in acute cerebral damage. J Neurol Neurosurg Psychiatry. 2001;71:448–54.
28. Broessner G, Beer R, Lackner P, et al. Prophylactic, endovascularly based, long-term normothermia in ICU patients with severe cerebrovascular disease: bicenter prospective, randomized trial. Stroke. 2009;40:e657–65.
29. Saloheimo P, Ahonen M, Juvela S, et al. Regular aspirin-use preceding the onset of primary intracerebral hemorrhage is an independent predictor for death. Stroke. 2006;37:129–33.
30. Dowlatshahi D, Butcher KS, Asdaghi N, et al. Poor prognosis in warfarin-associated intracranial hemorrhage despite anticoagulation reversal. Stroke. 2012;43:1812–7.
31. Al-Khindi T, Macdonald RL, Schweizer TA. Cognitive and functional outcome after aneurysmal subarachnoid hemorrhage. Stroke. 2010;41:e519–36.
32. Frontera JA, Claassen J, Schmidt JM, et al. Prediction of symptomatic vasospasm after subarachnoid hemorrhage: the modified fisher scale. Neurosurgery. 2006;59:21–7.
33. Hunt WE, Hess RM. Surgical risk as related to time of intervention in the repair of intracranial aneurysms. J Neurosurg. 1968;28:14–20.
34. Teasdale GM, Drake CG, Hunt W, et al. A universal subarachnoid hemorrhage scale: report of a committee of the World Federation of Neurosurgical Societies. J Neurol Neurosurg Psychiatry. 1988;51:1457.
35. Degen LA, Dorhout Mees SM, Algra A, et al. Interobserver variability of grading scales for aneurysmal subarachnoid hemorrhage. Stroke. 2011;42:1546–9.
36. Jaja BN, Cusimano MD, Etminan N, et al. Clinical prediction models for aneurysmal subarachnoid hemorrhage: a systematic review. Neurocrit Care. 2013;18:143–53.
37. Jaja BNR, Saposnik G, Lingsma HF, et al. Development and validation of outcome prediction models for aneurysmal subarachnoid haemorrhage: the SAHIT multinational cohort study. BMJ. 2018;360:j5745.
38. Mocco J, Ransom ER, Komotar RJ, et al. Preoperative prediction of long-term outcome in poor-grade aneurysmal subarachnoid hemorrhage. Neurosurgery. 2006;59:529–38.
39. Rosen DS, Macdonald RL. Grading of subarachnoid hemorrhage: modification of the World Federation of Neurosurgical Societies scale on the basis of data for a large series of patients. Neurosurgery. 2004;54:566–75.
40. Claassen J, Bernardini GL, Kreiter K, et al. Effect of cisternal and ventricular blood on risk of delayed cerebral ischemia after subarachnoid hemorrhage: the Fisher scale revisited. Stroke. 2001;32:2012–20.
41. Howington JU, Kutz SC, Wilding GE, et al. Cocaine use as a predictor of outcome in aneurysmal subarachnoid hemorrhage. J Neurosurg. 2003;99:271–5.
42. Lasner TM, Weil RJ, Riina HA, et al. Cigarette smoking-induced increase in the risk of symptomatic vasospasm after aneurysmal subarachnoid hemorrhage. J Neurosurg. 1997;87:381–4.
43. Ohman J, Servo A, Heiskanen O. Risks factors for cerebral infarction in good-grade patients after aneurysmal subarachnoid hemorrhage and surgery: a prospective study. J Neurosurg. 1991;74:14–20.
44. Harrod CG, Bendok BR, Batjer HH. Prediction of cerebral vasospasm in patients presenting with aneurysmal subarachnoid hemorrhage: a review. Neurosurgery. 2005;56:633–54.
45. De Rooij NK, Rinkel GJ, Dankbaar JW, et al. Delayed cerebral ischemia after subarachnoid hemorrhage: a systematic review of clinical, laboratory, and radiological predictors. Stroke. 2013;44:43–54.
46. Larsen CC, Astrup J. Rebleeding after aneurysmal subarachnoid hemorrhage: a literature review. World Neurosurg. 2013;79:307–12.
47. Tang C, Zhang TS, Zhou LF. Risk factors for rebleeding of aneurysmal subarachnoid hemorrhage: a meta-analysis. PLoS One. 2014;9:e99536.
48. Van Donkelaar CE, Bakker NA, Veeger NJ, et al. Predictive factors for rebleeding after aneurysmal subarachnoid hemorrhage: rebleeding aneurysmal subarachnoid hemorrhage study. Stroke. 2015;46:2100–6.
49. Chen S, Luo J, Reis C, et al. Hydrocephalus after subarachnoid hemorrhage: pathophysiology, diagnosis, and treatment. Biomed Res Int. 2017;2017:8584753.
50. Wilson CD, Safavi-Abbasi S, Sun H, et al. Meta-analysis and systematic review of risk factors for shunt dependency after aneurysmal subarachnoid hemorrhage. J Neurosurg. 2017;126:586–95.

16 Rehabilitation After Hemorrhagic Stroke: From Acute to Chronic Stage

Yun-Hee Kim

16.1 The Aim and Principles of Rehabilitation After Hemorrhagic Stroke

The aim of stroke rehabilitation is to reduce disability resulting from ischemic or hemorrhagic stroke. As a result of increasing evidence for its efficacy, it is now recommended that all patients with hemorrhagic stroke should have access to multidisciplinary rehabilitation [1]. However, in the absence of well-studied clinical data guiding specific practice, the rehabilitation of hemorrhagic stroke is mainly based on general principles learned from rehabilitation of ischemic stroke patients [2] (Fig. 16.1).

Stroke is a complex syndrome, and the rehabilitation process therefore requires a carefully planned and integrated program. General principles have evolved over time to form the basis of stroke rehabilitation. Multidisciplinary team care is the basis for the delivery of stroke rehabilitation. The multidisciplinary team includes medical, nursing, physical, and occupational therapy, speech and language pathology, and social work staff who provide rehabilitation input and coordinate their work through regular meetings. Evidence suggests that a well-functioning multidisciplinary team approach is more effective than the previous pathway [3]. Setting goals that replicate the specific rehabilitation aims of an individual can also improve functional outcomes. For motor function recovery, task-specific training is a well-accepted principle. Training should target the tasks that are relevant for the needs of individual patients and involve repeated practice. It is believed that rehabilitation should begin as soon as possible after stroke stabilizes and that intensive training improves recovery.

16.1.1 Rehabilitation in Acute Stages

Numerous studies have provided evidence that dedicated stroke units provide improved outcomes compared with general medical units [3]. It is important that rehabilitation is not a separate phase of medical care but an integral part of medical management and continues longitudinally through acute care, post-acute care, and community care. Patients who are managed in organized stroke units in the acute phase of both ischemic and hemorrhagic stroke experience fewer immobility-

Y.-H. Kim (✉)
Department of Physical and Rehabilitation Medicine, Sungkyunkwan University School of Medicine, Seoul, South Korea

Center for Prevention and Rehabilitation, Heart Vascular Stroke Institute, Samsung Medical Center, Seoul, South Korea

Samsung Advanced Institute for Health Science and Technology, Sungkyunkwan University, Seoul, South Korea
e-mail: yun1225.kim@samsung.com; yunkim@skku.edu

S.-H. Lee (ed.), *Stroke Revisited: Hemorrhagic Stroke*, Stroke Revisited,
https://doi.org/10.1007/978-981-10-1427-7_16

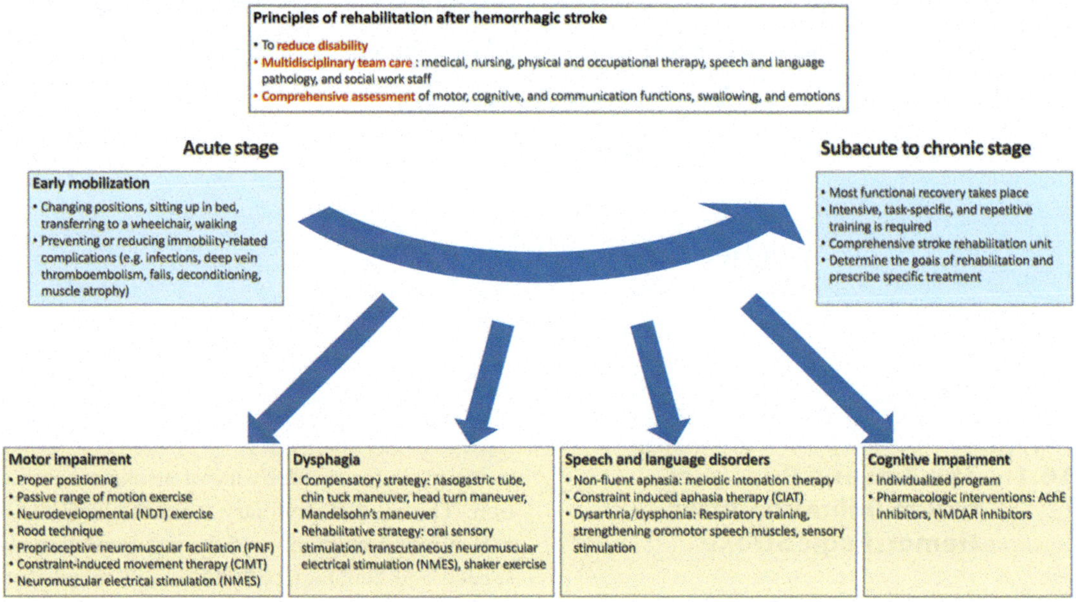

Fig. 16.1 A conceptual diagram of principles of rehabilitation after hemorrhagic stroke. *AchE* acetylcholinesterase, *NMDAR* *N*-methyl-D-aspartate receptor

related complications; this has been attributed to earlier and better management, including early mobilization and early rehabilitation.

Mobilization in stroke rehabilitation involves a set of physical activities that may be started passively but quickly progress to active participation by the patient. These activities include changing positions, sitting up in bed, transferring to a wheelchair, and walking. Early mobilization may be beneficial by preventing or reducing immobility-related complications, such as infections, deep vein thromboembolism, and falls. Secondary changes associated with stroke-related inactivity include deconditioning and muscle atrophy. Bedside or active exercises, early gait training, training in the performance of activities in daily living (ADLs), and swallowing training can be initiated during the acute poststroke phase.

Preclinical research has demonstrated a critical period of enhanced neuroplasticity early after stroke. Studies of ischemic stroke have shown that animals exposed to locomotor exercise beginning 24–48 h after stroke have better behavioral outcomes and smaller ischemic volumes than control animals who receive delayed or no exercise training [4]. There is strong evidence that early rehabilitation increases dendritic sprouting and levels of brain-derived neurotrophic factor (BDNF) protein, decreases expression of inflammatory cytokines, tightens the blood-brain barrier, suppresses apoptosis, and promotes neurogenesis [5]. Rehabilitation efficacy declines over time, suggesting that earlier initiation of training may enhance recovery.

The above results provide a biological basis for early training in humans, but recent results from the phase III AVERT (A Very Early Rehabilitation Trial for Stroke) trial raised controversy about the role of very early mobilization [6]. AVERT is a large-scale, multicenter, randomized controlled trial (RCT) that aims to assess the effectiveness of frequent high-intensity very early mobilization after stroke. Results of the AVERT study suggested that a higher intensity and very early mobilization protocol was associated with reduced odds of a favorable outcome at 3 months. However, the limitation of high-intensity, frequent out-of-bed mobilization does not indicate that early rehabilitation is harmful in stroke patients. In fact, even in the "usual care" group, which was the control group in the AVERT study, the median time of first mobilization was

22 h. It should also be noted that the AVERT trail included both ischemic and hemorrhagic stroke. Recently, a study from China reported the effect of early rehabilitation in patients with intracerebral hemorrhage (ICH) [7]. This article showed that commencing rehabilitation within 48 h of intracerebral hemorrhage improves survival and functional outcomes 6 months after stroke in hospitalized patients.

In aneurysmal subarachnoid hemorrhage (SAH), early mobilization is both feasible and safe [8]. In SAH patients with clip ligation or endovascular coiling, early mobilization reported to produce a favorable outcome as measured by the Hunt and Hess scale [9]. Some clinicians believe that total bed rest for 4–6 weeks is a basic intervention to avoid rebleeding in SAH patients who are not candidates for surgical treatment or who prefer conservative management. However, according to a recent Cochrane review that examined delayed mobilization in terms of rebleeding in these patients, there is no evidence to support or against staying in bed for at least 4 weeks after symptom onset in patients with aneurysmal SAH who were not eligible for surgical treatment of aneurysm [10]. To establish the optimal timing of rehabilitation in this group, further study is needed. Dose-response analysis of the efficacy of rehabilitation after hemorrhagic stroke also needs to be investigated.

16.1.2 Rehabilitation in Subacute to Chronic Stages

The subacute phase of stroke is the period when most functional recovery takes place; therefore, intensive, task-specific, and repetitive training is required at this time. Although the care of stroke survivors is organized in a variety of different systems around the world, it is recommended that stroke patients be admitted or transferred to a dedicated stroke rehabilitation unit where comprehensive rehabilitation intervention can be provided. Comprehensive rehabilitation in an organized multidisciplinary stroke unit improves patient survival and their ability to return home and regain independence in daily activities compared with treatment in general wards [3]. Comprehensive stroke rehabilitation occurs in specific systems of care based on the patient's symptoms and severity. Thus, before starting comprehensive and intensive rehabilitation, a detailed assessment should be performed for various aspects of function. Most stroke survivors experience impairment in motor, language, and cognitive function and a decline in ADLs; however, these symptoms manifest in various patterns and severity. Therefore, the physician should determine the goals of rehabilitation and prescribe specific treatment that helps each patient achieve them based on scientific evidence and experience. Prediction of functional recovery and long-term outcome after stroke is important in determining the appropriate treatment and timing of rehabilitation. Demographic and clinical factors including lower initial Barthel index, older age, severe paresis or paralysis, swallowing problems, ideomotor apraxia, ideational apraxia, visuospatial construction problems, and stroke-related complications such as extraparenchymal bleeding and cerebral edema are negative prognostic factors for ambulation and ADLs after stroke [11]. More recently, neurophysiological markers and neuroimaging biomarkers that predict functional recovery and long-term outcomes after stroke have been suggested. Accumulated evidence supports motor evoked potential (MEP) status as a useful biomarker for predicting upper limb motor recovery and outcomes. Neuroimaging biomarkers of corticomotor tract integrity, such as fractional anisotropy of corticospinal tract in diffuse tensor imaging, can also predict motor outcomes [12]. However, there is currently no consensus regarding the optimal neuroimaging measures.

16.2 Rehabilitation of Specific Symptoms After Stroke

16.2.1 Motor Impairment

Motor impairment is one of the most common consequences following stroke, affecting as many as 77.4% of patients with acute stroke [13]. Motor impairment after stroke affects the patient's mobility and limits ADLs, participation in society, and their chance of returning to professional activities. Strength, motor control and coordination, muscle tone, joint laxity, and balance may all be affected by stroke. Motor recovery begins within hours to days after stroke. Most of the spontaneous recovery occurs during the first 3–6 months after stroke; however, there is evidence that recovery may continue for many years [14].

In the acute phase of stroke, the hemiparetic limbs may be completely paralyzed, which might increase the risk for the development of contractures. Rehabilitation in this phase should consist of proper positioning of the patient in bed and support of the arm in a bed or wheelchair when sitting. All affected joints should go through gentle passive range of motion exercise at least once daily to prevent contractures, especially of the shoulder, wrist, fingers, hip, and ankles. The use of static resting splints for hand and ankle can help prevent contractures and maintain functional position in these joints.

A variety of approaches have been advocated to facilitate and enhance motor recovery. Traditional rehabilitation approaches include neurodevelopmental (NDT) exercises, the Rood technique, and proprioceptive neuromuscular facilitation (PNF). Neurodevelopmental (NDT) exercise inhibits abnormal postures and movement and aims to facilitate isolated muscle control. Rood proposed a technique that incorporates cutaneous stimuli to facilitate movement. Proprioceptive neuromuscular facilitation (PNF) relies on quick stretching and manual resistance of muscle activation of the limbs in functional directions. Although accumulating evidence over many years has validated conventional rehabilitation, nearly half of patients with stroke exhibit long-term motor impairment and dependence for ADL living.

Constraint-induced movement therapy (CIMT) was developed to overcome upper limb impairments after stroke. CIMT involves performing supervised structured tasks with the affected limb for 6 h a day for 10 days over a 14-day period, in addition to wearing a restrictive mitt or sling for 90% of waking hours. CIMT has been shown to be an effective means of stroke rehabilitation regardless of the level of initial motor ability, amount of chronicity, or infarct location. However, CIMT is only applicable to patients who are able to perform voluntary wrist and finger extension in the involved hand for the duration of the treatment.

Neuromuscular electrical stimulation (NMES) over a muscle induces muscle contractions. NMES can be delivered via electrodes placed near the peripheral nerve or near the muscle motor point and can be used to elicit simple muscle contractions without user effort and without being triggered by the user. In addition, NMES can be proportionally linked to user effort via electromyography (EMG) activity; when the stroke patient attempts the task and the EMG signal of the voluntary contraction exceeds a preset threshold, electrical stimulation is delivered to the target muscle to develop movement through to full range. NMES can be considered for both upper extremity and lower extremity. In the upper extremity, NMES and mental practice combined with repetitive and intense motor practice of functional tasks should be considered. In the lower extremity, NMES can be recommended as an adjunctive treatment for patients with impaired muscle contraction, specifically for patients with impaired gait due to ankle/knee motor impairment [15]. NMES can be utilized for individuals with acute or chronic deficits after stroke.

16.2.2 Cognitive Impairment

After stroke most patients experience some disturbance in cognitive function, and many have enduring difficulties in specific cognitive domains, such as attention, memory, spatial awareness, and executive function. Cognitive impairment has a significant impact on ADL and is one of the most difficult impairments to manage. Cognitive impairment is associated with size and location of the lesion and the presence of premorbid factors such as age, education, prior stroke, and dementia.

A bedside mental status assessment should be performed in all stroke patients. The mini-mental state examination (MMSE) is the most widely used tool to screen cognitive function in stroke patients; however, it does not provide full cognitive assessment. Thus, patients with detected cognitive impairment during the screening process should be further examined with formal neuropsychological tests.

Cognitive rehabilitation is a specialized treatment procedure that aims to help cognitively impaired patients recover normal functioning or compensate for cognitive deficits. Cognitive rehabilitation provides an individualized program of skills training according to each patient's specific needs. Clinical and laboratory evidence supports the effect of cognitive rehabilitation in attention deficit, memory deficit, spatial neglect, and perceptual disorders [3]. Pharmacologic interventions may also be recommended in patients with cognitive impairment. Acetylcholinesterase inhibitors, specifically galantamine, donepezil, and rivastigmine, should be considered in patients with vascular dementia or vascular cognitive impairment in the doses and frequency used for Alzheimer's disease. NMDA receptor inhibitors, such as memantine, have also attracted attention for use in patients with vascular dementia or vascular cognitive impairment.

16.2.3 Speech and Language Disorders

Approximately half of stroke survivors experience disorders in speech and language. Impairment of language is called aphasia and occurs when the dominant hemisphere is affected. Speech is a term that refers to the motor mechanism involved in the production of spoken words. The most common speech disorders in stroke are dysphonia and dysarthria.

Aphasia and speech disorders cause communication difficulties between patients and rehabilitation staff or caregivers in the early stage of stroke, resulting in difficulty in comprehensive assessment of the patient. Aphasias can be classified based on fluency, comprehension, and repetition. All patients are assumed to have impaired naming and some paraphasic errors. First, aphasias are divided into two main categories: fluent aphasias (able to produce connect speech, and sentence structure is relatively intact but lacks meaning) and nonfluent aphasias (speech production is halting and effortful, and grammar is impaired, but content words may be preserved). Impaired fluency, impaired comprehension, and impaired repetition are referred to as global aphasia. A patient with normal fluency and comprehension but impaired repetition has conduction aphasia. Broca's aphasia is characterized by impaired fluency and repetition, while comprehension is relatively spared. In contrast, Wernicke's aphasia is fluent, but repetition and comprehension are both impaired. Individuals with impaired fluency and normal comprehension, as in Broca's aphasia, but with spared repetition have transcortical motor aphasia. Individuals with normal fluency but impaired comprehension, as in Wernicke's aphasia, but with intact repetition have transcortical sensory aphasia. In patients with mixed transcortical aphasia, fluency and comprehension are both impaired, as in global aphasia, but repetition is intact. Finally, patients with normal fluency, normal comprehension, and normal repetition but some naming difficulties have anomic aphasia.

Although aphasia and speech disorders recover spontaneously as time elapses after stroke onset, in a substantial number of patients, persistent residual disability leads to difficulties returning to daily life and society. Therefore, patients with stroke in the dominant hemisphere or suspected communication problems after stroke should consider standardized language evaluation performed by a speech-language therapist. A number of strategies and techniques have been developed for the treatment of aphasia. Melodic intonation therapy is a language production therapy for severely nonfluent aphasic patients that use non-injured functioning neural pathways in the non-dominant hemisphere to restore language. Constraint-induced aphasia therapy (CIAT) is a relatively new technique to improve aphasia in stroke patients. CIAT consists of three components: (1) patients are strongly encouraged to use verbal communication approaches rather than nonverbal methods like gestures; (2) there is a massed practice of targeted language skills; (3) and the difficulty of required tasks is gradually increased according to patients' functional performance [16]. For dysarthria and dysphonia, respiratory training, strengthening oromotor speech muscles, and sensory stimulation may be helpful. An individualized rehabilitation plan should be established according to the subtypes and severity of aphasia and speech disorders.

16.2.4 Evaluation and Treatment of Dysphagia

Dysphagia is found up to 78% of patients with stroke and is an important risk factor for aspiration pneumonia [17]. It generally has a favorable prognosis but may be more severe and persistent in patients with brainstem lesions or with bilateral hemispheric stroke [18]. There are many reasons for dysphagia in patients with stroke, such as reduced laryngeal elevation, insufficient upper esophageal sphincter (UES) opening, vocal fold weakness, and severe weakness in oropharyngeal muscles. Dysphagia after stroke is often underdiagnosed because silent aspiration occurs in up to two-thirds of patients with dysphagia after stroke. To maximize recovery and minimize negative consequences, early detection of dysphagia must be followed by proper management.

16.2.4.1 Bedside Swallowing Evaluation

Protection against aspiration (and resulting pneumonia) includes avoiding oral feeding in patients who are not alert. Even in alert patients, the ability to swallow should be assessed carefully before starting oral intake of fluids or food. This is achieved through a bedside screening assessment that can be efficiently completed by the physician or nursing staff. The process generally includes giving the patient a small drink of water and observing for signs for aspiration. A wet voice and spontaneous cough after swallowing are predictors of high aspiration risk. Several standardized screening tests for stroke have been developed, such as the Gugging Swallowing Screen test or the Toronto Bedside Swallowing Screening Test [19, 20]. If patients have signs of aspiration such as cough or fail on a screening test, a video fluoroscopic swallowing study (VFSS) or flexible endoscopic evaluation of swallowing (FEES) should be performed to confirm the diagnosis.

16.2.4.2 Treatment of Dysphagia

Approaches for management of dysphagia can be differentiated into compensatory and rehabilitative strategies. Compensatory strategies aim to keep patients safe when eating, whereas rehabilitative strategies aim to promote the recovery process. Compensatory strategies include pharyngeal bypass, dietary modifications, and postural techniques. In the acute phase, a nasogastric (NG) tube should be considered as a primary choice for compensation of dysphagia in stroke patients. Patients who are lying flat in bed are at significant risk for regurgitation and aspiration; therefore, the head of the bed should be kept elevated during tube feeding. Patients with swallowing difficulty should start feeding with modification of the consistency of food. In general, thinner fluids are more easily aspirated.

Swallowing maneuvers may decrease the risk of aspiration during swallowing. The chin tuck maneuver can reduce aspiration by bringing the epiglottis and the aryepiglottic fold closer together, thus closing the airway during swallowing. The head turn maneuver involves rotating the head to the paretic side. In unilateral pharyngeal weakness, turning the head to the paretic side can divert the bolus to the intact side. Mendelsohn maneuver is a voluntary prolongation of hyolaryngeal elevation at the peak of the swallow, leading to UES opening and airway closure.

In addition, rehabilitative strategies, such as oral sensory stimulation, transcutaneous neuromuscular electrical stimulation (NMES), or indirect techniques, may improve swallowing physiology. A number of dysphagic stroke patients have decreased oral sensory awareness. Thus, techniques such as thermal/tactile simulation of pharyngeal swallow can increase sensory awareness in the oral cavity pre-swallow and reduce the delay between the oral and pharyngeal swallow. NMES has become quite popular; however, there is not enough evidence supporting this practice. Clinical guidelines of the American Heart Association (AHA)/American Society of Anesthesiologists (ASA) state that NMES treatment in stroke dysphagia has uncertain benefit and is currently not recommended [21]. Shaker exercise is an isotonic-isometric neck flexion exercise performed in the supine position. This exercise improves sphincter opening and thereby reduces post-swallow pharyngeal residue [22].

16.3 Novel Therapies in Stroke Rehabilitation

An increasing number of researchers are pursuing the use of new technologies to improve the efficacy of rehabilitation. Over the last decade, numerous devices for robotic-assisted training have been developed to move the patient's limbs under the supervision or help of a therapist. The types of robotic devices used for motor training can be parsed into two broad categories of end-effector type and exoskeleton type, each with their own strengths and weaknesses. End-effector devices work by applying mechanical forces to the distal segments of limbs and offer the advantages of easy setup and a relatively large degree of freedom but also limit control of the proximal joints of the limb, which could result in abnormal movement patterns. In contrast, exoskeleton-type robotic devices have the robot axes aligned with the anatomical axes of the wearer. These robots provide direct control of individual joints and gait cycle, which can minimize abnormal posture or movement [23]. Thus, the benefits or disadvantages of each device should be considered when they are applied to stroke patients.

Robots enhance conventional poststroke rehabilitation by allowing patients to perform early, intensive, and task-oriented exercises [24]. A recent Cochrane review reported that patients who receive robot-assisted gait training in combination with physiotherapy after stroke are more likely to achieve independent walking than those who receive gait training without these devices [25]. Specifically, stroke patients within the first 3 months after onset and those who are not able to walk seem to benefit most from this type of intervention. In addition, robot-assisted therapy for arm and hand training after stroke might improve the patient's ADLs, arm and hand function, and arm and hand muscle strength [26]. However, the results should be interpreted with caution because the quality of evidence was low to very low in arm and hand training.

Noninvasive brain stimulation has recently gained attention due to its effectiveness and safety. Repetitive transcranial magnetic stimulation (rTMS) and transcranial direct current stimulation (tDCS) are the best-known noninvasive brain stimulation techniques that modulate human brain function. rTMS modulates cortical excitability, and the effect depends on the pacing rate: high-frequency stimulation ($\geq$5 Hz) increases cortical excitability, whereas low-frequency stimulation ($\leq$1 Hz) decreases cortical excitability. Numerous studies have provided evidence that high-frequency rTMS over the ipsilesional primary motor cortex improved motor function in both acute and chronic stroke patients [27]. Another study demonstrated that the stimulation effect persisted even 3 months after the intervention [28]. In addition, rTMS enhances the effect of training on cognitive impairment, aphasia, dysphagia, and depression [29]. tDCS delivers weak polarizing direct currents to the cortex via paired electrodes placed on the scalp. At the neuronal level, it causes a polarity-dependent shift of resting membrane potential. Anodal stimulation increases the cortical excitability, and cathodal stimulation decreases the cortical excitability. The tDCS device is relatively cheap, portable, and easy to apply. Thus, it could be used as a stand-alone technique or as an add-on technique to enhance cortical excitability during rehabilitation. Anodal tDCS on the motor cortex has been shown to increase corticomotor excitability and improve motor function in stroke patients [30]. Also, the latest Cochrane review demonstrated that tDCS enhances ADL function in stroke patients, but there is limited evidence for enhanced speech-language therapy [31, 32]. However, there are many ongoing trials that could change the quality of evidence in the future.

Virtual reality (VR) has emerged as a new treatment approach in stroke rehabilitation. The advantage of VR therapy is that it can provide the opportunity to practice activities that cannot be practiced within the clinical environment. Moreover, VR therapy can also give a sense of immersion in the simulated environment and may provoke motivation in stroke patients. Evidence for the effectiveness of VR in improving arm function and ADLs has been accepted; however, the effectiveness of VR in walking or global function has not been established [33].

Emerging evidence supports improved outcomes and the potential clinical implications of novel therapies in stroke rehabilitation. Ongoing research will need to investigate the optimal treatment dose, timing of intervention, duration of intervention, and ideal patient population for these therapies.

16.4 Early Supported Discharge and Outpatient Rehabilitation Service

Once patients are medically stable and require less intensive management, the patient can be transitioned to another level of rehabilitation care. Early support discharge is defined as accelerated discharge of patients with stroke from the hospital and provision of an equivalent rehabilitation program in their home. Evidence shows that early supported discharge results in patients returning home earlier with a reduced need for long-term institutional care. Moreover, these patients show an increased likelihood of regaining independence in ADL. These services seem to be most effective in patients with mild to moderate disability.

Many stroke patients need rehabilitation after their discharge from hospital. Outpatient rehabilitation systems are organized differently around the world, and rehabilitation services can be provided through a clinic or day hospital or even in the patient's home. However, there is no clear information on the optimum intensity and duration of outpatient rehabilitation. Although some patients do not seem to show functional improvement, they may still need rehabilitation for many years. Late issues may include joint contracture, musculoskeletal pain, depression, deconditioning, spasticity, and osteoporosis. Patients with substantial residual disability from a stroke are likely to benefit from periodic assessment in an outpatient rehabilitation clinic.

16.5 Prevention and Management of Stroke Complications

Complications following stroke are common and are associated with poor clinical outcomes, increased length of stay in hospital, increased cost of care, delayed time to rehabilitation, and increased mortality [34]. These complications include seizure, hydrocephalus, venous thromboembolism, genitourinary complications, infections, pressure sore, musculoskeletal pain, and depression. The role of the rehabilitation department is rapid identification and initial workup of these stroke complications.

16.5.1 Seizure and Seizure Prophylaxis

Patients with hemorrhagic stroke are exposed to a substantial risk of seizures. The incidence of seizure and epilepsy in hemorrhagic stroke varies, in part because of differences between ICH and SAH. In ICH, the largest published series showed a 30-day risk of clinical seizures of 8.1% [35]. Literature on SAH has reported the seizure rate to be as high as 27% [36]. Fewer than 10% of patients with ischemic stroke develop seizure. Seizures occur at various time points after hemorrhagic stroke but most occur within the first week. Late-onset seizures occur at least 2 weeks after a stroke and are commonly encountered 6 months to 2 years after stroke but can occur several years later. The rate of development of chronic epilepsy is higher in patients with late-onset seizures.

Administration of prophylactic antiepileptic drugs (AEDs) for hemorrhagic stroke patients has been considered. AEDs may possess neuroprotective effects against hemin toxicity; however, they may also have adverse effects such as cognitive dysfunction. Recent studies have shown that prophylactic use of AED results in unchanged or worse outcomes and does not prevent long-term seizures. Thus, administration of an AED in all hemorrhagic stroke patients is now discouraged by the AHA. In a rehabilitation setting, AEDs should be tapered off in hemorrhagic stroke patients without a history of seizure or high-risk factors for epilepsy, including cortex involvement, lobar ICH, young age, and severe stroke. Future trials are needed to identify patients who may benefit from prophylactic antiepileptic drug use. Until then, the management of seizures after stroke should be similar to the management of seizures in other neurologic illnesses.

16.5.2 Hydrocephalus

Hydrocephalus after hemorrhagic stroke can occur in both SAH and ICH, although it is better known as a consequence of SAH. Hydrocephalus may develop immediately after SAH due to obstruction of the ventricular system from intravenous hemorrhage or after several weeks as a late complication resulting from arachnoiditis from blood in the cerebrospinal fluid (CSF). In ICH, hydrocephalus is usually associated with intraventricular extension (IVE) of the hemorrhage or CSF outflow obstruction from mass effect.

Recent studies have shown that hydrocephalus is a predictor of poor outcome in hemorrhagic stroke [37]. Chronic hydrocephalus, typically normal pressure hydrocephalus (NPH), usually occurs during rehabilitation treatment in stroke patients. When NPH occurs during the rehabilitation phase, it interferes with recovery because of impairments to rehabilitation therapy. It is very important for clinicians to diagnose NPH as soon as possible; otherwise functional recovery may be delayed or less than expected. There is no doubt that patients with high-pressure hydrocephalus must be treated through CSF diversion with a ventriculoperitoneal shunt (VPS). However, the optimal treatment of NPH is currently undetermined. In a recent study, the authors reported that patients with NPH might benefit more from VPS placement and rehabilitation than from rehabilitation alone [38]. Further study is needed to provide evidence for the standard treatment protocol for NPH after stroke.

16.5.3 Venous Thromboembolism

The incidence of venous thromboembolism (VTE) is as high as 50% for deep vein thrombosis (DVT) and 13% for pulmonary embolism (PE) among all stroke patients [39]. DVT may limit participation in rehabilitation and can lead to potentially fatal PE. Therefore, all patients with significant immobility related to stroke should receive DVT prophylaxis. For patients presenting with a hemorrhagic stroke, intermittent pneumatic compression devices should be used on the day of admission. Once cessation of bleeding is confirmed, a low dose of low-molecular-weight heparin or unfractionated heparin can be considered for patients with restricted mobility after 1–4 days post-event. Prophylactic use of low-dose subcutaneous heparin or low-molecular-weight heparin reduces the incidence of DVT, PE, and total mortality. In particular, in cases of hemorrhagic stroke, treatment with low-dose low-molecular-weight heparin reduced the risk of DVT without an increase in the risk of major intracranial or extracranial hemorrhage. In a meta-analysis of 1000 ICH patients, early heparin prophylaxis for VTE was associated with a significant reduction in PE, a nonsignificant reduction in DVT or mortality, and a nonsignificant increase in hematoma enlargement [40]. AHA guidelines for ICH management indicate that after documentation of hematoma stability, low-dose subcutaneous low-molecular-weight heparin may be initiated 1–4 days after ICH for prevention of VTE [1].

In patients who cannot safely take these medications, intermittent pneumatic compression combined with elastic stockings is an effective alternative, particularly in the acute hospital phase. Graduated compression stockings alone are ineffective in preventing DVT in patients with ischemic or hemorrhagic stroke. The optimal duration of prophylaxis remains uncertain, although it is recommended to discontinue its use once patients are able to walk significant distances on a frequent basis.

All patients with suspected DVT should undergo prompt investigation by venous duplex ultrasound imaging. Routine screening examinations are not generally used in this population at present. In patients who develop VTE following hemorrhagic stroke, systemic anticoagulation with low-molecular-weight heparin is recommended. In patients with recent hemorrhage or hematoma instability, an inferior vena cava filter should be inserted to prevent PE.

16.5.4 Genitourinary Complications

Urinary function can be affected in several ways by stroke, including urinary tract infection, urinary retention, and urge incontinence. In acute stroke, the most common reason for incontinence after stroke in uninhibited evacuation of bladder. Urinary retention can occur in one-third of stroke patients. This is caused by altered mental status or direct effects of the stroke on the neurological control of micturition and is associated with cortical stroke, diabetes, aphasia, and cognitive impairment. Catheterization, often with an indwelling catheter, is common during the acute management stage of the stroke survivor. Although this alleviates acute urinary retention, it may lead to urinary infection and interferes with reestablishment of a normal voiding pattern. Indwelling catheters should be removed as quickly as possible and substituted with intermittent catheterization for individuals unable to void spontaneously. Noninvasive measurement of bladder volume using ultrasound is often helpful when managing individuals with impaired bladder function after stroke.

Although urinary retention generally resolves quickly in affected stroke survivors, many develop urinary urgency and/or incontinence. Disinhibition of the bladder detrusor is common and leads to urinary frequency and urgency that may result in incontinence in some individuals. Timed voiding is the primary treatment strategy for patients with persistent uninhibited bladder. This strategy is approached by scheduling regular voiding before the urge to urinate occurs. In these patients urodynamic study is usually not necessary, but noninvasive measurement of bladder volume using ultrasound can be helpful. If residuals are high, the use of an α-blocking agent such as tamsulosin may promote complete voiding. If the voiding is complete, anticholinergic medications such as oxybutynin chloride or tolterodine are useful to inhibit bladder contraction, but in this case, the patient should be monitored for sign and symptoms of urinary retention. Also, these medications may cause anticholinergic side effects such as dry mouth or confusion.

16.5.5 Infections

Infection is a common complication in the acute phase after stroke that greatly affects morbidity and mortality in stroke patients. The most common sources of poststroke infection include pneumonia and urinary tract infection (UTI). A recent study reported that respiration infection was the most common infection in ICH, followed by UTI (17% and 16%, respectively) [41]. Pneumonia occurs in about one-third of patients with stroke, although the incidence is higher in the subset of patients who have SAH. Dysphagia can cause aspiration and result in pneumonia. Also, immobility and atelectasis can lead to the development of pneumonia. Thus, early mobilization and sufficient pulmonary care should be encouraged to prevent pneumonia. Prophylactic antibiotics for prevention of pneumonia are proven to be ineffective in stroke patients [42].

Patients with stroke are at a particularly high risk for developing UTI, whether catheterized or not. Urinary tract infections occur up to 24% of patients with stroke and are most often seen during the first 5 days of hospitalization although they can occur up to 3 months after stroke. Variables associated with an increased likelihood of UTI after stroke include female sex, older age, functional dependence before stroke, poor cognitive function, and catheterization [43]. Urinary tract infection is an independent factor for unfavorable outcomes and prolonged hospitalization. Thus, reducing UTI after stroke could improve outcomes, reduce length of stay, and decrease the cost of care. Clinicians should minimize the use of catheters in stroke patients; catheters should only be placed in patients with stroke in case of acute urinary retention or a patient who requires strict monitoring of fluid status due to a critical medical illness. The catheter should be removed as soon as possible, and intermittent catheterization can be applied to decrease infection risk.

16.5.6 Pressure Sores and Ulcerations

Pressure sore and ulceration are substantial problems that may occur in patients with decreased mobility. Stroke patients who are hemiplegic, lethargic, or incontinent are at high risk for developing pressure ulcers. Stroke rehabilitation guidelines recommend that a thorough assessment of skin integrity be completed upon admission with monitoring at least daily thereafter. Deliberate strategies should be followed to prevent skin breakdowns, including proper positioning, turning, and transferring techniques and judicious use of barrier sprays, lubricants, special mattresses, and protective dressings and padding to avoid skin injury due to maceration, friction, or excessive pressure.

16.5.7 Musculoskeletal Pain and Complex Regional Pain Syndrome

Shoulder and arm pain is a common complication in stroke survivors that restricts patients' daily life after stroke. It tends to develop early, at several weeks to 6 months after stroke. Previous studies found that almost one-third of stroke patients developed shoulder pain after stroke onset, the majority with moderate to severe pain. There is an increased risk of shoulder pain for patients with impaired arm motor function, sensory impairment, duration of hemiplegia, and decreased shoulder range of motion [44].

Shoulder pain in stroke survivors results from varying combinations of glenohumeral subluxation, spasticity, and contraction. Among these, subluxation is the most common cause. Shoulder subluxation in hemiplegia refers to increased translation of the humeral head relative to the glenoid fossa and occurs in almost half of stroke patients with shoulder pain [45]. Shoulder subluxation is evident on physical examination, and imaging studies are not necessary in most situations. Neuromuscular electrical stimulation to the deltoid and supraspinatus muscles delivered via electrodes placed on the skin surface can reduce shoulder subluxation and pain [46].

Complex regional pain syndrome (CRPS) type 1 is a constellation of symptoms. The incidence of CRPS remains controversial. The diagnosis can be made by medical history and physical examination; however, the gold standard method is three-phase bone scintigraphy in which radionuclide uptake is seen in a typical pattern involving the shoulder, wrist, and hand. Initial treatments are oral prednisolone and exercise. Preventative measures, including frequent passive range of motion and desensitization with massage, may contribute to the reduction in the occurrence of this syndrome.

16.5.8 Depression

Depression is an important and common complication of stroke, with reported frequencies ranging from 10 to 40% [47, 48]. The natural history of poststroke depression (PSD) is dynamic, although symptoms most frequently develop in the first year. Known predictors of PSD include physical disability, stroke severity, underlying depression before stroke, and cognitive impairment.

While no clear evidence indicates that improvement of PSD is independently associated with functional improvement, untreated depression can negatively impact the patient's ability to participate in rehabilitation and result in delayed recovery and poorer outcome. Several studies have shown that not only poststroke major depression but also mild depression or even depressive symptoms have a negative influence on the functional recovery of patients after stroke [49]. Active treatment should be considered for all patients with significant clinical depression. Patients with PSD generally respond well to standard antidepressant medications, with selective serotonin reuptake inhibitors (SSRIs) being commonly prescribed. The AHA recommends that the use of antidepressant should be continued for at least 6 months after recovery of depressed symptoms [50]. Stimulant medications, such as methylphenidate, may also be applied to boost the response and achieve more rapid improvement.

16.6 Suggestions from Clinical Practice Guidelines

The current state of evidence for rehabilitation after hemorrhagic stroke is limited; therefore, most rehabilitation methods for hemorrhagic stroke follow general principles acquired from evidence in ischemic stroke rehabilitation. However, it is clear that all patients with hemorrhagic stroke should start early rehabilitation after stabilization of medial and neurological status. Patient motor function, cognitive function, language and communication ability, swallowing, and emotional status should be evaluated as early as possible. Comprehensive rehabilitation provided by a multidisciplinary stroke care team is recommended for hemorrhagic stroke patients, although optimal rehabilitation parameters including content, onset time, dose, intensity, and duration still need to be established for this specific group. Early- and late-phase complications may negatively affect the functional outcome of survivors after hemorrhagic stroke. Thus, prevention and management of stroke complications are essential components of stroke rehabilitation.

References

1. Hemphill JC 3rd, Greenberg SM, Anderson CS, et al. Guidelines for the management of spontaneous intracerebral hemorrhage: a guideline for healthcare professionals from the American Heart Association/American Stroke Association. Stroke. 2015;46:2032–60.
2. Saulle MF, Schambra HM. Recovery and rehabilitation after intracerebral hemorrhage. Semin Neurol. 2016;36:306–12.
3. Langhorne P, Bernhardt J, Kwakkel G. Stroke rehabilitation. Lancet. 2011;377:1693–702.
4. Zhang P, Xianglei J, Hongbo Y, et al. Neuroprotection of early locomotor exercise poststroke: evidence from animal studies. Can J Neurol Sci. 2015;42:213–20.
5. Coleman ER, Moudgal R, Lang K, et al. Early rehabilitation after stroke: a narrative review. Curr Atheroscler Rep. 2017;19:59.
6. Bernhardt J, Langhorne P, Lindley RI, et al. Efficacy and safety of very early mobilisation within 24 h of stroke onset (AVERT): a randomised controlled trial. Lancet. 2015;386:46–55.
7. Liu N, Cadilhac DA, Andrew NE, et al. Randomized controlled trial of early rehabilitation after intracerebral hemorrhage stroke: difference in outcomes within 6 months of stroke. Stroke. 2014;45:3502–7.
8. Olkowski BF, Devine MA, Slotnick LE, et al. Safety and feasibility of an early mobilization program for patients with aneurysmal subarachnoid hemorrhage. Phys Ther. 2013;93:208–15.
9. Shimamura N, Matsuda N, Satou J, et al. Early ambulation produces favorable outcome and nondemential state in aneurysmal subarachnoid hemorrhage patients older than 70 years of age. World Neurosurg. 2014;81:330–4.
10. Ma Z, Wang Q, Liu M. Early versus delayed mobilisation for aneurysmal subarachnoid haemorrhage. Cochrane Database Syst Rev. 2013;5:CD008346.
11. Meijer R, Ihnenfeldt DS, De Groot IJ, et al. Prognostic factors for ambulation and activities of daily living in the subacute phase after stroke. A systematic review of the literature. Clin Rehabil. 2003;17:119–29.
12. Stinear CM. Prediction of motor recovery after stroke: advances in biomarkers. Lancet Neurol. 2017;16:826–36.
13. Lawrence ES, Coshall C, Dundas R, et al. Estimates of the prevalence of acute stroke impairments and disability in a multiethnic population. Stroke. 2001;32:1279–84.
14. Yekutiel M, Guttman E. A controlled trial of the retraining of the sensory function of the hand in stroke patients. J Neurol Neurosurg Psychiatry. 1993;56:241–4.
15. Management of Stroke Rehabilitation Working G. VA/DOD clinical practice guideline for the management of stroke rehabilitation. J Rehabil Res Dev. 2010;47:1–43.
16. Pulvermuller F, Neininger B, Elbert T, et al. Constraint-induced therapy of chronic aphasia after stroke. Stroke. 2001;32:1621–6.
17. Martino R, Foley N, Bhogal S, et al. Dysphagia after stroke: incidence, diagnosis, and pulmonary complications. Stroke. 2005;36:2756–63.
18. Horner J, Massey EW, Brazer SR. Aspiration in bilateral stroke patients. Neurology. 1990;40:1686–8.

19. Trapl M, Enderle P, Nowotny M, et al. Dysphagia bedside screening for acute-stroke patients: the Gugging swallowing screen. Stroke. 2007;38:2948–52.
20. Martino R, Silver F, Teasell R, et al. The Toronto bedside swallowing screening test (TOR-BSST): development and validation of a dysphagia screening tool for patients with stroke. Stroke. 2009;40:555–61.
21. Winstein CJ, Stein J, Arena R, et al. Guidelines for adult stroke rehabilitation and recovery: a guideline for healthcare professionals from the American Heart Association/American Stroke Association. Stroke. 2016;47:e98–e169.
22. Shaker R, Easterling C, Kern M, et al. Rehabilitation of swallowing by exercise in tube-fed patients with pharyngeal dysphagia secondary to abnormal UES opening. Gastroenterology. 2002;122:1314–21.
23. Chang WH, Kim YH. Robot-assisted therapy in stroke rehabilitation. J Stroke. 2013;15:174–81.
24. Morone G, Paolucci S, Cherubini A, et al. Robot-assisted gait training for stroke patients: current state of the art and perspectives of robotics. Neuropsychiatr Dis Treat. 2017;13:1303–11.
25. Mehrholz J, Thomas S, Werner C, et al. Electromechanical-assisted training for walking after stroke. Cochrane Database Syst Rev. 2017;5:CD006185.
26. Mehrholz J, Pohl M, Platz T, et al. Electromechanical and robot-assisted arm training for improving activities of daily living, arm function, and arm muscle strength after stroke. Cochrane Database Syst Rev. 2015;6:CD006876.
27. Hummel FC, Cohen LG. Non-invasive brain stimulation: a new strategy to improve neurorehabilitation after stroke? Lancet Neurol. 2006;5:708–12.
28. Chang WH, Kim YH, Bang OY, et al. Long-term effects of rTMS on motor recovery in patients after subacute stroke. J Rehabil Med. 2010;42:758–64.
29. Fregni F, Pascual-Leone A. Technology insight: non-invasive brain stimulation in neurology-perspectives on the therapeutic potential of rTMS and tDCS. Nat Clin Pract Neurol. 2007;3:383–93.
30. Bastani A, Jaberzadeh S. Does anodal transcranial direct current stimulation enhance excitability of the motor cortex and motor function in healthy individuals and subjects with stroke: a systematic review and meta-analysis. Clin Neurophysiol. 2012;123:644–57.
31. Elsner B, Kugler J, Pohl M, et al. Transcranial direct current stimulation (tDCS) for improving activities of daily living, and physical and cognitive functioning, in people after stroke. Cochrane Database Syst Rev. 2016;3:CD009645.
32. Elsner B, Kugler J, Pohl M, et al. Transcranial direct current stimulation (tDCS) for improving aphasia in patients with aphasia after stroke. Cochrane Database Syst Rev. 2015;5:CD009760.
33. Laver KE, Lange B, George S, et al. Virtual reality for stroke rehabilitation. Cochrane Database Syst Rev. 2017;11:CD008349.
34. Ingeman A, Andersen G, Hundborg HH, et al. In-hospital medical complications, length of stay, and mortality among stroke unit patients. Stroke. 2011;42:3214–8.
35. Passero S, Rocchi R, Rossi S, et al. Seizures after spontaneous supratentorial intracerebral hemorrhage. Epilepsia. 2002;43:1175–80.
36. Lin YJ, Chang WN, Chang HW, et al. Risk factors and outcome of seizures after spontaneous aneurysmal subarachnoid hemorrhage. Eur J Neurol. 2008;15:451–7.
37. Xi G, Strahle J, Hua Y, et al. Progress in translational research on intracerebral hemorrhage: is there an end in sight? Prog Neurobiol. 2014;115:45–63.
38. Chen Z, Song W, Du J, et al. Rehabilitation of patients with chronic normal-pressure hydrocephalus after aneurysmal subarachnoid hemorrhage benefits from ventriculoperitoneal shunt. Top Stroke Rehabil. 2009;16:330–8.
39. Kelly J, Rudd A, Lewis R, et al. Venous thromboembolism after acute stroke. Stroke. 2001;32:262–7.
40. Paciaroni M, Agnelli G, Venti M, et al. Efficacy and safety of anticoagulants in the prevention of venous thromboembolism in patients with acute cerebral hemorrhage: a meta-analysis of controlled studies. J Thromb Haemost. 2011;9:893–8.
41. Lord AS, Langefeld CD, Sekar P, et al. Infection after intracerebral hemorrhage: risk factors and association with outcomes in the ethnic/racial variations of intracerebral hemorrhage study. Stroke. 2014;45:3535–42.
42. Westendorp WF, Vermeij JD, Zock E, et al. The preventive antibiotics in stroke study (PASS): a pragmatic randomised open-label masked endpoint clinical trial. Lancet. 2015;385:1519–26.
43. Poisson SN, Johnston SC, Josephson SA. Urinary tract infections complicating stroke: mechanisms, consequences, and possible solutions. Stroke. 2010;41:e180–4.
44. Turner-Stokes L, Jackson D. Shoulder pain after stroke: a review of the evidence base to inform the development of an integrated care pathway. Clin Rehabil. 2002;16:276–98.
45. Lindgren I, Jonsson AC, Norrving B, et al. Shoulder pain after stroke: a prospective population-based study. Stroke. 2007;38:343–8.
46. Faghri PD, Rodgers MM, Glaser RM, et al. The effects of functional electrical stimulation on shoulder subluxation, arm function recovery, and shoulder pain in hemiplegic stroke patients. Arch Phys Med Rehabil. 1994;75:73–9.
47. Morris PL, Robinson RG, Raphael B. Prevalence and course of depressive disorders in hospitalized stroke patients. Int J Psychiatry Med. 1990;20:349–64.
48. Gainotti G, Azzoni A, Marra C. Frequency, phenomenology and anatomical-clinical correlates of major post-stroke depression. Br J Psychiatry. 1999;175:163–7.
49. Robinson RG, Jorge RE. Post-stroke depression: a review. Am J Psychiatry. 2016;173:221–31.
50. Hackett ML, Kohler S, O'brien JT, et al. Neuropsychiatric outcomes of stroke. Lancet Neurol. 2014;13:525–34.

The manufacturer's authorised representative in the EU is Springer
Nature Customer Service Centre GmbH, Europaplatz 3, 69115 Heidelberg,
Germany. If you have any concerns regarding our products, please
contact ProductSafety@springernature.com

Printed and bound by CPI Group (UK) Ltd, Croydon, CR0 4YY
30/09/2026
02225445-0018